ORIENTATION TO HOME CARE NURSING

Carolyn J. Humphrey, RN, MS
Associate Professor
School of Nursing and Health Sciences
Spalding University
Principal
C.J. Humphrey Associates
Louisville, Kentucky

Paula Milone-Nuzzo, RN, PhD
Associate Professor and Chairperson
Specialty Care and Management Division
Yale University School of Nursing
New Haven, Connecticut

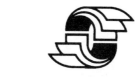

AN ASPEN PUBLICATION®
Aspen Publishers, Inc.
Gaithersburg, Maryland
1996

The authors have made every effort to ensure the accuracy of the information herein. However, appropriate information sources should be consulted, especially for new or unfamiliar procedures. It is the responsibility of every practitioner to evaluate the appropriateness of a particular opinion in the context of actual clinical situations and with due consideration to new developments. Authors, editors, and the publisher cannot be held responsible for any typographical or other errors found in this work.

This publication is designed to provide accurate and authoritative information in regard to the Subject Matter covered. It is sold with the understanding that the publisher is not engaged in rendering legal, accounting, or other professional service. If legal advice or other expert assistance is required, the service of a competent professional person should be sought. *(From a Declaration of Principles jointly adopted by a Committee of the American Bar Association and a Committee of Publishers and Associations.)*

Library of Congress Cataloging-in-Publication Data

Humphrey, Carolyn J., 1947-
Orientation to home care nursing / Carolyn J. Humphrey, Paula Milone-Nuzzo.
p. cm.
Student condensed version of: Manual of home care nursing orientation.
Includes bibliographical references and index.
ISBN 0-8342-0706-0
1. Home care services—United States. I. Milone-Nuzzo, Paula.
II. Humprhey, Carolyn J., 1947-.
Manual of home care nursing orientation. III. Milone-Nuzzo, Paula.
IV. Humprhey, Carolyn J., 1947-. Manual of home care nursing orientation.
V. Home care nursing. VI. Title.
[DNLM: 1. Home Care Services—United States. WY 115 H926o 1996]
RA645.35.H862 1996
362.1'4'0973—dc20
DNLM/DLC
for Library of Congress
95-21181
CIP

Editorial Resources: Jane Colilla

Printing and Manufacturing: Terri Miner

Copyright © 1996 by Aspen Publishers, Inc.

All rights reserved. Aspen Publishers, Inc., grants permission for photocopying for limited personal or internal use. This consent does not extend to other kinds of copying, such as copying for general distribution, for advertising or promotional purposes, for creating new collective works, or for resale. For information, address Aspen Publishers, Inc., Permissions Department, 200 Orchard Ridge Drive, Gaithersburg, Maryland 20878.

Orders: (800) 638-8437
Customer Service: (800) 234-1660

Library of Congress Catalog Card Number: 95-21181
ISBN: 0-8342-0706-0

Printed in the United States of America

3 4 5

To Jonathan Evan Humphrey Gross—the light of my life.

Carolyn

To my father, John M. Milone, Sr.,
who touched so many lives in such a special way.
He is truly missed.

Paula

Contents

Contributors

Lazelle E. Benefield, RN, PhD
Associate Professor
Harris College of Nursing
Texas Christian University
Forth Worth, Texas
Principal
L. Benefield Associates
Colleyville, Texas

Lazelle lent her expertise in many home care areas to the entire work. From her doctoral work she contributed to the material on productivity and to the material that describes the knowledge and abilities needed to hire and orient a new nurse.

Judith Benson, RN, BSN, MBA
National Director of Clinical Support Services
NMC Home Care, Inc.
Waltham, Massachusetts

Judy contributed her excellent knowledge of and experience in high-tech home care in revising the high-tech section of Chapter 11 for this edition.

Mary M. Friedman, MS, RN, CRNI
Principal and Home Care Consultant
Home Health Systems, PC
Marietta, Georgia

As a Joint Commission on Accreditation of Healthcare Organizations surveyor and consultant, Mary was able to bring a wonderful perspective to the accreditation information in Chapter 1 and to the performance improvement content in Chapter 6.

John C. Gilliland II, JD
Attorney
The Law Offices of John C. Gilliland II
Crestview Hills, Kentucky
Elizabeth Zink-Pearson, JD
Attorney
The Law Offices of John C. Gilliland II
Crestview Hills, Kentucky

John and Elizabeth contributed current home care legal issues and revised the original material regarding the legal aspects of home care practice. The original contribution of Susan Westrick Killion, RN, MS, JD, to the first edition of this work is acknowledged.

Gail L. Grammatica, RN, MS
Supervisor of Project Development and Training
Tufts Associated Health Plans
Waltham, Massachusetts

Gail revised her original work on pediatric home care for this edition, integrating new strategies for this growing home care area.

Donna M. Hird, RN, MSN
Clinical Education Coordinator
VNA Health Care, Inc.
Waterbury, Connecticut

The complex regulations and requirements of infection control are a challenge for all practitioners. Donna was able to take the complex information in Chapter 3 and help make it understandable and practical for the home care nurse.

Ruth Galten Irwin, RN, CSN
Director of Regulatory and State Affairs
National Association for Home Care
Washington, DC

Bringing a national home care perspective and her vast understanding of Medicare, Ruth contributed a great deal to the significantly revised and updated Medicare information found in Chapters 4 and 5.

Ruth N. Knollmueller, RN, PhD
Visiting Professor
University of Kentucky College of Nursing
Hazard, Kentucky

Ruth used her wealth of experiences as a clinical director to revise the supervision material (found in Chapter 9) that she contributed to the first edition.

Cheryl M. Leslie, RN, MPH
Director of Reimbursement Services
Connecticut Association for Home Care
Wallingford, Connecticut

Management information systems are an important, growing aspect of the home care nurse's role. Cheryl significantly contributed to the development of that material in Chapter 8.

Mary Joyce Pfaadt, RN-C, BSN
Manager of Quality Improvement/Education
Caretenders of Louisville
Louisville, Kentucky

Laurel A. Benson, RN-C, PHN, BSN
Assistant Manager of Education
Caretenders of Louisville
Louisville, Kentucky

Missy and Laurel, as an education team, helped reorganize the Medicare and documentation material from the first book to become Chapters 4 and 5 in this edition.

Acknowledgments

Since we wrote our initial orientation book in 1989, the health care delivery system and the practice of home care nursing have changed significantly. We have worked very hard to make this product a comprehensive resource for nurses transitioning to a new career in home care, for the more experienced home care nurse, for nursing students, practicing nurses, managers, and others who wish to increase their knowledge of this challenging nursing specialty.

We've heard from many who have used the information we presented in our first book, *Home Care Nursing: An Orientation to Practice,* and also have heard from the various people we have met as we speak and work with agencies around the country on this important topic. We want all of you to know how much we value and appreciate your ideas, comments, and suggestions. The great support from colleagues, family, friends, and students has always made us see our efforts as an ongoing work in progress that needs constant evaluation and feedback.

Many individuals have given a great deal of support to us both professionally and personally and have helped us complete the work by writing and reviewing important sections. Debra Hapner, RN, BS, as a certified case manager and national consultant, wrote the case management section of Chapter 8 in a simple, easy to understand way. Terrye Fairly, RN, BSN, an author

and consultant herself, gave great input to Chapter 6 on quality management. Terrye's wit and wisdom always bring us a smile when we are working on this complex subject. Thanks also go to Debbie Holt, Diane Caldwell, and Sonya Johnson.

We also want to thank our colleagues at Spalding University and Yale University who have provided support and assistance with this project. Dr. Marjorie Perrin, Dean of the School of Nursing and Health Sciences at Spalding, provided the support necessary to complete this work. A special thanks goes to Donna Epps, who assisted with typing, and to Ruth Langlais, who provided research support. Many, many thanks go to Jane Garwood, the senior nursing editor at Aspen, who always listens, and to Jane Colilla, who with her tough editorial support made the work look good and our words make more sense.

And now, a special word for our families—what would we do without them? To Fred and Jonathan Gross, who missed many good times enjoying my glowing personality and suffered through many not-so-good times when my patience was short because of deadlines and late night writing spells, all my love and thanks.

To Joe, JohnPaul, and Jessica Nuzzo, thanks for understanding when I was too busy to always listen, understand, and do the things I really wanted to. A special thanks also goes to Pauline Milone, my mom, for her support.

We also both want to thank each other for the laughs when the computer broke down; the encouraging words on the fax, voice mail, and phone; understanding when one did not have the time to complete the assigned work; and most of all for remaining best friends through it all.

Carolyn J. Humphrey
Paula Milone-Nuzzo

How To Use This Text

Each chapter begins with the Objectives and Key Concepts covered in the chapter, as well as a list of the Agency-Specific Material needed to complete a stage of the orientation program. Before you read each chapter, the agency material listed should be assembled for the orientee's easy reference as the information is covered. At the end of each chapter are Test Yourself questions designed to allow the new staff nurse to review the content of the chapter and discuss the material learned with the supervisor or preceptor. This format is helpful to the nurse new to home care as well as the experienced home care nurse who is being oriented to a new agency.

Throughout this text, the terms *client* and *patient* have been used synonymously to identify the individual recipient of care. *Family* and *significant other* have been used to describe the patient support systems with whom the home care nurse works to deliver care. For convenience, the pronouns *her* and *she* have been used to refer to the home care nurse throughout the text. The terms *orientation coordinator* and *supervisor* have been used to identify the person(s) responsible for planning and implementing the home care nurse's orientation. *Home health agency* refers to any agency providing professional home care services, regardless of the type of agency, method of reimbursement, or geographical location. *Home* refers to the client's place of residence.

Chapter 1 gives an overview of the development and current status of the home care system in the United States. A discussion of the internal and external influences on home care, and of the types of providers and staff working in a home health agency with their roles and functions, gives the new staff nurse a broad overview of the home care system and the personnel working in it. This chapter provides a framework for the remaining chapters, which are specific to home care nursing.

Chapter 2 begins with the definition of home care nursing and discusses the specific roles and functions of the home care nurse, including coordination of the plan of care. The nursing process in the home care setting is outlined, focusing on the unique aspects of its use in the home.

Chapter 3 details two of the most important concepts in home care nursing: infection control and the home visit. Home visiting steps, safety, and bag technique are included in the section on how to do a home visit. Infection control includes the Occupational Safety and Health Administration (OSHA) regulations regarding bloodborne pathogens and tuberculosis. In addition, measures for the immunocompromised client are included.

Chapter 4 discusses the Medicare home care benefit. Because the majority of home care is reimbursed by Medicare, an understanding of the Medicare home care benefit is essential. Also included are the criteria for Medicare reimbursement of professional and paraprofessional home care providers.

Chapter 5 discusses documentation of the nursing care provided, as it is an essential component of home care nursing practice. The general principles of home care documentation are covered, as is an introduction to how home care documentation differs from that in other practice areas. Documentation to satisfy Medicare regulations and how to write Health Care Financing Administration (HCFA) Forms 485, 486, and 487 are also discussed in detail.

Chapter 6 includes a discussion of quality management in home care. Every home care agency must be concerned about the quality of care it provides. In addition to defining a current model used to assess quality, this chapter provides an in-depth discussion of performance improvement and its relationship to the Joint Commission on Accreditation of Healthcare Organizations standards.

Chapter 7 details the teaching-learning process and its application in home care. Client teaching is frequently used in home care practice. Because teaching is one of the most important intervention strategies in home care, a detailed description of development, implementation, and documentation of the teaching-learning process is included.

Chapter 8 details strategies for effective clinical management. Contracting and critical paths are described, followed by a detailed description of case management. The home care nurse will often have to work with a case manager as she provides home care to clients. Management information systems allow home care agencies to collect, store, and retrieve the important information they need. This chapter concludes with a discussion of how a home care nurse works with a management information system.

Chapter 9 addresses home care nursing strategies for success. Descriptions of types of home care delivery systems, productivity issues, and time and stress management techniques give the new nurse an understanding of how to use these strategies to become a more efficient and effective member of the staff. An extensive discussion of how the home care nurse can work with her supervisor is included. Case studies are provided to facilitate an understanding of important concepts. Strategies for professional growth are included to encourage the home care nurse to set professional goals and develop in home care and in nursing.

Chapter 10 covers legal issues relevant to home care nursing practice. It examines such basic legal considerations as confidentiality, witnessing documents, and risk management. This material is basic to practice and should be covered in the initial orientation. The section on liability issues in home care nursing provides a more detailed examination of the situations confronting home care nurses as they practice. This material will be more meaningful to the new nurse after several weeks of home care experience and should be included later in the orientation period. It should also be available for future reference. Ethical issues in home care, including advance medical directives, and the American Nurses Association (ANA) scope of practice are also included in this chapter.

Chapter 11 looks at the special considerations of high-tech home care, pediatric home care, hospice care, early newborn discharge programs, and psychiatric mental health programs. These important home care services may not be provided directly by all home health agencies, but basic information about these services should be covered as part of initial orientation. All home care nurses either will work with these clients and their families in direct service or in collaboration with other agencies or will need to understand the services to make appropriate referrals.

At the end of the text are several appendixes that can be used to clarify material covered in the chapters. There are three glossaries included in the appendixes: Appendix L defines general home care terms; Appendix M defines terms specific to Medicare; and Appendix N defines legal terminology. The reader should refer to these glossaries to further define the material in this text. Also included is a list of additional resources, Appendix P, that can be helpful to the orientation coordinator, new staff nurse, and student nurse.

Organization of the Home Care System

OBJECTIVES

Upon completion of this chapter, the reader will be able to identify:

1. The development and current status of home care in the United States
2. The structure and human resource aspects of home health agencies
3. Internal and external forces that affect the provision of home care
4. Rights and responsibilities that affect the client and agency relationship
5. Organizations that influence and represent home care services
6. Home care certification, licensure, and accreditation
7. The nurse's role and responsibilities regarding home care licensure, certification, and accreditation

KEY CONCEPTS

- **Definitions of home care**
- **Differences between technical and professional home care**
- **Roles of home care providers**
- **Types of home care reimbursement**
- **Home care organizations**
- **Client Bill of Rights and Responsibilities**
- **Nurse's role in licensure, Medicare certification, and accreditation**

AGENCY-SPECIFIC MATERIAL NEEDED

- Mission statement
- Agency brochure
- Organizational chart
- Orientee's job description
- Any paperwork associated with licensure, accreditation, and certification that would be helpful to the orientee
- Client Bill of Rights and Responsibilities

INTRODUCTION

The 1980s witnessed a rapid increase in the need for home care by all segments of the U.S. population with resulting growth in the number, type, and variety of organizations that provided health services in the home. As the 1990s unfold, the rapid rate of change in the overall health care system is resulting not only in continuing growth in the number of home care providers and the increased variety of services provided but also in a dramatic shift in the reimbursement for home and community-based services. These dramatic changes in the health care delivery system, including the increasing focus on legislation and reimbursement, have been as confusing for health care providers as they have been for consumers. This chapter outlines the major aspects encompassing the broad field of home care. Definitions of home care and the various internal and external components that affect home care are discussed.

In no area of nursing practice is the understanding of the "big picture" more important than in home care. The nurse must understand how the day-to-day activities performed in the agency affect and are affected by the larger health care delivery system. By the end of this chapter, the reader will better understand the field of home care and how it fits into the larger health care system. The remaining chapters of this work examine the unique aspects of home care nursing practice.

THE HISTORICAL DEVELOPMENT OF HOME CARE

Home Care—The Past

The root of home care is found in the practice of visiting nursing, which had its beginnings in the United States in the late 1800s. The modern concept of providing nursing care in the home was established by William Rathbone of Liverpool, England, in 1859. Rathbone, a wealthy businessman and philanthropist, set up a system of visiting nursing after a personal experience in which nurses cared for his wife at home before her death. In 1859, with the help of Florence Nightingale, he started a school to train visiting nurses at the Liverpool Infirmary, the graduates of which focused on helping the "sick poor" in their homes (Clemen-Stone, Eigsti, & McGuire, 1995).

In the late 1800s, the U.S. cities experienced rapid growth, and the waves of immigrants who came to America seeking opportunity played a large role in this change. These two social factors were the underlying reasons for the development of visiting nursing in the United States. As in England, home nursing care focused, from its inception, on the poor. At that time, dismal living and working conditions gave rise to problems with hygiene and increases in various illnesses. Visiting nurse associations (VNAs) in the United States, like their English counterparts, were established by groups of people who wanted to assist the poor to improve their health. Buffalo, New York, Boston, and Philadelphia developed visiting nurse services during 1885 and 1886 and focused on caring for the middle-class sick as well as the poor (Clemen-Stone et al., 1995).

During World War II, as physicians made fewer home visits and focused instead on their offices and hospitals, the home care movement grew, with nurses providing most of the health and illness care in the home. In 1946, Montefiore Hospital in New York City developed a posthospital acute care program and initiated convalescent home care (Mundinger, 1983).

From these early beginnings through the mid-1960s, VNAs were developed in major cities, small towns, and counties throughout the country. During that period much of their work focused on providing health and illness services to the poor in their homes with most of the acute care given to clients in a hospital setting. With the passage of Medicare legislation through the Social Security Act in 1965, home care, almost solely provided by VNAs, became more frequently used because it was a benefit provided to elderly clients who participated in the Medicare program. This change in the delivery of home care services brought about a change in the organization of home health agencies and an increase in the number of for-profit home health care providers (Roberts & Heinrich, 1985).

Home Care—The Present

In the early 1980s, to curb the increasing hospital costs incurred by the Medicare program and the increasing numbers of elderly clients needing hospitalization, diagnosis-related groups (DRGs) were phased in over a four-year period in hospitals nationwide. Two results of the implementation of the DRG system were a decrease in a client's length of stay in the hospital and an increase in the use of home care services to these clients. Also, because Medicare would not cover hospitalization for some conditions, many clients were not admitted to a hospital, and the needed care was provided in the home by a home health agency. Following the federal government's lead with the Medicare program, Medicaid programs (which are administered individually by the states), private insurance companies, and other payers who cover home health services also began restricting payments for hospitalizations, thus increasing the need for home care services. This activity brought about a record increase in the number of providers who deliver home care services.

As of March 1994, the National Association for Home Care (NAHC) identified a total of 15,027 home care agencies in the United States. Of this number, 7,521 are Medicare-certified home health agencies; 1,459 are Medicare-certified hospices; and 6,047 are home health agencies, home care organizations, and hospices that do not participate in Medicare. The growth of these agencies since the late 1980s has been significant as evidenced by Table 1–1.

Despite the cost-saving efforts of the recent past regarding utilization of institutional care, as the 1990s unfold, health care costs throughout the nation continue to increase while fewer individuals are being covered by some form of health insurance. The financial crisis and human suffering that have resulted from the combination of these factors make some kind of political and economic solution to the problem a necessity. Throughout the debate that continues to evolve, one thing is certain. Health care provided in the home is an essential component of a reformed health care delivery system, and nursing will continue to be an integral part of home care.

DEFINITIONS OF HOME CARE

Home care, home health care, and *home health agency* can be confusing terms, both to the providers and consumers of the care. The following list represents definitions of home care developed by leading professional and trade associations who are active in the home health field.

- *Medicare Definition.* Illness care.
- *NAHC Definition.* "Services to the recovering, disabled or chronically ill person providing for treatment and/or effective functioning in the home environment. Home care can also assist in the provision of services to adults and children in danger of abuse or neglect. Generally, home care is appropriate whenever a person needs assistance that cannot be easily or effectively provided only by family members or friends on an ongoing basis for a short or long period of time" (National Association for Home Care, 1987).
- *American Hospital Association Definition.* "Services providing nursing, therapy and health-related homemaker or social services in the client's home" (American Hospital Association, 1992).
- *American Medical Association Definition.* "The provision of nursing care, social work, therapies, vocational and social services and homemaker-health aide services may be included as basic components of home health care. The provision of these needed services to the client at home constitutes a logical extension of the physician's therapeutic responsibility. At the physician's request and under his or her medical direction, personnel who provide these home health care services operate as a team in assessing and developing the home health care plan" (American Colleges of Physicians, Health and Public Policy Committee, 1986).
- *Consumer's Union Definition.* "People care at home. It is diagnosis, treatment, monitoring, rehabilita-

Table 1–1 Home Care Agencies: Certified Home Health Agencies, Certified Hospices, and Others, 1989–1994

| Year | Total | Certified Agencies | | |
		HHAs	Hospices	Other
1989	11,097	5,676	597	4,824
1990	11,765	5,695	774	5,296
1991	12,433	5,780	898	5,755
1992	12,497	6,004	1,039	5,454
1993	13,959	6,497	1,223	6,239
1994	15,027	7,521	1,459	6,047

Source: Reprinted with permission from *Basic Statistics about Home Care*, National Association for Home Care, © 1994.

tion and supportive care provided at home, rather than in an impersonal hospital, nursing home or other institution. At best, home care is holistic, providing in-home health, social and other human services that can help you as a whole person, not just as a 'patient'" (Nassif, 1985).

Although the home care definitions presented thus far may tend to confuse the reader, they do represent the divergent opinions of home care and leave room for further discussion and clarification. This broad notion of exactly what home care involves indicates that home care is constantly evolving and that providers, payers, and clients have far to go in clarifying the role and function of home care and home care providers.

The terms *home care* and *home health care* have been used synonymously by those working in the field and are used throughout this text in that context. *Home care* is used in this text as the term that describes the broad spectrum of professional and technical services delivered in the home. The authors do believe, however, that there is a distinct difference between the professional and technical home care services that are provided to clients.

THE DIFFERENCE BETWEEN PROFESSIONAL AND TECHNICAL HOME CARE

Professional home care is practice driven, that is, the boundaries of practice are determined by professional standards with a basis in scientific theory and research. The foundation for this type of practice is provided by professionals with licenses, certifications, or specific qualifications. These professionals work for home care organizations that are licensed, often are accredited, and have internal standards as well as external standards that guide the provision of their services. Nursing, therapy, social work, and paraprofessional services, such as services provided by home care aides, are examples of professional home care practice.

Technical home care is more product driven, often with a focus on bottom-line profits, that may affect the clear delineation of client and family needs. Although providers of this care may have reimbursement standards, they are not necessarily required to have professional standards or regulations that govern the services they provide. Professional and ethical home care companies that provide technical home care do exist and the consumer of these services needs to evaluate closely the services and the prices. Durable medical equipment (DME) suppliers, oxygen providers, and other equipment home delivery providers make up this category (Humphrey, 1988).

This text focuses on the professional practice of home care and home care nursing, and the technical aspects of home care are referred to only briefly. Professional services that (1) are provided for acutely and chronically ill clients and for well clients and families and (2) that are skilled, short-term, and intermittent are the emphasis of this text.

In the delivery of a professional model of home care, nursing is the foundation of the delivery system. How the nurse functions in that system is discussed in the subsequent chapters. It is up to the home care nurse to examine the various roles used in working with clients continually and determine how this specialized field of nursing should be practiced in the larger home care and health care system and within the scope of ever-changing professional clinical and organizational practice.

THE HOME HEALTH AGENCY

Home care agencies of various types have been providing high-quality, in-home service throughout the United States for over a century. When Medicare was enacted in 1965, the home health industry's growth was greatly increased because skilled nursing and therapy of a curative or restorative nature were made available to the elderly. Beginning in 1973, these same services were provided to certain disabled younger Americans. The significant increase in the number of agencies providing home care meant that there were more variations on the types of agencies that were providing home care services.

The Medicare Conditions of Participation for Home Health Agencies define a home health agency as "a public agency or a private organization . . . primarily engaged in providing skilled nursing services and other therapeutic services" (Conditions of Participation, 1991). Medicare terms that are used throughout the text can be found in Appendix M. The following gives an overview of the many types of agencies that provide home health care.

TYPES OF HOME HEALTH AGENCIES

Not-for-Profit Agencies. These agencies are given this status based on their exemption from taxation on profits or excess income under Section 501 of the Internal Revenue Code of 1954. Any excess the agency has at the end of its fiscal year is put back into the organization, and no part of the net earnings can be used for the private benefit of owners, partners, or share-holders.

For-Profit or Profit-Making Agency. This is also a designation for tax purposes. These agencies are not eligible for tax exemption and pay all business and corporate taxes any other business pays.

Free-Standing Agency. This means that the home health agency (HHA) is not affiliated with any other institution such as a hospital or nursing home. Usually this also means that it is a local agency serving a defined geographical area.

Voluntary Agencies. These are HHAs that do not depend on state and local tax revenues but are financed primarily with nontax funds, such as donations, endowments, United Way contributions, and third-party payment (Medicare, Medicaid, private insurance). Voluntary agencies are usually governed by a volunteer board of directors and are considered to be community based because they provide services within a well-defined geographic location or community. An example of a voluntary agency is a VNA. VNAs are free-standing, voluntary, nonprofit organizations governed by a board of directors and usually financed by tax-deductible contributions as well as by revenue gained from the provision of direct services. Before home care gained the status it has currently, voluntary agencies were assured of receiving almost all the home care referrals in their community. The proliferation of other agencies has eroded their traditional referral base and put the agencies in a competitive mode with other home care providers.

Proprietary Agencies. These are free-standing, for-profit home health agencies. Proprietary agencies may be owned by individuals, groups, or corporations. Many of the large proprietary agencies are part of national chains that are administered through corporate headquarters. Proprietary agencies plan to make a profit on the home care services they provide, either for the private individuals who own them or for their stockholders. Some proprietary agencies participate in the Medicare program and some do not. Although revenues are generated by some proprietary agencies through third-party payers, such as Medicare and private insurance, others rely on "private pay" clients who use their own money to pay for services.

Hospital-Based Agencies. These agencies are operating units or departments of a hospital. Agencies that have working arrangements with a hospital or perhaps are even owned by a hospital but operate as separate entities, are usually classified as free-standing agencies. The majority of referrals to this type of agency usually come from the sponsoring institution although it accept referrals from anyone.

Official, Public Agencies. These are government agencies operated by a state, county, city, or other unit of local government having a major responsibility for preventing disease and for providing community health education. Traditional public health nursing services provided through a public agency are communicable disease investigation, health promotion, disease prevention, and environmental health services, as well as maternal-child health and family planning. These agencies may also provide home care services as part of their mission.

Combination Agencies. These are combined public and voluntary agencies. Such agencies are sometimes included with statistical counts for VNAs. Home health services are frequently provided by the nursing divisions of local health departments and may or may not combine the home care services (care of the sick) with their traditional public health nursing (preventive) services.

Homemaker-Home Care Aide Agencies. Agencies that provide homemaker-home care aide services exclusively are usually private and derive their reimbursement from direct payment by the client or private insurance policies. They may also be governed by individual owners or corporate headquarters.

Hospice. A hospice is a specialized program of health care for terminally ill patients and their families. The goals of hospice care are directed toward palliation of pain and control of other symptoms rather than toward curative measures. Hospice care is appropriate only for those patients for whom cure is no longer possible. A more in-depth discussion of hospice is found in Chapter 11.

Other Home Care Organizations. Other types of home care services, different than the ones mentioned earlier, can be provided by companies that perform a technical, house call function rather than a professional home care one. Usually these companies provide DME, high-technology services (e.g., ventilators, total parenteral nutrition) and other services to assist clients in their homes. Oxygen companies usually have respiratory therapists available to work with clients as contractors or as employees. Additionally, DME suppliers may have therapists who are available to go into a client's home to measure for equipment such as pull bars and other assistive devices and enterostomal therapists who can assist the client and nurse in planning for dressing and incontinent supplies. These home care providers do not provide any professional "hands on" clinical services in the home like those delivered by traditional home health agencies, such as nursing; physical, speech, or occupational therapy; social work; or home care aide services.

HOME HEALTH AGENCY PERSONNEL

The organizational structure of a home health agency varies by type, size, geographical location, and levels of accountability. The following discussion describes briefly the positions, functions, and roles of the typical positions found in the three areas of a home health agency: administration, management, and staff. A more in-depth discussion of clinical roles and functions and coverage guidelines for nursing, therapy, and social work can be found in Chapters 2 and 4.

Administration

The following three positions make up the basic administrative personnel of a home health agency. Various titles can be given to the positions, but the responsibilities remain almost the same. If the agency is very large, there may be more top administrators with various roles identified.

Executive Director or Chief Executive Officer (CEO). The CEO is responsible for the total administration of the agency and reports to the board of directors, owner, or corporate headquarters.

Assistant Director or Chief Operating Officer (COO). The COO is responsible for the day-to-day operations of the agency and is usually someone with a professional clinical background in one or more of the services provided by the agency. Most often that background is nursing, since most of the service provided is nursing. The COO reports to the CEO.

Finance Director or Chief Financial Officer (CFO). The CFO is responsible for the total financial operations of the agency. This administrator usually supervises the business office and reports to the CEO.

Management

The various management roles in a home health agency are the ones most determined by the size, type, and programs delivered by the agency. If programs or services are offered beyond the basic ones found in most home health agencies (e.g., nursing; physical, speech, and occupational therapy; social work; home care aide services), there will be a management person assigned to each program. The following is a list of typical management positions related to the clinical functions of a home health agency. The business office role and functions are covered at the end of this section.

Director of Clinical Services. The professional in this top management position, who oversees the personnel delivering the various program services of the agency,

is really the clinical supervisor's supervisor and may have several program directors and clinical supervisors reporting to him or her. The responsibility for maintaining the agency's professional standards of client care and compliance with various regulatory guidelines lies with this position. This director is comparable to the hospital director of nursing who reviews every aspect of the agency operations that affect patient care. In smaller agencies, this function may be assumed by the clinical nursing supervisor(s).

Nursing Supervisor or Clinical Coordinator. This supervisor is comparable to the head nurse in a hospital who usually assigns and schedules professional personnel and oversees and helps coordinate the care given by the nursing staff. The supervisor monitors the care given by all staff members working in the patient's care plan and is the link between staff and higher-level management and administration.

Intake Coordinator or Home Care Coordinator. The manager at this level sees that initial requests to the agency for home care are processed according to agency policy. This person is usually a nurse, with clerical and secretarial support provided to this function.

Home Care Aide Supervisor. Most agencies employ someone in this management position to oversee the overall personnel activities related to the home care aides. Instruction and supervision of a home care aide on direct client care in the home are provided by the home care nurse assigned to the clients. The home care aide supervisor works with the home care nurses to coordinate and evaluate client care provided by the paraprofessionals and also directs the inservice, scheduling, and personnel-related issues of the home care aides.

Special Supervisors. As mentioned earlier, there may be supervisors of special programs and services provided by a home health agency. Typically, individuals are named who supervise the services delivered by the therapy and social work departments; these individuals are usually called therapy supervisors or coordinators and social work supervisors. If the agency provides special programs to patient groups such as maternal-child health services, AIDS, and mental health, one supervisor may be assigned to oversee all those programs depending on the size of the agency and its client population.

Clinical Staff/Nurses

Because the clinical staff of a home health agency is determined by the type of services provided, the size of the agency, and the specific type of diagnoses the clients have, the following list discusses the clinical staff that might be found in a typical home health agency, regardless of type.

In home care the nurse plays a pivotal role in the care a client receives. Most agencies use a primary nurse and/or team model to deliver nursing care. Regardless of the model used, the nurse is the coordinator of the total care provided for all clients in coordination with the physician, client, family, other disciplines, and community resource agencies. There are a few clients in a caseload for whom physical and/or speech therapy is the only service needed and ordered. In this case, the nurse makes an initial visit, and if no nursing needs are found, the nurse remains available for consultation throughout the time the client is on service. The following description of nurse positions describes the various roles nurses can play in a home health agency.

Registered Nurse. These nurses may have associate degrees, diplomas, or BSN degrees, with responsibilities often tied to their level of education. Most HHAs feel that nurses with BSNs are best prepared to deliver the broad scope of skilled nursing services to their clients. Most agencies also require that a nurse have at least one year of clinical experience, preferably in medical/surgical nursing, before coming to home health. These nurses function in the mode of delivery determined by the agency, that is, primary care, team, or case management. Many registered nurses (RNs) have specialized skills that enable them to work with high-tech clients or clients who need long-term rehabilitation in the home.

Nurse Practitioner/Clinical Specialist. These nurses may provide total client care, supervise others in difficult cases related to their specialty, or direct a special program. For example, a pediatric nurse practitioner may not only deliver direct care to the agency's pediatric clients but may act as a consultant to staff RNs to develop a care plan for their pediatric clients. These specialty nurses may come from all fields; perinatal, cardiac, diabetic, and mental health are the most prevalent.

Enterostomal Therapist (ET). An agency may have an ET on staff who will provide direct care to clients or act as a consultant to staff members whose clients have bowel or bladder problems or wound management problems.

Licensed Practical Nurse (LPN). These nurses are called licensed vocational nurses (LVN) in California and Texas. The specific skills that an LPN can deliver to a home care client and the type of reimbursement are governed by the state nurse practice acts, state licensure laws for home health agencies, the policies of various reimbursement sources, and the policies of the home health agency.

A brief discussion of other providers can be found in the following section. The Medicare coverage criteria for these services and more elaboration about the types of services they deliver can be found in Chapter 4 and Transmittal 222 in Appendix O.

Therapists

Physical Therapist (PT). The PT delivers skilled care that involves assessment for assistive devices relative to rehabilitation and safety that can be used in the home, performs therapy procedures for the client, and teaches the client or family to assist in treatment. The PT usually works with a client who has limited mobility and is unable to go out of the home for therapy. The client's diagnosis must reflect the need for PT services.

Speech Therapist (ST). The ST provides speech therapy for clients whose diagnosis or condition indicates a need for such therapy.

Occupational Therapist (OT). This therapist provides care that is concerned with peak function, focusing on improving physical, mental, or social abilities. It is often difficult to decide when a client needs physical or occupational therapy, and the assessment should be made by the therapy department in collaboration with a nursing supervisor and the physician.

Social Worker (SW). Traditionally, social workers help clients and their families identify needs and make referrals to community resources. In home care the social work function also includes assisting with applications for services and providing financial assistance information.

Respiratory Therapist (RT). Some home health agencies work on a contractual basis with respiratory therapists for clients who have a diagnosis related to their respiratory function. This relationship is especially important with clients who are on ventilator support, and often the RT works with the DME supplier in providing not only the technical products and services (e.g., ventilator, oxygen) but also the professional treatment.

Dietitian. These staff members provide diet and nutrition counseling to clients with special needs. If an agency has this service available, it is usually on a contractual basis, since the direct service of a dietitian is not a reimbursable home care service.

Paraprofessionals

A home health agency usually provides the service of home care aides and, depending on the type of agency, homemaker services. Although these positions are separate, their functions overlap in many areas. The rule of thumb is that a home care aide may perform some of the duties of a homemaker (related to household tasks) but a homemaker is not qualified to provide the hands-on, personal client care a home care aide is trained to perform.

Home Care Aide (HCA). At most agencies a home care aide performs three general services: (1) personal care, (2) basic nursing tasks (as opposed to skilled), and (3) incidental homemaking. The home health agency will have a list of the "basic" personal care procedures a home care aide may perform, and the home care nurse needs to become familiar with these procedures to supervise the aides appropriately. Basic nursing care tasks include taking vital signs, conducting selected treatments, and assisting the client with self-administered medications. Most state laws prohibit aides from administering medications.

Homemaker (HM). The bulk of the work a homemaker provides is light housekeeping, such as washing the dishes, doing the laundry, preparing light meals, and changing the linens. Homemakers may also do grocery shopping and pick up medications for the client at the drugstore. Homemakers don't perform heavy housework and only under very strict guidance may assist the client directly with a minor aspect of personal care.

Business Office Staff

The business office of a home health agency is an integral part of the organization's ability to deliver services to clients. A home health agency cannot perform well without a business department that works closely with clinical staff. Never in your nursing career are you called upon to become involved with the financial aspects of your clients' care as you will be in home care. Throughout your orientation you will learn how to relate to the business department of your agency and what systems are in place for the processing of visit and financial information. As you look at the organizational structure, position titles, roles, and responsibilities of all departments in your agency, be sure to be clear also on the functions of the business office and personnel who work there; they will help you get your job done efficiently and effectively.

ENVIRONMENTAL INFLUENCES ON HOME CARE

Internal Influences

Mission

The internal environment of a home health agency is important because it provides the basic structure for the agency to reach its mission. Every agency should have a mission statement, sometimes called a purpose statement or list of objectives. This document outlines the population and services it has identified that it will deliver relative to home care. If the agency has a parent institution, then its mission statement should be reflected in the agency or unit objectives that relate to home health. You should review your agency's mission statement, goals and objectives, brochure, and any other printed materials given to the public or to clients. It is important that the nurse understands clearly the overall goals of the agency so she can assist in communicating them to others and ensure they are accomplished through the care provided.

Structure

The agency's administrative structure, found in its organizational chart, outlines the responsibilities each employee has to the organization. By reviewing this chart in orientation, the nurse can determine the type of agency as well as the roles and functions of the agency's personnel. Reporting responsibilities and the relationship of all employees to the client are outlined graphically in the organizational chart. Chapter 6 gives a more in-depth discussion of the various components of the structure and processes of a HHA in relation to measuring quality. Later in your orientation, you may want to read that section to better understand the various components of the internal influences of your agency and how they affect your daily practice.

Many factors outside of the internal organizational structure and the professional responsibilities of providers influence the way home care is provided. Because home care was initiated based on societal trends, it is important to look at the current social environment to understand how and why home care is practiced as it is today. The main external factors a nurse must be aware of to work in the home care field are (1) community and family aspects, (2) the political system, and (3) reimbursement.

External Influences

Community and Family Aspects

Home care begins with the individual client who has been identified as needing home care nursing or therapy. Although this is the initial focus, home care nurses must implement the nursing process using the principles of family and community health nursing. Usually the major base of client support comes from family, friends, neighbors, community resources, and religious affiliations who form the informal caregiving system so necessary to meet the client's needs at home. Even if the client lives alone and has no family nearby to assist, the home care nurse should look to this caregiving system as the family and apply many of the principles of family theory to the plan of care.

The community in which the client lives may assist or detract from the provision of professional home care and the attainment of home care goals. The ability to assess the client's community and its support of the client is a challenge for all home care nurses. Socioeconomic status, status in the community, cultural and ethnic background, religious practices, and the community's way of defining health, illness, and dying all impact on the client's home care plan and progress in meeting outcomes.

The Political System

Home care nursing is practiced within the context of the larger health care system. The nature of home care, providing care to individuals and families in their homes, dictates that there are many aspects in the external political environment that affect the way nurses are able to deliver care. Local, state, and federal laws that affect nursing practice, such as nurse practice acts, advance medical directives, and living wills, all have an impact on the way a nurse practices in home health. Simply because the client receives home health benefits that are payable under the federal programs of Medicare or Medicaid, those programs dictate a great deal of the ways nursing care is delivered in the home. Because reimbursement is such an important issue that affects home care practice, it is discussed further in the following section.

Reimbursement

Federal Government. Medicare (Title 18 of the Social Security Act) represents an effort by the federal government to provide national health insurance to an across-the-board population based on chronological age and other considerations, such as disability. It is an insurance program that almost everyone over 65 years of age is eligible for, regardless of income. It also includes persons under 65 years of age who are disabled for more than 24 months and are receiving Social Security benefits. Medicare is the largest single payer of home care services. In 1992, Medicare spending accounted for more than a third of total home care expenditures. Other funding sources for home care are listed in Table 1–2.

Although Medicare pays a large proportion of home health expenditures, the Medicare home health benefit represents only about 8% of total Medicare benefit pay-

Table 1–2 Sources of Payment for Home Care, 1992

Source of Payment	1992
Total	100.0%
Medicare	37.8%
Medicaid	24.7%
Private insurance	5.5%
Out-of-pocket	31.4%
Other	0.6%

Source: Reprinted with permission from *Basic Statistics about Home Care*, National Association for Home Care, © 1994.

ments in 1994. Over half of the estimated $167 billion Medicare benefit payments go to hospitals and nearly a quarter to physicians. Hospice payments account for less than 1% of total Medicare benefit payments (Health Care Financing Administration [HCFA], Office of the Actuary, unpublished information used for FY84 Board of Trustees Report).

The Medicare program is administered by HCFA, a branch of the Department of Health and Human Services. HCFA is responsible for overseeing the entire Medicare program, which governs how and what services are reimbursed by Medicare. The Medicare home health benefit is regulated by HCFA. The home health regulations set forth by HCFA have a great impact on how the home care nurse practices when caring for a Medicare client. The policies and regulations set by HCFA in the clinical and reimbursement areas are often followed by other payers, such as Medicaid and private insurance (Harris, 1994).

Although the administration of Medicare is controlled by HCFA, payments to agencies on behalf of the program are handled by a fiscal intermediary (FI). The FI is usually an insurance company that has a contract with HCFA to see that the regulations are carried out appropriately by providers (HHAs) and to issue payments on behalf of the Medicare beneficiary (the client). Chapters 4 and 5 outline Medicare requirements for home care, documentation necessary to indicate that care is covered, and how services are paid for by the FI.

State Government. Medicaid (Title 19 of the Social Security Act), a public assistance program, is a federally assisted state program that provides health care benefits to needy and low-income persons. Medicaid eligibility and coverage criteria vary from state to state and you should review the Medicaid home care regulations for your state during your orientation program.

The Medicaid program accounts for more than 20% of all HHA funding nationwide.

Commercial Insurance. Companies such as Blue Cross, AEtna, Prudential, and the Travelers provide varying degrees of home care coverage for the people they insure. The health insurance industry is rapidly recognizing the savings that can be realized by the use of home care services instead of institutional care, but getting coverage for clients who have private insurance is often as difficult as it can be for other types of payments, such as Medicare. Because commercial insurance coverage varies so much from client to client, the agency has a process to determine exactly what home care coverage the client has upon admission to the HHA. Review the agency's policy for dealing with private insurance clients.

Indigent Care. Delivering home care to clients who have no payment source has long been the mission of nonprofit HHAs, such as VNAs. Often called free or subsidized care, it is important that you, as a home care nurse, understand that the care is not free—someone is paying for it, just not the client. If an agency lets the amount of care exceed the financial resources available for that purpose, the agency can face a potentially catastrophic financial loss, which could jeopardize the future of the agency. Check your agency's policy on free and reduced fee care.

Other Reimbursement Programs and Payment Sources. There are many other programs existing nationally and on state or local levels that have been designed to assist home care clients who fall between the cracks of the Medicare and Medicaid programs. These programs, however, account for only 5% to 10% of the total money spent nationwide for home care. Private cash payers make up another payment source to the home health agency, but only to a very limited degree for the traditional services provided (nursing; physical, speech, and occupational therapies; social work; and home care aide). Private pay clients usually pay for the services of a private duty RN or for a home care aide beyond what is covered by another payer. They also pay for other services desired by the client that go beyond what is covered by a third-party payer. Rarely do clients pay directly for the minimum traditional services provided when they are acutely ill.

ETHICAL STANDARDS FOR HOME CARE: THE NAHC CLIENT BILL OF RIGHTS AND RESPONSIBILITIES

The NAHC has established a national code of ethics for its membership with the goal of informing the general public as to what ethical conduct for home health agencies and their employees involves. Federal legislation mandates that home health agencies participating in the Medicare program have a "client bill of rights and responsibilities." National trends indicate that the federal government will soon mandate specific ethical standards that will guarantee consumers certain rights while protecting the quality of home care they receive. The NAHC Bill of Rights (Exhibit 1–1) is helpful in understanding the rights of clients and families to quality home care. A home health agency may add any other rights it feels are applicable to its clients and may add responsibilities that the client and family must assume to receive home care. Listing both client rights and responsibilities emphasizes the active role clients and families must play in home care. An example of a client's responsibility might be the requirement to have supportive coverage when agency personnel are not present.

HOME CARE ORGANIZATIONS

The National Association for Home Care

The NAHC is the major organization that represents the broad spectrum of home health services on a national level. The NAHC was formed in 1982 by a merger of the National Association of Home Health Agencies (NAHHA) and the Council of Home Health Agencies/Community Health Services (CHHA/CHS). In 1986, the NAHC's allied organization, the Foundation for Hospice and Homecare, acquired the assets of the National HomeCaring Council, which accredits home care aide services. These affiliations bring the NAHC close to its goal of unifying the industry and being the one voice for home care on a national level.

NAHC Mission

The NAHC summarizes its mission in one line: "We're bringing health care back home where it belongs." The NAHC's specific mission involves the following 15 purposes:

1. Serve as the unified voice for the home care and hospice community.
2. Provide direct needed services to the members.
3. Heighten the political visibility of home care and hospice interests.
4. Influence the legislative, judicial, and regulatory processes with respect to issues of importance to hospice and home care.
5. Sponsor research and gather and disseminate home care and hospice data.

Exhibit 1–1
HOME CARE BILL OF RIGHTS

Home care clients have a right to be notified in writing of their rights and obligations before treatment begins and to exercise those rights. The client's family or guardian may exercise the client's rights when the client has been judged incompetent. Home care providers have an obligation to protect and promote the rights of their clients, including the following rights.

Clients and Providers Have a Right to Dignity and Respect

Home care clients and their formal caregivers have a right to not be discriminated against based on race, color, religion, national origin, age, sex, or handicap. Furthermore, clients and caregivers have a right to mutual respect and dignity, including respect for property. Caregivers are prohibited from accepting personal gifts and borrowing from clients.

Clients have the right:

- to have relationships with home care providers that are based on honesty and ethical standards of conduct
- to be informed of the procedure they can follow to lodge complaints with the home care provider about the care that is, or fails to be, furnished, and regarding a lack of respect for property. (To lodge complaints with us call _____)
- to know about the disposition of such complaints
- to voice their grievances without fear of discrimination or reprisal for having done so
- to be advised of the telephone number and hours of operation of the state's home health "hot line," which receives complaints or questions about local home care agencies. The hours are _____ and the number is _____

Decision Making

Clients have the right:

- to be notified in advance about the care that is to be furnished, the types (disciplines) of the caregivers who will furnish the care, and the frequency of the visits that are proposed to be furnished
- to be advised of any change in the plan of care before the change is made
- to participate in the planning of the care and in planning changes in the care, and to be advised that they have the right to do so
- to be informed in writing of rights under state law to make decisions concerning medical care, including the right to accept or refuse treatment and the right to formulate advance directives
- to be informed in writing of policies and procedures for implementing advance directives, including any limitations if the provider cannot implement an advance directive on the basis of conscience
- to have health care providers comply with advance directives in accordance with state law requirements
- to receive care without condition on, or discrimination based on, the execution of advance directives
- to refuse services without fear of reprisal or discrimination

The home care provider or the client's physician may be forced to refer the client to another source of care if the client's refusal to comply with the plan of care threatens to compromise the provider's commitment to quality care.

Privacy

Clients have the right:

- to confidentiality of the medical record as well as information about their health, social, and financial circumstances and about what takes place in the home
- to expect the home care provider to release information only as required by law or authorized by the client and to be informed of procedures for disclosure

continues

Exhibit 1–1 continued

Financial Information

Clients have the right:

- to be informed of the extent to which payment may be expected from Medicare, Medicaid, or any other payer known to the home care provider
- to be informed of the charges that will not be covered by Medicare
- to be informed of the charges for which the client may be liable
- to receive this information, orally and in writing, before care is initiated and within 30 calendar days of the date the home care provider becomes aware of any changes
- to have access, upon request, to all bills for service the client has received regardless of whether the bills are paid out-of-pocket or by another party

Quality of Care

Clients have the right:

- to receive care of the highest quality
- in general, to be admitted by a home care provider only if it has the resources needed to provide the care safely, and at the required level of intensity, as determined by a professional assessment; a provider with less than optimal resources may nevertheless admit the client if a more appropriate provider is not available, but only after fully informing the client of the provider's limitations and the lack of suitable alternative arrangements
- to be told what to do in the case of an emergency

The home care provider shall ensure that:

- all medically related home care is provided in accordance with physicians' orders and that a plan of care specifies the services and their frequency and duration
- all medically related personal care is provided by an appropriately trained home care aide who is supervised by a nurse or other qualified home care professional

Client Responsibility

Clients have the responsibility:

- to notify the provider of changes in their condition (e.g., hospitalization, changes in the plan of care, symptoms to be reported)
- to follow the plan of care
- to notify the provider if the visit schedule needs to be changed
- to inform providers of the existence of, and any changes made to, advance directives
- to advise the provider of any problems or dissatisfaction with the services provided
- to provide a safe environment for care to be provided
- to carry out mutually agreed responsibilities

To satisfy the Medicare certification requirements, the Health Care Financing Administration requires that agencies:

1. Give a copy of the Bill of Rights to each patient in the course of the admission process.
2. Explain the Bill of Rights to the patient and document that this has been done.

To minimize confusion, NAHC recommends that agencies have clients sign one form that shows that the client acknowledges all of the agency's policies and procedures (e.g., release of medical information, billing procedures).

Source: Copyright © 1993, National Association for Home Care. Used with permission.

6. Promote home care and hospice services as a viable component of the health care delivery system.
7. Foster, develop, and promote high standards of patient care in home care and hospice services.
8. Provide expert advice and assistance to members with respect to management, legal, or operational issues.
9. Disseminate information to the media and the general public to promote the acceptance of home care and hospice services and to support family/informal caregivers.
10. Expand private health insurance and other third-party sources for financing hospice and home care services.
11. Promote collaboration among national, state, and local organizations relating to home care and hospice services and issues.
12. Initiate, sponsor, and promote educational programs.
13. Represent the interests of caregivers (nurses, homemaker-home care aides, physicians, and therapists) who work in the home care field, and encourage individuals to choose a career in home care and hospice services.
14. Protect the legal rights of hospice and home care beneficiaries and those of the organizations and their employees who provide consumers with such services.
15. Promote independence and contribution by potential home care clients, thereby shattering the myth that dependence is a necessary state for the aged and disabled in America.

In addition to serving as the home care community's voice before Congress, regulatory agencies, courts, and the media, the NAHC provides the following services to its members: legislative, regulatory, and legal assistance; research, clinical, and policy information; insurance benefits; discounts on registration at NAHC-sponsored meetings; publications; educational, training, and public relations materials; and eligibility to participate in policy-changing focus groups. The NAHC produces several periodicals including a monthly magazine called *Caring*; a monthly newsletter called *Homecare News*; a monthly newsletter called *Caregiver*; a biweekly newsletter called *Hospice Forum*; a weekly legislative, regulatory, and legal "hot sheet" called *NAHC Report*; and *Health Care Reform Update*, a bulletin published twice a week to keep members up to date on the latest developments in health care reform.

NAHC Membership

The association primarily consists of home care and hospice provider agencies. The following eight categories of membership allow broad participation by a host of organizations and individuals interested in home care and hospice delivery.

1. *Provider members* are organizations whose primary purpose is to deliver health and social services directly to the sick and disabled in their own homes.
2. *Corporate membership* is available for the headquarters of multientity providers. It may include any home care provider that controls one or more additional legal entities in the home care field.
3. *Subcorporate membership* is open to branch offices of a corporate member.
4. *State association members* are state home care and hospice associations that collectively constitute the Forum of State Associations that is very active in working with the NAHC.
5. *Associate members* are for-profit entities that provide products or services to home care agencies, such as commercial suppliers, consultants, and vendors.
6. *Subcorporate associate members* are branch offices of associate members.
7. *Allied membership* is available for related not-for-profit health groups involved in home care, such as nursing schools, medical libraries, and other associations.
8. *Individual membership* is open to persons employed by a NAHC member agency and those interested in home care and hospice services, yet ineligible for membership in any other category. Individuals are grouped into special interest forums to build networks among industry members.

NAHC Affiliate Organizations

The NAHC has established special affiliate organizations to focus attention on specific areas of importance to the home care and hospice field (National Association for Home Care, 1994). These affiliates provide vehicles for communication, special interest dialogue, education, and training on issues relating to the specialties.

Hospice Association of America (HAA). This organization was founded in 1985 to give hospice providers a voice before Congress. HAA represents the full range of hospice programs, including free-standing, community- and coalition-based home care and hospital-based hospice programs. It is dedicated to promoting hospice as a concept of caring for the terminally ill rather than merely creating a place to die. The majority of hospice services are provided in the home.

Forum of State Associations. This group was established in 1985 as an entity for dialogue and information exchange among state associations representing home care and hospice. It aims to develop consensus and promote networking and communication throughout the home care community.

National Association for Physicians in Home Care (NAPHC). This association was created in 1986 to support the growing involvement of physicians in home care and hospice resulting from advances in home-specific medical technology and changes in hospital discharge policy. It serves as an advocate for home care and hospice physicians before Congress and the Administration and promotes education and information sharing within the profession.

The Center for Health Care Law. This is a nonprofit public interest law firm founded in 1987 to help protect the rights of Medicare patients and other vulnerable groups, such as the disabled and chronically ill.

World Organization for Care in the Home and Hospice (WOCHH). This organization was established in 1992 in response to requests by more than 70 countries that the NAHC be the moving force behind an international association. The goals of this association are to share information; influence public policy; provide education, training, and quality assurance; and enhance public awareness of the universal shift from institutional to home and community-based care.

National Home Care and Hospice Congressional Network (NAHC NET). This network was founded in early 1994 to serve as a national legislative grassroots network comprised of NAHC and State Forum members who are home care and hospice providers. It supplies participants with federal legislation information and educational tools to help them lobby members of Congress on critical hospice and home care issues.

Hospital Home Care Association of America (HHCAA). HHCAA was established in 1994 to focus on issues pertinent to hospital and home care service operation and integration. It aims to assist hospital- and nonhospital-based providers in managing agencies successfully within the changing health care environment.

VNA of America

VNA of America (VNAA) is a national organization that represents a sector of home care providers, the VNA. The VNAA is a national network of over 500 community-based, nonprofit, Medicare-certified home health agencies serving virtually every part of the country. VNAA, started in 1982, provides membership programs, educational events, business development, managed care marketing and contracting, communications, national imaging, and group purchasing services for its members.

State and Local Organizations

Most states have one or more home care organizations that have similar goals as the NAHC with a focus on local and state issues. These organizations may work with the national association(s) but additionally represent their members with the state legislature, state Medicaid program, and other state legislative and regulatory bodies that deal with home care. A large benefit of the state associations is their ability to provide local and regional meetings that provide updates on current issues affecting the industry as well as inservice educational offerings for all home health personnel. The opportunity to network with peers and share ideas, as well as ways to address problems, makes membership in the state home health association a must for most agencies.

With the progression of managed care and health care reform, many home health agencies and other health organizations have come together to form local and regional networks. Your agency may be a member of these and may share the information that pertains to your specific responsibilities in orientation.

CERTIFICATION, LICENSURE, AND ACCREDITATION

Medicare Conditions of Participation

The regulations that certify a home health agency to participate in the Medicare program are called Conditions of Participation. In order for a home care organization to receive Medicare Part A or Medicaid reimbursement, the home care organization must be surveyed and certified by a state agency as complying with the Conditions of Participation developed by HCFA (Conditions of Participation, 1991).

As a staff nurse your main responsibility is to know these conditions exist and to understand that policies, procedures, and billing practices are often dictated by these regulations. Although the responsibility for adherence to the conditions is ultimately up to the managers and administrators of your agency, it is up to everyone on staff, especially the home care nurse, to see that policies are followed.

State Licensing Laws

Thirty-nine states have licensure laws for home health agencies that set specific requirements about staffing, policies, and practices and set minimal operating standards for various services and programs. The licensure requirements are closely linked to Medicare's Conditions of Participation. If a state has a licensure law, an agency must be licensed before applying for Medicare certification.

Agencies are required to be surveyed not later than 15 months after the date of the previous standard survey for certification (and licensure, where required) on a surprise basis as mandated by the Omnibus Budget Reconciliation Act of 1987. Frequently, the individual state health department has a contract with the HCFA to conduct the certification survey. This means that an agency can become both certified for Medicare and state licensed at the same time by this same survey. You will likely be involved in some aspect of the licensure visit under the direction of your supervisor.

If a home health agency meets the requirements put forth in the licensure law, it will receive a license. If not, the agency may be given a certain period of time to reach compliance, or if the problems are severe, the agency will not be permitted to operate until the standards in the laws are met.

Accreditation

Accreditation is a voluntary process that allows the home care organization to demonstrate to the public and its customers that it provides coordinated, integrated, quality home care services delivered by proficient, competent health care professionals and para-professionals. The process of accreditation allows an objective, third-party operational review to occur that is conducted by surveyors from the accrediting organization. The decision to become accredited and by what organization is determined by the home care organization; it is not a requirement for participation in either Medicare or Medicaid. The accreditation process is always in addition to the licensing and Medicare

Conditions of Participation review process outlined earlier.

Why Home Care Organizations Seek Accreditation

Many home care organizations have or are currently seeking accreditation as insurers and case managers are recognizing voluntary home care accreditation as a requirement to be a part of preferred provider contracts and referral arrangements or health care networks. Voluntary accreditation has become an industry measure that indicates the home health agency provides high quality home care services. Some home care organizations that are functionally and organizationally related to a Joint Commission on Accreditation of Healthcare Organizations (Joint Commission) accredited organization, such as a hospital, are also required to be accredited based on Joint Commission internal policies. The result of accreditation is similar to receiving the "Good Housekeeping Seal of Approval" for the home care organization. Once home care accreditation has been achieved, a continuous commitment to improving the organization's performance and maintaining substantial compliance with the standards is paramount.

MAJOR HOME CARE ACCREDITING BODIES

The three major accrediting bodies for home care organizations are the Joint Commission; the Community Health Accreditation Program (CHAP), through the National League for Nursing (NLN); and the National HomeCaring Council.

Joint Commission on Accreditation of Healthcare Organizations

The Joint Commission has been accrediting home care organizations since the inception of its Home Care Accreditation Program in 1988. The accreditation process begins with an application and deposit submitted to the Joint Commission. The home care organization is then scheduled for an on-site review within four to six months of the application date. The duration of the survey is a minimum of one day, but is increased depending on the volume of the services provided, the number of branches, and their distance from their main office. Additionally, the variety of services provided by the home care organization directly or indirectly through a contract will influence the length of the survey process.

The focus of the on-site survey process includes a review of the activities and responsibilities of the governing body and management, staff interviews, home visits, documentation review, clinical record review, and as applicable, a review of equipment, warehouse, and delivery vehicles and pharmacy operations.

The accreditation decision is based on the home care organization's demonstration of compliance with the standards in the *Accreditation Manual for Home Care.* Compliance with the standards is measured using a scoring system of one to five. Upon completion of the survey, the surveyor will review the findings during an exit conference held with staff and management and will submit a report to the Joint Commission. These findings are reviewed to ensure national consistency in the interpretation of the standards, and the final report will recommend an accreditation decision to the Joint Commission Accreditation Committee.

The outcome of the accreditation visit results in the home care agency being placed in one of five categories: (1) accreditation with commendation, (2) accreditation with or without recommendations, (3) conditional accreditation, (4) provisional accreditation, and (5) not accredited. Except for provisional accreditation, the accreditation decision is awarded for three years. One-day, unannounced surveys are conducted to a random sampling of 5 percent of accredited organizations approximately midpoint in the triennial accreditation time period. The home care organization is contacted 24 hours in advance if it is to be surveyed on selected standards that were found to be problematic for home care organizations on a national basis. The results of the random, unannounced survey may change the organization's overall accreditation status; therefore, it is essential for an agency to always keep up with the accreditation standards.

Community Health Accreditation Program

CHAP is a subsidiary of the NLN. CHAP has been accrediting home care organizations since 1965. Accreditation by CHAP involves a four-step process. The accreditation process begins with an application submitted to CHAP and a contract returned to the home care organization outlining the fees and the specific elements of the three-year contract. The home care organization then completes a self-study guide that is a preparation for the on-site visit (National League for Nursing, 1993). The self-study is a self-assessment of the organization that allows the organization to compare itself against the CHAP standards in clinical and business aspects, fiscal viability, and focus on the consumer of services.

After the self-study is received, plans are made for an on-site visit. The on-site visit is conducted by a team of surveyors who remain on site an average of four to five days, as determined by the size and complexity of the organization. The surveyors review appropriate documents to ensure the quality of clinical services, financial stability, and the appropriateness of the organization's strategic plan. Considerable time in the survey is spent on home visits and staff and governing body interviews, as well as telephone surveys to clients and the others in the community who work with the organization. Findings of the site visit are discussed at an exit conference with management and staff, and consultation from the surveyors is available regarding specific findings.

A cumulative look at the completed self-study prior to the on-site survey and a review of findings from the survey team is done by a CHAP board of review to determine the accreditation status of the home care organization. Once accredited, the home care organization receives a focused visit annually and an on-site total accreditation visit from a survey team on a three-year cycle.

National HomeCaring Council

The National HomeCaring Council, a division of the Foundation for Hospice and Home Care, has been accrediting home care aide services since 1971. The process of seeking accreditation begins with the home care organization. Similar to the CHAP process, the home care organization must complete a six-month self-study and related community organization and consumer questionnaires that are then sent to the council. A two-day on-site visit by one or two surveyors is scheduled to review the home care organization's operations. At the conclusion of the site visit, an exit conference is conducted to share findings and any recommendations.

An unbiased review of the survey findings is conducted by the accreditation commission by coding each report to allow anonymity. The accreditation commission then reviews and acts on the report by granting full accreditation for three years with an interim review, provisional accreditation for one year to conform to the standards, or denial of accreditation.

DEEMED STATUS

As mentioned earlier, HCFA requires home health organizations to comply with the Medicare Conditions of Participation. If a national accrediting organization such as the Joint Commission or CHAP provides HCFA reasonable assurance that the home care organization it accredits meets the federal Conditions of Participation, HCFA may "deem" the home care organization as meeting the certification requirements. Thus, the home care organization undergoing an annual unannounced survey could have "deemed status" and would not have to undergo the Medicare certification review. Deemed status may not eliminate the requirement for state licensure surveys, however.

Seeking deemed status through accreditation is optional and may be conducted by the Joint Commission or CHAP. The home care organization may choose to continue with the usual state survey process and not pursue deemed status. Regardless of which survey method is selected, to continue Medicare certification, the home care agency must undergo an annual, unannounced survey process that examines the agency's compliance with the Conditions of Participation.

The home care accreditation programs discussed in this section have established standards of excellence for home care organizations. These standards demonstrate to the public and the home care organization's customers and staff that it delivers quality home care services that can be measured and validated.

THE STAFF NURSE'S ROLE IN THE ACCREDITATION AND SURVEY PROCESS

The staff nurse is increasingly asked to participate in survey and accreditation visits to a home care organization. This section outlining the staff nurse's role and responsibilities in these various processes has been developed to examine all the potential experiences a staff nurse may have based on the various accreditation and certification processes discussed previously. Specific references are made to Joint Commission requirements because many home health organizations are seeking Joint Commission accreditation and the number of hospital-based home health agencies is rising rapidly. If your agency is not accredited by the Joint Commission or CHAP or if you are not chosen to participate in the survey process, this material can still be helpful. An understanding of the large amount of information a staff nurse is expected to know will assist you in fulfilling your responsibility to the organization, yourself, and the client and family and additionally help you understand why the orientation process is so essential to your successful functioning in the home health agency.

1995 Joint Commission Orientation Content Requirements for Staff Nurses

In the *Accreditation Manual for Home Care* (Joint Commission, 1995a, 1995b), the Joint Commission outlines the minimal topics that must be addressed during the nurse's orientation. Exhibit 1–2 includes the minimal content staff nurses are responsible for knowing and applying to their assigned responsibilities.

Other standards that may pertain to the knowledge and skills of the staff nurse depend on how the nurse's job description, duties, and responsibilities have been determined. An important aspect of a staff nurse's duties centers on the management of information. The Joint Commission standards require individuals to understand the principles of information management if they generate, collect, analyze, and use data and information. The staff nurse may need to understand the following important areas affecting principles of information management in a HHA:

- ensuring security and confidentiality of data and information
- using measurement instruments, statistical tools, and data analysis methods
- collecting unbiased data and assisting in interpreting the data
- using data and information to assist in decision making
- educating and supporting the participation of clients and families in the care processes and using indicators to assess and improve systems and processes over time

This information may be provided to the HHA staff in the initial orientation or may be provided on a just-in-time basis, such as when the staff nurse participates in the measurement phase of a process improvement team and must understand statistical tools and techniques.

In the *Accreditation Manual for Home Care* (Joint Commission, 1995a, 1995b), the standard requires that the organization comply with applicable laws and regulations. This standard applies to the Occupational Safety and Health Administration (OSHA) bloodborne pathogen regulations and the airborne pathogen regulations. These regulations require that staff receive training upon hire and annually thereafter. Prior to performing care the staff member must be determined to be proficient in the skills relative to these issues. Equipment set-up standards for home care nurses are shown in Exhibit 1–3.

Exhibit 1–2
JOINT COMMISSION TOPICS TO BE ADDRESSED DURING NURSES' ORIENTATION

The staff nurse must demonstrate the following skills and knowledge:

- an understanding of the types of care or services to be delivered in the client's environment
- equipment management, including safe and appropriate use of equipment as applicable to the care or service provided: Individuals responsible for maintaining equipment must demonstrate knowledge and competence in appropriate maintenance procedures for all equipment, and when required by the manufacturer, individuals responsible for preventive maintenance must successfully complete the manufacturer's training program or another training program with equivalent content
- home safety issues including bathroom, fire, environmental, and electrical safety
- storage, handling, and access to supplies, medical gases, and drugs appropriate to the care or service provided
- identification, handling, and disposal of hazardous or infectious materials and wastes in a safe and sanitary manner and in accordance with law and regulation
- principles of infection control, including personal hygiene, precautions to be taken, aseptic procedures, communicable infections and appropriate cleaning, disinfection and/or sterilization of equipment and supplies
- confidentiality of client information
- appropriate policies and procedures
- community resources as applicable to the care or service provided
- guidelines for appropriate referrals, which include timeliness
- appropriate actions in unsafe situations
- any specific tests or procedures to be performed by the staff
- policies and procedures regarding advance directives
- organizational policies and procedures regarding death and dying
- screening for abuse and neglect, appropriate to the staff member's role and responsibility
- emergency preparedness
- any other client care responsibilities
- information regarding the care or service to be provided by other members of the staff to better coordinate care and appropriately refer the client

Source: Adapted from "Management of Human Resources," in *Accreditation Manual for Home Care, Volume II: Scoring Guidelines*, Joint Commission on Accreditation of Healthcare Organizations, 1995.

Exhibit 1–3
JOINT COMMISSION EQUIPMENT SET-UP STANDARDS FOR HOME CARE NURSES

Home care nurses who are involved in equipment set-up need to demonstrate competency in the following areas:

- arrangement of the home to accommodate the physical, electrical, and other needs of the equipment
- duties of unpacking, assembling, and performing needed operational checks of equipment
- verification of appropriate considerations for equipment adaptation or fitting when applicable
- correct use, operation, storage, maintenance, and cleaning and/or disinfecting of equipment and related supplies in the home according to the manufacturer's guidelines

Source: Adapted from "Environment of Care," in *Accreditation Manual for Home Care, Volume II: Scoring Guidelines*, Joint Commission on Accreditation of Healthcare Organizations, 1995.

Survey Process

Staff Interview

In the past, home care surveyors sat in a conference room looking at agency documents and client records. In the current environment of active quality management, the current survey process is interactive and outcome oriented. As part of this interactive survey process, staff members will be randomly selected for the surveyor to interview. This interview may take place in the car driving back and forth from home visits, in a group setting, or individually in the home care office. The scope of the interview will parallel the applicable accreditation standards and explore how the home care organization meets those standards.

Some issues that would be appropriate for a surveyor to discuss with a staff nurse include a review of the processes for care and service planning and coordination between nursing and pharmacy, client and family training and documentation for equipment management, interventions used by the nurse for medication administration, emergency procedures, and hazardous waste management in the home. The staff nurse's knowledge and processes will be evaluated by the surveyor regarding safe use of equipment, electrical safety, handling hazardous drugs, disposal of hazardous drugs and management of spills, as well as the nurse's management of adverse drug reactions. To be successful in the interview process, the staff nurse should be familiar with the procedures and general policies of the home care organization. During orientation, the staff nurse is exposed to all documents that support the home care organization's processes. This is the critical first step in understanding their implementation and being able to recount that to a surveyor during the accreditation process.

Home Visits

The surveyor is required to make home visits and will randomly select clients for whom care will be ob-
served and the client and family will be interviewed. Surveyors may select clients who are receiving the following services: an admission visit; wound care; specialty or high-risk clients; multidisciplinary services; and high-volume or low-volume service. During the home visit, the surveyor will be reviewing the environment of care to determine if all risk factors have been identified and if the home is suitable for care. The education of the client and family is assessed to determine if training specific to the client's and family's needs and abilities is provided and if the educational process is interdisciplinary, if that is appropriate to each client's plan of care.

Infection control measures in the home will be assessed by the surveyor to ensure that clinical practice is conducted according to the home care organization's policies and procedures and applicable laws and regulations. The nurse's vehicle will be monitored for storage of supplies, hazardous waste, and ways of ensuring confidentiality of client records carried in the field. The nurse's bag will be inspected to determine if prescription drugs are carried and, if they are carried, that they are properly dispensed and labeled. The surveyor will determine if the client and family have been informed of their rights and responsibilities, if they are knowledgeable regarding how to voice complaints or grievances, and if they understand how to contact the home care organization after normal business hours.

CONCLUSION

It is important that the new home care nurse understand generally the many aspects involved in the home care system. This chapter has outlined the major aspects common to all home care agencies (e.g., types of agencies, personnel, and environmental influences that affect practice). This information sets the stage for the rest of the work, which examines in detail the role and function of the home care nurse as she works in the larger home health system.

TEST YOURSELF

1. Discuss aspects of the development of home care in the United States discussed in this chapter that you found interesting.

2. Based on your reading, develop your own definition of home care.

3. In what type of home health agency do you work?

4. How does your job fit into the mission of the agency?

5. Name two types of home care reimbursement mechanisms and the populations they serve.

6. Does your agency belong to NAHC? If yes, what are the benefits you/they derive?

7. Discuss the similarities and differences between the NAHC Bill of Rights and Responsibilities and your agency's.

8. Is your agency licensed? Certified? Accredited? If yes, by whom? When is the next scheduled visit(s)?

REFERENCES

American Colleges of Physicians, Health and Public Policy Committee. (1986). Home health care position paper. *Annals of Internal Medicine, 105,* 454–460.

American Hospital Association. (1992). *Hospital statistics, 1993–1994 edition.* Chicago: Author.

Clemen-Stone, S., Eigsti, D., & McGuire, S. (1995). *Comprehensive community health nursing family, aggregate, and community practice* (4th ed.) St. Louis: Mosby.

Conditions of Participation, 42 C.F.R. §484 (1991).

Harris, M.D. (1994). *Handbook of home health care administration.* Gaithersburg, MD: Aspen Publishers.

Humphrey, C.J. (1988). The home as a setting for care—clarifying the boundaries of practice. *Nursing Clinics of North America, 223,* 305–314.

Joint Commission on Accreditation of Healthcare Organizations. (1995a). *Accreditation manual for home care, Volume I: Standards.* Oakbrook Terrace, IL: Author.

Joint Commission on Accreditation of Healthcare Organizations. (1995b). *Accreditation manual for home care, Volume II: Scoring guidelines.* Oakbrook Terrace, IL: Author.

Mundinger, M. (1983). *Home care controversy: Too little, too late, too costly.* Rockville, MD: Aspen Publishers.

Nassif, J.F. (1985). *The home health care solution.* Mount Vernon, NY: Consumers Union.

National Association for Home Care. (1987). *How to choose a home care agency.* Washington, DC: Author.

National Association for Home Care. (1994). *About NAHC: A profile of the National Association for Home Care.* Washington, DC: Author.

National League for Nursing. (1993). Policies and procedures. In *Standards of excellence for home care organizations.* (pp. 2–11). New York: Author.

Roberts, D., & Heinrich, J. (1985). Public health nursing comes of age. *American Journal of Public Health, 75* (10), 162–167.

The Specialty of Home Care Nursing

OBJECTIVES

Upon completion of this chapter, the reader will be able to identify:

1. The definition of home care nursing
2. Issues involved in moving from hospital to home care nursing
3. The purpose of home care standards
4. Aspects of becoming a certified home care nurse
5. Roles and functions of the home care nurse
6. How the nursing process is implemented in home care nursing practice
7. Criteria used to determine a client's discharge from home care

AGENCY-SPECIFIC MATERIAL NEEDED

- New staff nurse's job description
- Standardized care plans (if used)
- Home care aide job description
- Community resource file
- Case conference documentation form, if used
- Criteria for discharge and discharge summary procedure
- Intra- and interagency referral form
- Listing of community resources with phone numbers
- Local telephone book, including Yellow Pages

KEY CONCEPTS

- **Definition of home care nursing**
- **Considerations in moving from the hospital to home care**
- **Home care nursing as a specialty practice area**
- **Supervision of paraprofessionals**
- **Steps of the nursing process applied to home care**
- **The home care nurse as coordinator of service**
- **Effects of reimbursement on home care nursing practice**
- **Setting client-centered goals and priorities**
- **Discharging the client from service**

INTRODUCTION

Chapter 1 outlines the many aspects of home care as a broad field that provides both technical and professional services to people in their homes. This chapter serves as an introduction to the focus of this text, that is, the provision of professional home care nursing services. Home care nursing is a specialized practice area within nursing, and this chapter outlines the numerous components of the role and function of a home care nurse, the nursing process applied to home care, and how to do a home visit. Before exploring the many aspects of the home care nursing role, it is important to answer the question: What is home care nursing?

HOME CARE NURSING—WHAT IS IT?

Home care nursing is a unique field of nursing practice that focuses on caring for the sick in the home. This unique field of practice requires a synthesis of community health nursing principles with the theory and practice of medical/surgical, maternal-child, and mental health nursing. Home care nursing is provided to clients experiencing an illness outside the confines of an acute care hospital. Home care nurses care for acute and chronic clients of all ages, those who have procedures and treatments conducted in their homes, and those who wish to live out the final stages of life in their homes rather than in an institution.

Home care nursing, especially since the inception of Medicare, has become known as the provision of care to ill persons in the home as evidenced by the definitions outlined in Chapter 1. Many agencies call the home care program, Care of the Ill (COI), to denote this specific kind of client as compared with those clients who are primarily receiving health promotion/illness prevention interventions. Clearly, home care nursing is much more than just the provision of medical/surgical nursing in the home.

The client cared for by the home care nurse is the individual client, his or her family, and significant others. Caring for an ill individual at home is complex and requires that the nurse consider numerous factors related to the client's family, home, and community. Also, to care for a home care client professionally, the nurse must understand how the environmental, psychosocial, economic, cultural, and personal health-related factors affect the client's illness and his or her ability to meet the goals outlined in the plan of care. This broad approach of caring for individuals, families, and communities is the cornerstone of community health nursing practice.

Community health nurses are experts on intervening with families and communities to maximize the effect of the medical and nursing regimen on the client's care. To deliver home care services effectively, the nurse must be familiar with principles of community health nursing and with the principles underlying medical/surgical, maternal-child, and mental health nursing practice. These practice areas are used together by the home care nurse to provide comprehensive quality nursing services to clients in their homes.

In the current regulatory and economic climate in health care, it is increasingly difficult for the home care nurse to practice the community health nursing role with clients. Reimbursement sources focus on medical diagnoses and often are not supportive of what they perceive is the "extra" care (beyond basic medical/surgical care) a client may need. For example, a client who needs a dressing change may also be having difficulty coping with his or her diagnosis and prognosis and should be able to discuss it with the nurse with the possibility of being referred to other agencies for the necessary counseling. The extra time needed to integrate this supportive care is difficult to deliver when the nurse is asked to justify reimbursement for service by focusing on the direct care given to the wound. Intervention in areas other than wound care are not supported by reimbursement sources and often not by others in the home care area.

It is important that, in this environment, the home care nurse continue to provide a comprehensive approach to client care (relating to all areas of nursing practice) and act as a client advocate in justifying this care as essential, not extra. The focus of nursing care is the treatment of human responses. Home care nursing demands that the varied human responses seen in home care clients are addressed in a holistic framework so the client and family can be assisted to reach their goals.

Definition of Home Care Nursing

Although many sources discuss the aspects of home care nursing, there is no consensus on a definition. For the purpose of this text, the following definition will be used:

> Home care nursing is the provision of nursing care to acute, chronically ill, and well clients of all ages in their homes while integrating community health nursing principles that focus on health promotion and on environmental, psychosocial, economic, cultural, and personal health factors affecting an individual's and family's health status.

Transitioning from Hospital to Home Care Nursing

Many nurses come to home care with experience exclusively in an institutional setting. Because home health agencies typically require at least one year of experience in an acute care setting prior to employment, even nurses who have had home care as part of their educational preparation have adjustments to make in this new specialty area of practice. If new nurses are to make a successful transition to home care, it is important that they identify the major differences in the two areas of practice and seek out ways to learn this information. Additionally, there are also commonalties faced by all nurses who move from a structured institutional setting to home care. To move through the transition more comfortably, it can be helpful for nurses to realize they are not the only ones who are having these feelings. The following differences between hospital and home care nursing have been identified.

Assessment Skills

In the hospital, the nurse mainly focuses on applying physical and psychological assessment skills to the individual in the structured institutional environment. In home care, the nurse also conducts a complete physical and psychological assessment, but additionally assesses social, economic, environmental, home safety, and family issues that affect the client's care.

Autonomy

Even when an institution has a primary care nursing focus of delivering client care, nurses care for clients on only one shift (8–12 hours). There is always another shift that comes on and considers the nursing needs of the client for those other hours of the day. In home care, the client's 24-hour care must be considered in the care plan. Time management is a critical aspect of a successful home care nurse. The nurse must plan the day, balancing travel and visit time, professional activities, and paperwork to maximize time.

Communication with the Physician

The client and nurse see a physician at least daily in the hospital, and specific orders are written based on their assessments. Because the nurse can talk directly with the physician, there are opportunities for face-to-face communication and collaborative problem solving. Clients receiving home care may not have seen a physician for several days or weeks. The physician relies on the nurse to make skillful assessments and communicate concisely and in a timely manner regarding significant changes in the client's condition. This means the home care nurse must learn how to communicate with the physician concisely and paint a picture of the client over the telephone to the physician.

Determining Frequency and Duration of Care

The discharge date of a hospitalized client is determined predominantly by the physician, the hospital's utilization review department, and the insurer. In home care, the nurse, in collaboration with the physician, uses the Medicare coverage criteria and the client's needs to determine the frequency (how many visits a week) and the duration (for how many weeks) of care.

Direct Care

The technical skills provided to the client in the hospital center around interpreting laboratory values, using high-technology equipment, and providing hands-on care that focuses on the acutely ill. In home care, nurses have to be able to improvise equipment for clients with limited resources, understand the various aspects of home visiting, use the nursing bag appropriately, and teach a variety of skills to clients and their caregivers.

Documentation

The hospital nurse focuses client documentation on improvement that is being made with an eye toward a quick discharge to another level of service. Because home care is usually the last service delivered before the client is left to self-care, the goals and relative documentation need to be comprehensive. Such documentation covers anticipatory guidance to prevent future problems, provision of direct treatments of current conditions such as wounds, and client teaching. The documentation should focus on those areas in which the home care nurse can affect change in collaboration with the client and be specific on how this is measured.

Patient Teaching

No matter how much the nurse loves to teach clients, the health care system demands that clients be discharged from the hospital before adequate teaching can be completed. Teaching is a skilled service that is Medicare reimbursable and is one of the main roles of the home care nurse.

Referral to Community Resources

While the client is in the hospital, the social service department and the discharge planning department primarily assess and coordinate the client's need for external referrals, including home care. As the coordinator of the client's care, the home care nurse is responsible for identifying the needs *and* ensuring that the client and family are aware of what might be helpful. This means the home care nurse must develop knowledge, over time, of the community resources available both locally and nationwide.

Reimbursement

In the hospital, the admission and billing offices, in conjunction with the physician, handles all the client's financial information. Although home health agencies have similar departments in the office, the nurse validates and discusses these issues with the client and family in the home and verifies the client's eligibility for home care services with the physician.

Safety

In the hospital, workplace issues center on the Occupational Safety and Health Administration (OSHA), hospital security, and implementation of internal clinical safety practices. These are present in home care also, but because the nurse travels away from the office to see clients, she must be able to read a map, manage home visiting safety issues, and assess troublesome situations.

Work Environment

In the hospital, the client is always there, usually in the bed or in the room. Everything is familiar and handy for the nurse, and she is supported with a myriad of departments such as dietary, lab, X-ray, pharmacy, laundry, and housekeeping. If something goes wrong with the client, the nurse can call others to assist. In home care, the nurse is always a guest in the client's home and often has to adjust to variations in a client's environment. The family is present and should be included in the plan of care where appropriate. If, on a visit, the client is found to need further assistance, the nurse must rely on her assessments to make clinical judgments in collaboration with others via the telephone, if available.

Home Care Nursing Standards

An essential aspect of home care nursing that sets it apart from the services of technical home care providers is that of a practice based on professional standards. The American Nurses Association (ANA) has produced *Standards for Home Health Nursing Practice* (ANA, 1986b) to fulfill the profession's obligation to provide a means

of improving the quality of care provided to consumers. Standards reflect the current state of knowledge in the field and are the basis for characterizing, measuring, and providing guidance in achieving quality care. The home care standards are based on the ANA *Standards of Community Health Nursing Practice* (ANA, 1986a) and are to be used with that document to base nursing service practice in home health agencies. The standards, without their interpretive statements, are found in Exhibit 2–1.

The standards reflect two levels of practice: that of the generalist prepared at the baccalaureate level and that of the specialist prepared at the graduate level. In the absence of the specialist, the generalist may assume aspects of the comprehensive role of the specialist. These standards outline levels of professional nursing practice to be achieved by the nurse and should be reviewed with your supervisor early in your orientation. As the home care nurse goes through the orientation, she should look for the ways her agency integrates the standards in the many areas of practice and the agency's policies.

Home Care Nursing Certification

Nurses from many specialty areas, including home care, can have a tangible indicator of their excellence in practice by becoming certified by the ANA. In 1973, the ANA established the ANA certification program to provide recognition to nurses who have demonstrated professional achievement in a defined functional or clinical area of nursing. The American Nurses Credentialing Center (ANCC), a division of the ANA, was formed to develop and administer the credentialing programs for nurses. The goal of the ANCC is to promote and enhance the public health by certifying nurses who perform nursing care based on the standards of practice for their profession.

Certification can be obtained in both general and specialty areas of nursing practice. The areas of general practice in which nurses can become certified include:

- psychiatric and mental health nursing
- medical/surgical nurse
- gerontological nurse
- college health nurse
- perinatal nurse
- pediatric nurse
- high-risk perinatal nurse
- maternal-child nurse
- community health nurse
- school nurse

Exhibit 2–1
ANA STANDARDS FOR HOME HEALTH NURSING PRACTICE

Standard I. Organization of Home Health Services
All home health services are planned, organized, and directed by a master's-prepared professional nurse with experience in community health and administration

Standard II. Theory
The nurse applies theoretical concepts as a basis for decisions in practice.

Standard III. Data Collection
The nurse continuously collects and records data that are comprehensive, accurate, and systematic.

Standard IV. Diagnosis
The nurse uses health assessment data to determine nursing diagnoses.

Standard V. Planning
The nurse develops care plans that establish goals. The care plan is based on nursing diagnoses and incorporates therapeutic, preventive, and rehabilitative nursing actions.

Standard VI. Intervention
The nurse, guided by the care plan, intervenes to provide comfort, to restore, improve, and promote health, to prevent complications and sequelae of illness, and to effect rehabilitation.

Standard VII. Evaluation
The nurse continually evaluates the client's and family's responses to interventions in order to determine progress toward goal attainment and to revise the database, nursing diagnosis, and plan of care.

Standard VIII. Continuity of Care
The nurse is responsible for the client's appropriate and uninterrupted care along the health care continuum, and therefore, uses discharge planning, case management, and coordination of community resources.

Standard IX. Interdisciplinary Collaboration
The nurse initiates and maintains a liaison relationship with all appropriate health care providers to ensure that all efforts effectively complement one another.

Standard X. Professional Development
The nurse assumes responsibility for professional development and contributes to the professional growth of others.

Standard XI. Research
The nurse participates in research activities that contribute to the profession's continuing development of knowledge of home health care.

Standard XII. Ethics
The nurse uses the code for nurses established by the American Nurses Association as a guide for ethical decision making in practice.

Source: Reprinted with permission from *Standards for Home Health Nursing Practice*, American Nurses Association, © 1986.

- staff development
- home health care
- cardiac rehabilitation
- general nursing practice
- informatics

Certification in a specialty practice usually requires advanced education or continuing education in a specialized area of nursing. The areas of specialty practice in which a nurse can become certified include:

- pediatric nurse practitioner
- school nurse practitioner
- adult nurse practitioner
- family nurse practitioner
- gerontological nurse practitioner
- psychiatric and mental health clinical specialist—adult
- psychiatric and mental health clinical specialist—child and adolescent

- medical/surgical clinical specialist
- gerontological clinical specialist
- community health clinical specialist
- nursing administration
- nursing administration—advanced

The number of nurses in the specialty of home care nursing has grown in the last several years in response to shortened hospital stays, increased use of community-based health services, and client preference for home care. In 1993, the first home care certification exam was administered by the ANCC, establishing home care nursing as a specialty area of practice. The home care nurse certification exam is based on the scope of home health care practice and the standards of practice for home health care nursing developed by the ANA. Certification of home care nurses provides a way to ensure that standards of quality in home health nursing practice are maintained. Nurses working in home care can choose to become certified in home health care or any other area of nursing where they meet the specific practice and continuing education requirements.

In order for a nurse to become certified by ANCC in home health care, she must meet certain practice and continuing education requirements. In addition, the nurse must sit for and successfully pass the written certification exam. All certification exams are multiple choice and cover knowledge, application, and understanding of professional nursing theory and practice. The home health nurse certification exam includes questions on program management, concepts and models of home health care practice, clinical management of the client in the home, and trends, issues, and research in home health care. Included in these broad categories are questions related to case management, continuous quality improvement, reimbursement, home health care delivery systems, patient teaching, client needs assessment, management of common health problems, high-technology issues, legal and ethical issues research in home care, and future trends in home health care delivery. Certification is valid for a period of five years, and recertification is obtained by providing evidence of continuing education or by retaking the certification exam.

ROLE AND FUNCTION OF THE HOME CARE NURSE

Although there is a great deal of similarity between the nursing practice of home care nurses and their colleagues who work in a hospital, there are many roles and functions a home care nurse must assume that are different from the nursing roles assumed in an institutional setting. This section examines the roles and functions of the home care nurse (i.e., determining financial coverage, providing direct care, coordinating care and service, supervising paraprofessionals, ensuring continuity of care, and being a client advocate), focusing on the uniqueness of home care practice.

Determining Financial Coverage

A unique feature of home care nursing is that the nurse must be involved constantly in the reimbursement aspects of the client's care. When a client is admitted to a hospital, most frequently the nurse does not know how the client is paying for his or her hospitalization, and all financial concerns are given to the business office. In home care, the nurse must determine who is going to pay for the services from the first visit until the time of discharge.

At the initial assessment, the home care nurse determines the type of service needed based on assessment of the client and the physician's orders. As these aspects of the initial plan are completed, the home care nurse must also determine if the payment source (private insurance, Medicare, Medicaid, other) will cover the specific type(s) of care necessary. The nurse must work with her supervisor, billing office staff, the physician, and other care and service providers, if ordered, to develop the plan of care and discuss with the client what is and is not covered by payers. This is especially important because, if some needed services are not covered, the nurse must talk with the client and family to determine how these serv-ices are to be paid for.

This involvement with payment sources is very foreign and not always a desirable topic for new or experienced home care nurses. Your agency should have a policy that deals with fee setting, specific forms to have clients sign relating to financial information, and procedures that outline who specifically is to handle various aspects of the financial plan for the clients' care. Chapters 4 and 5 outline many of the restrictions and regulations involving financial coverage for home care services. Your agency should also have information about some payment sources that might be unique to your area.

Providing Direct Care

Direct care is defined as the actual nursing interventions delivered in the home visit. Direct care activities include assessing the client, performing procedures, and teaching. Assessing a client's cardiovascular status, changing a dressing, or teaching the client and family about a new diet or medication would be examples of the three direct care activities.

Consideration of the client's home care needs must cover a 24-hour period; therefore, the focus of direct care in home care nursing integrates the client, family, and any other caregivers who might be involved in providing direct care. Because home care is provided on a short-term, intermittent basis, the home care nurse's direct care always involves the participation of the client and caregivers so that care can be provided while the nurse is not present. The home care nurse develops the care plan considering short- and long-term goals, which again take into consideration the need to instruct the client, family, and caregiver to assume responsibility for learning the procedures, medications, and other aspects of the client's care plan.

Third-party payers, such as Medicare, expect that the home care nurse will identify a competent caregiver for the client and instruct him or her about the client's care. Not only does this approach ensure comprehensive coverage of the client's needs, but it can significantly decrease the number of home care visits that need to be done by home health agency personnel, resulting in lower costs. For example, after the home care nurse taught a spouse to do daily care for a peripheral vascular ulcer, daily nursing visits were decreased to twice weekly. The focus of the nurse's visits went from directly doing the procedure daily to seeing the client semiweekly and (1) determining the extent of wound healing, (2) assessing for signs and symptoms of infection, (3) determining if the procedure was being completed appropriately, and (4) coordinating and communicating questions and progress reports with the client's primary physician.

The home care nurse is not routinely involved in the client's personal care, such as bathing, hair washing, or changing linen. Although these activities are essential to the client's recovery, if the client needs assistance with these beyond what the family may give, these tasks can be accomplished by a home care aide. This is not to say that the home care nurse should never get involved in the personal care of clients. During the course of a home visit, you may be in a situation that requires you to bathe a client or help him or her change clothing. You should perform these duties so that you can move on to provide the skilled nursing activities related to the client's direct care that are the purpose of your home visit. If you find that every time you visit a particular client, there is a question of his or her receiving adequate personal care, you should evaluate the client's needs for the services of a home care aide or, if the client has one, if there needs to be an increase in the amount of time the aide spends with him or her. You will also want to discuss your observations with the client's caregiver and determine strategies that will assist him or her in caring for the client. You may determine that the client needs more care than the family or caregiver is able to provide. In this instance, you would want to discuss other options, such as nursing home care, day care, or other structured living arrangements.

Coordinating Services

In addition to providing direct care, the home care nurse is also responsible for the coordination of other professional and paraprofessional services involved in the client's care, even if not all these services are directly provided by the home health agency. Central to the role of coordinator of care is the ability to assess the client's needs, set priorities regarding problems that affect the recovery and independence of the client, identify how and if those needs can realistically be met, and develop a plan of action that can meet these needs. Also,

the home care nurse is the main contact with the client's physician, both reporting pertinent changes in the client's condition and securing needed changes in the plan of care.

Referral to Other Resources

To function as a coordinator of services, you must be knowledgeable about the services offered by your own agency and the many resources available in the community. It is important that you have a clear understanding of the roles of other providers within your agency, such as physical therapist (PT), speech therapist (ST), occupational therapist (OT), and home care aide (HCA), and as part of your orientation program you should spend some time with these other people to learn more about their roles and functions and how you can work with them. You must also have a working knowledge of the services provided by those community resources outside your agency.

A community resource is any agency, organization, program, or service that delivers a service to residents of your community. The American Cancer Society, American Heart Association, American Red Cross, and Meals on Wheels are some of the well-known community resources with which you might work. There are usually many more resources, depending on the size of your community and the specific needs of your clients. Your agency should have a list of often-used community resources and an explanation of the services they provide. Another community resource information source is the Yellow Pages of your telephone book. In your community, there may also be an organization that coordinates and ensures easy access to these resources for professionals and consumers. Talk with your supervisor about what is available in your area.

As you explore your community, it is helpful to keep the information you gain about each resource on a 3 × 5 index card and keep the cards in a small box. In this way, you begin a resource file that will be very helpful in your future work with various clients. Exhibit 2–2 provides an outline for recording information about a community resource. Use this to gather the information for your 3 × 5 cards.

Case Conferences

As the client's care coordinator, the home care nurse must have up-to-date information regarding the services provided by all caregivers in the home. The sharing of information among these various providers is a difficult but not impossible task and is accomplished through the use of a case conference. At regularly sched-

Exhibit 2–2
COMMUNITY RESOURCE INFORMATION

Name of Agency
Contact Person/Administrator
Address
Telephone Number
Hours of Operation
Services Provided
Eligibility Requirements
Cost of Services

uled times (usually at least every 60 days) and as needed on an informal or formal basis, the home care nurse and others involved in the client's care discuss the client's response to the treatment plan and develop modifications to future goals. For example, the home care nurse may chair a case conference about a 65-year-old woman with the diagnosis of a right-sided cerebrovascular accident (CVA). Also present at the case conference are the physical therapist, the speech therapist, and the home care aide coordinator.

In this meeting, the physical therapist shares his or her assessment that the client has progressed satisfactorily with gait training and that the therapist is anticipating the client's discharge from physical therapy within the next two weeks. The speech therapist also feels that the client's speech has progressed so well that the two-week discharge date is appropriate for that discipline also. The nurse, considering this information, plans that diet teaching and ongoing cardiovascular assessment goals can be reached also in the next two weeks if the client's condition doesn't change. From the case conference, it becomes clear that the client will be ready for discharge in two weeks and should be informed immediately so that plans can be made for the home health agency to discharge the client. Also, it is important for the client to understand that because the covered services for Medicare (skilled nursing, physical therapy, and speech therapy) are going to be terminated in two weeks, the home care aide visits will also need to be discontinued and that the client and family will have to explore other health aide services, if necessary.

All case conferences should be documented in the client's home care record. Sometimes, case conferences can occur over the telephone, mainly with caregivers who are not directly affiliated with the agency. For example, a case conference between the home care nurse and the client's primary physician might occur via telephone following a client's last physician visit. This may

be necessary in order to determine the results of the physician's visit and to make any changes in the plan of care. If the client is receiving a service such as occupational therapy from another agency, the nurse would want to schedule a conference with that service provider relating to the client's care and record the telephone conference in the record, adjusting the plan of care appropriately.

Supervision of Paraprofessionals

HCAs are increasingly significant workers in the home care agency. The care provided by the home care aide is essential to home care and, without it, the skilled nursing interventions necessary would be greatly limited. Clients receiving this care are often dependent on the HCA and are deeply grateful for this assistance, as they are often in a state of limited physical ability. The new staff nurse is responsible for the supervision of these paraprofessionals and needs to learn how to work with, instruct, and supervise them.

It is the staff nurse's responsibility to supervise the work of the HCA. The home care nurse or therapist, as appropriate, will develop written instructions for the HCA and instruct on how to implement them. Third-party payers usually have specific criteria for the activities of the HCA. For example, Medicare requires that the HCA give personal care to the client in order to qualify for reimbursement, and in some states a HCA may not perform errands or shopping for a Medicaid client. Because states vary in their requirements, the home care nurse should become familiar with agency policies governing HCA practice and reimbursement.

The HCA is supervised by the staff nurse after completing a required number of hours of classroom and supervised practical training totaling at least 75 hours. Once the requirements have been fulfilled, the licensed and Medicare-certified home health agency can hire the person as a certified home care aide. In 1991, Medicare regulations required that HCA competency and training measures be implemented in all agencies. This means that your agency has an evaluation system to assess the HCA's ability to perform specific tasks and skills from initial employment and on an annual basis every year thereafter. For example, the HCA must annually demonstrate that he or she can read and record temperature, pulse, and respirations. Medicare requires that certified HCAs have 12 hours of inservice training each year of their employment. The training that the home care aide receives and the continuing inservice education that is part of the employment arrangement are closely linked with the direct supervision the nurse provides to the aide in the home.

The activities a HCA can perform, as outlined in the Medicare Conditions of Participation, include the following (Conditions of Participation, 1991):

- using communication skills
- observing, reporting, and documenting client status and the care or service furnished
- reading and recording temperature, pulse, and respiration
- using basic infection control procedure
- knowing basic elements of body functioning and changes in body function that must be reported to an aide's supervisor
- maintaining a clean, safe, and healthy environment
- recognizing emergencies and knowing of emergency procedures
- recognizing the physical, emotional, and developmental needs of and ways to work with the populations served by the HCA, including the need for respect for the client, his or her privacy, and his or her property
- using appropriate and safe techniques in personal hygiene and grooming that include: bed, sponge, tub, or shower bath; shampoo in sink, tub, or bed; nail and skin care; oral hygiene; and toileting and elimination
- using safe transfer techniques and ambulation
- understanding normal range of motion and positioning
- understanding adequate nutrition and fluid intake
- performing any other task that the nurse may choose to have the HCA perform

The scope of work carried out by the HCA under the supervision of the staff nurse includes all of the preceding but are not limited to just these activities. The HCA can also provide some home management activities such as:

- marketing, meal planning, and meal preparation
- cleaning and tidying home (bedroom, bathroom, kitchen, living room)
- dusting and vacuuming living area
- performing floor care
- assisting with or doing laundry, washing dishes
- assisting with errands (e.g., banking, mailing, grocery shopping, picking up medications)
- performing child supervision (e.g., bathing, meals, homework, recreation, bedtime)

All of the above activities should be listed and identified by the nurse on a written worksheet, often called the HCA plan of care. The nurse can then acquaint the aide with the activities to be completed and the plan of care can be left for the aide in the home. The staff nurse should evaluate the aide's performance every two weeks in the home to determine that the care is provided appropriately. Any changes in the care plan can be made at these times or anytime during care over the phone by the staff nurse or the HCA supervisor.

A common pitfall for the staff nurse overseeing the HCA is the temptation to focus on the tasks to be done, neglecting teaching the aide important concepts and family dynamics that will assist the aide in implementing all aspects of the care plan. Like the nurse, the aide likes to be given information to increase the knowledge base needed to care for the client. Although the HCA may not have had as much formal education as the nurse, the nurse should regard the aide as a partner in the client's care, explain the care, and relate what needs to be done in the client's plan of care. The staff nurse must provide the aide with specific guidelines to note when observing client changes. For example, specific temperature or pulse ranges may need to be outlined so the aide will understand when there is a deviation from the client's normal range. Working along with the HCA during a home visit can be a good way for the nurse to teach the aide and to continue to assess and evaluate the client's needs.

Some HCAs may possess only basic reading and writing skills. The supervising nurse must work with agency staff to develop communication methods that can inform the aide without causing embarrassment. This can be done through a one-to-one demonstration and return demonstration of a procedure or through pictures. Simple descriptive words are appropriate in this situation. When English is the second language of the aide, it is important to be sensitive to the manner and choice of vocabulary used to explain a procedure or activity in the home. Speaking quickly, especially on the telephone, is to be avoided and the use of body language when speaking in person is useful for more complete understanding. The nurse should bear in mind how she would feel if English were not her first language.

If there is any concern regarding the paraprofessional's literacy level, many cities offer literacy programs that can provide the agency with tools and methods for dealing with this special situation. These tools can include literacy screening material that assists in determining the paraprofessional's proficiency in reading and writing and guides to assist the agency develop forms and records so that the person with limited literacy skills can communicate successfully. The nurse must use verbal exchange, direct observation, and client review of the HCA's work in the home to determine that the HCA's care is safe and follows the care plan.

Some home care agencies have home maintenance or home help services through which assistance is provided for doing some seasonal or heavy housework, such as washing curtains and windows and cleaning cabinets. Other work might include washing floors, cleaning the bathroom fixtures, dusting and vacuuming, caring for house plants, some shopping, and meal preparation. These activities are not supervised by the nurse.

Ensuring Continuity of Care

Continuity of care can involve seeing that optimal care is given on a 24-hour basis within one agency, that optimal care continues if the client is transferred to another agency, or that if there is more than one agency delivering services, all involved understand their roles.

Coordinating Care on a 24-Hour Basis

Aside from the client's home care record, verbal reporting among professionals is very important. Communication between professionals within the agency should be concise, stress the individual needs of the client, and indicate any special considerations for care. Such reporting should give the other professional a clear picture of what needs to be done for the client and how the care must be individualized so that the next professional has direction in providing the care. Clients can become very frustrated when they deal with a variety of caregivers, each of whom treats them differently or is confused about procedures and the plan of treatment.

In a home care agency, the chart may not be readily available at times other than regular office hours. For very ill clients, who may call when the office is closed, an abbreviated chart containing information on diagnoses, care needed, and support systems for the client should be given to the "on call" nurse so she can handle any phone call or make a home visit with some knowledge of the client and care plan. For scheduled visits after regular office hours, an abbreviated chart, often called an in-home log, which includes flowsheets with procedures and descriptions of objective data, can be left in the home. Nurses could chart on the home-based record as well as the office chart. Agency policy dictates if this home-based record is an official part of the record or a worksheet used for communication among disciplines; in either case, a specific policy should outline how this written information is to be handled.

When a Client Is Transferred

If a client is being transferred to another home health agency, hospital, nursing home, or other health facility, written and verbal communication is required. The new agency needs to know such things as the client's diagnoses, the care that has been given, what future goals are identified, the status of the client's advance medical directives, and specific orders, such as diet, treatments, and medications.

When More than One Agency Is Delivering Services or the Client Is Contracting with an Outside Agency/Person

If a client is being seen by two home health agencies for different services, it is essential that the personnel from both agencies communicate and decide which will be the primary agency. This situation often happens if one agency is engaged for nursing and physical therapy and another agency provides the HCA. The primary agency is usually responsible for the written orders and the supervision of the care given in the client's home. Certain states have regulations guiding such relationships between agencies.

If the client or family contracts with individuals such as a homemaker to care for the client at various times while a home health agency is caring for the client, the agency must determine the relationship it is to have with the individuals employed by the client. Each agency should have a policy governing the role that the nurse is to play in this situation and how the nurse shall interact with these persons. In this situation, it is essential that the family and client understand completely that they have the primary responsibility for the work performed by those persons.

Client Advocacy

Although the nurse's role as client advocate is not unique to home care, the way the nurse implements that role involves different knowledge and skills. When a home care nurse visits clients in the home following hospitalization, sometimes the most important issue for the clients is how to access their insurance systems so that they can pay the many bills that have accumulated from their inpatient stays. Often these bills can be in a confusing format, without explanation of specific information, and can cause great anxiety in both the client and family. Helping clients negotiate the complex system of health care insurance, or guiding them to someone who can, is an important advocacy role for the home care nurse.

The stress caused by these financial matters can prohibit clients from learning what they need to know for the successful completion of their care plans. Again, community resource referral becomes an important advocacy role for the home care nurse. Clients may lack knowledge of the many community agencies that may be able to assist them. As the home care system grows, it becomes difficult for professionals to keep informed of available services. Imagine how complex the system appears for a layperson! Assisting the client and family in identifying community resources is an important role of the home care nurse.

At times, a referral to another health professional or organization may be necessary to provide the client with the most effective care. For example, if you find that a client is living in poverty and has many unpaid medical bills, the client may qualify for a state assistance program. In this case, you would make a referral to a social worker, either in your agency or one at the local assistance office, who can assist the client in the application process. Some clients and families will resist the idea of seeing a social worker, and it is up to you as their home care nurse to help them understand that he or she is the professional with the skills needed to provide the proper care. Helping the client and family gain access to the most appropriate professional to meet their needs is another important advocacy role.

In summary, nurses in home care carry out a variety of roles and functions that build on traditional nursing skills. Providing direct care, coordinating client care and services, supervising paraprofessionals, ensuring continuing of care, determining financial coverage, and being a client advocate are all unique challenges that home care nurses must meet to be successful. The next section discusses the nursing process applied to home care and how it is similar to, yet very different from, institutional nursing practice.

THE NURSING PROCESS APPLIED TO HOME CARE

The nursing process is a framework that helps to organize and systematize the nursing care provided to clients. Home care nurses can use the steps of the nursing process as a guide to the practice of professional nursing in the home. The nursing process is a deliberative, problem-solving approach that requires technical, cognitive, and interpersonal skills and is directed toward meeting the client/family needs. The five steps of the nursing process are as follows:

1. *Assessment* involves activities that focus on gathering information regarding the client, the family, or the community for the purpose of identifying the client's needs, problems, or strengths. Using a systematic approach, data are collected through interview, physical assessment, and review of reports from other health care providers.

2. *Diagnosis* is the second phase of the nursing process. Nursing diagnosis involves the critical appraisal and analysis of the data collected during the assessment phase. It is during this phase that the nurse identifies the needs, problems, and strengths of the client that form the basis for the remainder of the nursing process.

3. *Planning*, the third phase of the nursing process, involves the development of strategies that will alter the identified problem or support the identified strength. In the planning phase, the needs, problems, and strengths identified are organized according to priority so that the need that is most significant to the client is cared for first. Less significant needs can be addressed after the primary need is met. Following the establishment of priorities, short- and long-term goals are identified and nursing interventions are proposed that lead to the accomplishment of those goals.

4. *Implementation* is the fourth step of the nursing process and is defined as the initiation and completion of the designated activities that meet the goals outlined. In some cases, nurses may not be the exclusive providers of care during the implementation phase. The plan of care is used as a guide to the provider of care, whether the provider is the nurse, the client, or the family members. The implementation phase also includes recording the client care on the appropriate documents.

5. *Evaluation* is the fifth and final step of the nursing process. In this phase, the nurse determines which goals have been met and which goals have not yet been achieved. In collaboration with the client, the nurse tries to identify if goals continue to be realistic or need to be modified. If goals have not been achieved and continue to be important, perhaps a change in the plan of care to achieve the stated goals needs to be made. The identification of areas in the nursing care plan that require revision is an important part of this phase.

These steps help the home care nurse to organize the nursing care to meet the specific needs of the client. Using the nursing process benefits both the client and the family by encouraging their active participation in all phases of care. Also, continuity of care is ensured through a systematic process of delivering care to clients. When the client care record is organized and completed according to the steps of the nursing process, the individualized care provided to the client is described clearly. This enhances communication between home care nurses, justifies coverage to third-party payers, and allows the nurse and agency to document care that stands up legally and against standards and regulations. Although the nursing process is discussed as five distinct phases, it must be remembered that these phases, in practice, are very difficult to separate. The five phases of the nursing process are highly interdependent and interrelated. In the clinical setting, nurses are assessing the client's situation continually while at the same time they are developing some portions of the care plan and perhaps evaluating the attainment of other goals. The nursing process is also cyclical in nature. When you have completed the evaluation phase of the process, you often find that you need to go back to the assessment phase and collect more data so goals or interventions can be revised.

In home care, the nursing process is used as a framework or guide for providing care to the client. There are some unique characteristics that the nursing process assumes in the home care setting. In this section, each of the phases of the nursing process is again discussed, this time with special attention to the application of the nursing process in the home setting.

Assessment

Assessment is described as the organized and systematic process of collecting data from a variety of sources to make a determination about the health status of a client (Iyer, Taptich, & Bernocchi-Losey, 1986). In home care, assessments are being made continually to update previously collected information or collect data in a totally new area. Much of the information about the client is collected during the admission visit, which is the first home visit made by the home care nurse. Some information about the client and his or her clinical problems may be gathered during the telephone call to the client and the initial intake information, but most of the data will be collected during the first home visit.

In planning for the first home visit, there are several areas that need to be considered. Supervisory staff at the agency usually have the responsibility of giving assignments of new cases to home care nurses. When given a new client, the home care nurse needs to review all the information about this client that is provided on the referral form, or if the client has been seen by the agency previously, an old record may be available. Although old records are sometimes very useful, a client's physiological or psychosocial status may have changed dramatically since he or she was last seen by the agency. Use the old record as a beginning point of assessment, recognizing the need to validate pertinent information and collect new data.

After you have reviewed all the information provided, you will want to make an initial telephone call to the client to arrange for the home visit. The initial contact between the home care nurse and the client is very important because it sets the stage for the relationship between the client and the agency. The home care nurse should identify herself and the employing agency clearly. For example, the nurse may say, "Hello Mr. Jones, this is Nancy Smith, a nurse from the visiting nurse association of Metropolis. You have been referred for home care from Metropolis Hospital and I am calling to set up a visit for today." By identifying yourself, your agency, and the way in which the client was referred to your agency, the client can feel assured that the call is legitimate and that there is a purpose for scheduling a visit.

When arranging for your first visit on the telephone, there are certain issues you will want to address. First, you should be able to share with the client the purpose of the visit. Whether the client was referred to the agency for a procedure such as wound care, teaching, or monitoring, you can share the purpose of the visit with the client. In doing this, assessments can be made to determine if the client has sufficient supplies or equipment in the home to accomplish the designated task portion of the visit. For example, if the client needs wound care, you will want to ask him or her about the supplies available in the home. Most home care agencies have a policy on the acquisition of supplies for the performance of a procedure in the home. Some agencies require the client's family to obtain the supplies necessary for the nurse to perform a specific procedure. In other agencies, the home care nurse assumes responsibility for ordering supplies and having them delivered before the home visit. You need to know your agency's policy with regard to obtaining supplies.

It is often helpful to arrange to have a significant other, such as a family member, with the client on this initial visit. If teaching needs to be done, the nurse can teach both the client and the family member at the same time. The home care nurse may also assess that a procedure such as wound care may be able to be done by a family member and teaching of this procedure can begin on this first visit. A family member is often instrumental in helping the home care nurse find needed items or operate such home appliances as the stove.

It is helpful for the home care nurse to ask a few other specific questions during this initial telephone encounter. These questions include:

- Are there any landmarks or specific directions that will help me locate your house more easily?

- How will I be able to get into your home? (front door, back door, first floor, door open or locked, etc.)
- Do you have any pets that will be a danger for a stranger entering your home?

Following the preliminary review of information and telephone call, the home care nurse is ready to make the initial visit to the client. It will be helpful if you arrive at the client's home close to the predetermined time. If you are unable to visit clients at the scheduled time, make every effort to call and reschedule. This shows clients that you recognize that they are partners in their care and that their time is valuable. Clients will worry about your safety and the validity of the agency if communication is weak at the onset of care. Upon arrival at the client's home, you will spend the first few minutes of the visit in a social interaction with the client and his or her family. Introductions will be reinforced and the tone will be set for this and future home visits.

Much of the structure for this initial home visit will be dictated by the initial visit procedure of your agency. Many agencies will provide the nurse with a client care folder that includes many blank forms for the home care nurse to complete as part of the assessment process. These forms may include:

- physiological database
- psychosocial database
- financial database
- flowsheets, including a visit record
- medication sheet
- family roster
- agency information, such as Bill of Rights, hours of operation, telephone numbers, or services provided

Types of Data

As the data forms are filled out, the home care nurse should use all her senses to collect data to obtain a complete and accurate assessment of the client. The senses of smell, hearing, and touch may provide a wealth of information about the client, the family system of which he or she is a part, or the community in which he or she resides. For example, if you hear a great deal of arguing between family members during your home visit, you may question whether the client will be able to have a restful convalescence. Another situation may involve a client trying to recuperate from an exacerbation of emphysema in an industrial neighborhood with many pollutants in the air. A complete and accurate assessment of the client includes data that are objective, subjective, historical, and current.

Objective Data. These are the physical assessment and any other pieces of information observed or measured during the home visit. For example, objective data include such things as weight (176 pounds), blood pressure (126/46), or respiration rate (16).

Subjective Data. These are the perceptions or views of the client about the situation. Subjective information may include statements the clients make regarding their prognoses or their perceptions regarding the reasons they have particular problems. Examples of subjective data include "I think I'm going to be all right now that I've had the surgery," or "I have this rash because of nerves."

Historical Data. These are important to collect in order to establish a time frame for the current medical problem. Historical data involve information about the past medical history of the client and the significant behaviors that affected that past history.

Current Data. These are information that is relevant to the medical problem the client is presently experiencing. Clients may have a tendency to spend a great deal of time telling the story of their past medical history. Although some of the information is useful, the home care nurse may need to channel the interview to the current medical problems to avoid lengthy and time-consuming interviews. This can be done through the use of such very specific questions as:

- Can you tell me why you went into the hospital this time?
- What kind of diet were you on in the hospital?
- What happened just before you went into the hospital this time?

Methods of Data Collection in the Home

There are several methods of data collection the home care nurse must consider in the assessment stage. The three major methods of collecting data in the home are (1) interviews, (2) direct observation, and (3) physical examination. These three methods can be used together to provide the home care nurse with a full and accurate picture of the client situation.

Interviews. This method involves asking well thought out, relevant, open-ended questions. The home care nurse may ask the client some questions while other questions may be directed toward the significant other. Because the purpose of the interview is to gather some of the subjective information needed to make a total assessment, it will be important for the nurse to be an active listener. Note taking during the interview will be helpful for charting following the interview, but remember, it is difficult to have an open, frank discussion with someone who is looking down at a piece of paper. Jot down key words and phrases that will help you to remember the important parts of the story. Try to maintain as much eye contact as possible to show the client that you are interested.

Direct Observation. This method gives will give you the most information about the client. In home care, the nurse observes not only the client's physical status and affect, but also the home, family relationships, and how the client is integrated into the family environment. Using all the senses, the home care nurse gathers significant information that will add to the total assessment of the client. For example, the home care nurse may go to a home for an initial visit to find the smell of alcohol permeating the house. One of the initial determinations that must be made is whether the client or some other member of the family is drinking. If the client is living with a significant other who is drinking, data may need to be gathered regarding the safety of the nurse and the client in that situation.

Physical Examination. This method of collecting data involves a physical assessment of the client to gather information about the physical status of the client and validate subjective data gathered in the interviewing process. Many home care agencies will include a physical assessment form that can be used as a guide to collecting assessment information. Most approaches to physical assessment involve a head-to-toe assessment, using the techniques of inspection, palpation, percussion, and auscultation. If you are unsure about your physical assessment skills or need a refresher, there are many physical assessment texts and classes that may be helpful. You should discuss this with your supervisor.

In summary, much of the initial assessment of the client takes place during the first home visit. As the first step of the nursing process, assessment involves the collection of data about clients, their physical status, and the environment in which they live. The home care nurse uses a variety of skills in the collection of data during the assessment process. These skills include interviewing, observation, and physical assessment. All these data collection strategies are useful in obtaining a full picture of the client and are to be collected on your agency's data assessment form(s) of the client clinical record.

Diagnosis

The next step in the nursing process involves the development of nursing diagnoses. A diagnosis is a statement of a problem or potential problem experienced by a client. The diagnosis stems logically from the data that are collected through the assessment process and it mainly focuses on those areas that relate to independent nursing function. Independent nursing functions, those that do not require a physician's order, include such activities as teaching and assessment and nursing interventions, such as turning, encouraging fluids, or reality orientation.

In 1950, the term *nursing diagnosis* was introduced, and at that time the ANA did not support the concept. In the early 1970s, a group of nursing leaders recognized that nursing needed a method by which to label commonly seen health problems. In 1973, the first National Conference on the Classification of Nursing Diagnosis was held to begin to develop a list of accepted nursing diagnoses. This group has continued to meet annually to refine further the initial entries and develop a list that is inclusive of the types of problems nurses see in practice.

In 1982, the North American Nursing Diagnosis Association (NANDA) was developed from a task force of the 1973 conference. NANDA became an integral force in the development and refinement of a system of nursing diagnoses in the United States. Also, they have been involved in promoting research in the area of nursing diagnosis and sharing the results of research and programs related to nursing diagnosis. NANDA publishes a list of approved nursing diagnoses that can be used in clinical practice. The nursing diagnoses were developed using nine interactional patterns as the theoretical foundation. These interactional patterns, called human response patterns, are central to the care provided to clients by nurses. Exhibit 2–3 provides a list of the human response patterns that form the foundation of the diagnostic categories. This list now contains numerous diagnostic labels that have been approved for clinical use and testing. The overall NANDA list is found in Appendix A.

There are many definitions of nursing diagnosis in professional literature. Many nurse practice acts suggest that nurses have the responsibility for diagnosing human responses to actual or potential problems of the client. Early definitions of nursing diagnosis from the literature include:

- Nursing diagnosis is a statement of a client problem that is arrived at by making inferences from collected data. The problem is one that can be alleviated by nursing (Mundinger & Jauron, 1975).
- Nursing diagnoses made by professional nurses describe actual or potential health problems that nurses, by virtue of their education and experience, are capable and licensed to treat (Gordon, 1976).

Exhibit 2–3
HUMAN RESPONSE PATTERNS

- Exchanging—mutual giving and receiving
- Communicating—sending messages
- Relating—establishing bonds
- Valuing—assigning relative worth
- Choosing—selection of alternatives
- Moving—activity
- Perceiving—reception of information
- Knowing—meaning associated with information
- Feeling—subjective awareness of information

Source: Reprinted with permission from C. McFarland and E. McFarlane, *Nursing Diagnosis and Intervention*, Mosby-Year Book, © 1989.

For the purpose of this discussion, a nursing diagnosis is a statement of actual or potential health problems of a client that a nurse is legally able to treat. Whether the NANDA classification of identifying nursing diagnosis or another method is used, the purpose of writing nursing diagnoses is to communicate the client's problems to anyone who is reading the record. It also helps to organize the large volume of information that is collected during the assessment phase of the nursing process.

In some agencies, a classification system for writing nursing diagnoses is not used. Instead, nurses are asked to write nursing diagnoses of the client based on the information collected. A common method of writing nursing diagnoses is the PES system. Using this method, the home care nurse identifies the *problem, etiology,* and *symptoms* of the client.

The first part of the diagnosis statement, the problem, is defined as a short, concise statement of the client's health condition. For example, one problem experienced by a new diabetic may be lack of knowledge of foot care.

The second part of the nursing diagnosis is to determine the etiology. In this portion of the diagnosis, the factors that affect the existence of the problem are identified. Referring to the preceding example, the client may lack knowledge about foot care because the client, a newly diagnosed diabetic, has not yet attended any diabetic classes.

The third part of this diagnostic process relates to the signs or symptoms that provide evidence for the existence of the problem. Again using the previous example, the client's lack of knowledge about proper diabetic foot care may be determined by his or her verbalization of a lack of knowledge and the home care nurse's observations of the client walking barefoot in the house. The following are additional examples of nursing diagnoses, using the PES method:

- difficulty with accomplishment of activities of daily living (ADLs) because of immobility from fractured hip, as evidenced by client expression of difficulty and condition of house at time of home care nurse's visit
- difficulty breathing because of exacerbation of chronic obstructive pulmonary disease (COPD), as evidenced by shallow noisy respirations, diaphoresis, and extreme fatigue
- decubitus ulcer because of long-standing immobility and poor nutrition, as evidenced by 2" × 2" × 1" wound on coccyx

In summary, the diagnosis phase of the nursing process occurs when the data collected in the assessment phase are processed and organized into meaningful statements so that planning can begin. In home care, accurate and complete nursing diagnoses are critical to efficient communication between home care nurses and to providing a means for problem identification, which is a necessary element for reimbursement.

Planning

The planning phase of the nursing process begins after the formulation of the nursing diagnosis and concludes with the documentation of the plan of care. Planning involves the development of strategies designed to prevent, minimize, or correct the problems identified in the nursing diagnosis (Iyer et al., 1986). The planning component of the nursing process consists of two stages, which are discussed individually. They are (1) setting priorities and (2) writing goals.

Setting Priorities

There are many theoretical models that can be used to help the home care nurse develop priorities of care. One such model is Maslow's Hierarchy of Needs. Maslow's Hierarchy of Needs suggests that there are five levels of need experienced by humans. These levels are physiological, safety or security, social, self-esteem, and self-actualization. Maslow suggested that the physiological needs must be met before the client may be willing or able to meet the higher-level needs. For example, a home care nurse identifies two problems being experienced by the client, incontinence and social isolation. According to Maslow's hierarchy, the physiological problem of incontinence should have a higher priority than the upper-level problem of social isolation because once the physiological problem is addressed, the client will be better able to deal with that problem and the nurse can better assess and evaluate how the social isolation can be overcome.

Writing Goals

Following the identification of priorities of care, the home care nurse will develop goals or outcomes. Goals are statements defining specific behaviors that demonstrate that the problem has been corrected, minimized, or prevented (Iyer et al., 1986). They are derived from the nursing diagnoses identified in the previous phase of the nursing process. For example, if a nursing diagnosis identifies constipation as a problem for a specific client, the goals related to this diagnosis would identify the specific behaviors the client could demonstrate that would indicate that constipation was no longer a problem. In this case, a goal might be "The client will have a bowel movement within one day and every three days thereafter without straining." These statements will provide the mechanism for the evaluation of the effectiveness of the care provided.

Clearly written goals are essential to effective communication between home care nurses. Nurses unfamiliar with the client should be able to read the goals and understand what they mean. More important, the nursing staff member should be able to work toward this goal with the client when the primary nurse is unavailable. There are six rules or guidelines for developing meaningful and understandable goals (Iyer et al., 1986).

1. Goals should be client centered. Goals are always written in terms of what behaviors the client will achieve. For example, goals should always begin with "The client will . . ." and never with "The home care nurse will. . . ."
2. Goals should be clear and concise. Long, involved goals are frequently difficult to understand. In writing goals, try to use simple words and phrases with approved abbreviations.
3. Goals should be observable and measurable. In writing goals, the home care nurse is identifying what *the client* will do following the interventions. These behaviors must be observable and measurable so that it can be determined if the interventions were effective. Avoid goals that are too vague. For example, how can you measure a goal that states "the client will know about his COPD"? Can you observe or measure knowledge? This goal needs to be rewritten to reflect the measurable elements of the client's knowledge. These measurable elements may be:

    (a) The client will identify three factors that cause difficulty in breathing.
    (b) The client will list, in sequence, the steps he must take when short of breath.
    (c) The client will identify two safety measures associated with having oxygen in the home.
4. Goals should be time limited. A time frame for achievement of the goal should be clearly identified as part of the goal. Some goals will be achieved early in the care of the client, while others will be achieved by the time of discharge. A time frame allows the home care nurse to evaluate the necessity of certain nursing diagnoses as goals are met. For example, a goal that states "the client will lose two pounds in one week" determines when the home care nurse and the client will evaluate achievement of the goal. Without the time frame, there is no direction on when the goal should be evaluated.
5. Goals should be realistic. In writing goals in the home care setting, the nurse must take into account both the resources of the client and the home environment. It would be unrealistic for the home care nurse to write a goal that "the client will obtain a maid service to clean up the home environment" for a client living in poverty. A more realistic goal in this situation might be "within the next two days, the client will request help from his two children to clean up his home."
6. Goals should be mutually agreeable between the client and the nurse. Goals should be written by the home care nurse in collaboration with the client and his or her family. Following the identification of nursing diagnoses, the home care nurse and the client discuss the behaviors that will be achieved as a result of the interventions being specified. Contracting is a strategy that can be effective in determining goals and the methods to achieve them. This active participation between the nurse and the client allows for the validation of expectations and the sharing of unrealistic perceptions before the care plan is instituted.

Implementation

The implementation phase consists of two stages: (1) intervention strategies and (2) documentation. Well-planned and executed interventions can allow for effective and efficient accomplishment of goals as well as assist the nurse in documenting appropriately. The following sections outline how these two important phases can be carried out.

Intervention Strategies

Intervention strategies are those activities carried out with the purpose of helping the client achieve the identified goals. These activities are clearly defined approaches for meeting the client's goals. By documenting clearly the interventions that must be done, the nurse can avoid the need for long, drawn-out reports when someone unfamiliar with the case needs to fill in and see the client. In addition to the specific strategy, the home care nurse needs to consider who will work with the client to reach goals.

Some activities will be carried out exclusively by the nurse. For example, biweekly blood pressure assessment is an intervention done by the home care nurse. The home care nurse may assign certain responsibilities to the paraprofessionals in the agency, such as the home care aide. If a goal for a client was to have a weekly bath and the client was unable to accomplish this, a home care aide might be assigned to the case to help the client meet this goal. It must be remembered that although the home care aide has the responsibility for giving the client the bath, the home care nurse retains responsibility for all aspects of the client's care. Regular supervisory visits are indicated to ensure that the goals are being met through the use of the home care aide.

Other intervention strategies are carried out exclusively by the client. An example of this might be the client who takes full responsibility for insulin self-administration following instruction by the home care nurse. In some instances, the client and the home care nurse share responsibility for an intervention. An example of this might be when a home care nurse performs wound care on Tuesday and Friday while the client performs wound care on the rest of the days of the week. This arrangement is very useful in that it allows the nurse to assess the healing of the wound while the client maintains primary responsibility for the care of the wound. This can be a valuable approach for teaching the client wound care.

How does the home care nurse determine what interventions are appropriate for a particular client? It is most helpful to begin with the medical diagnosis furnished by the hospital and physician. There are certain interventions to be done for every client with a specific diagnosis. For example, an assessment of a client's peripheral vascular status and inspection of the feet are indicated for every diabetic. Similarly, for every cardiac client, assessment of the blood pressure and pulse would be performed on each visit. Some agencies provide flowsheets for specific illnesses or conditions that detail the basic interventions for a client with the identified illness. These are very useful in identifying the common interventions for all clients with a specific illness. You may want to see if your agency uses standardized flowsheets.

Other sources of information that can be useful to the home care nurse in developing the interventions for the client are the many books of standard care plans written for home care clients. These texts take a specific diagnosis, nursing or medical, and suggest interventions for the care of a client with that particular diagnosis. Again, these texts present the interventions generally so that they may be applicable to all clients with the identified diagnosis. An example of a standard care plan can be found in Appendix B.

Because both flowsheets and standard care plans are generic in nature (i.e., they do not take into account the unique needs of a particular client), the interventions must be personalized to reflect the needs and characteristics of the client and his or her environment. The home care nurse identifies the unique characteristics of the client during the assessment phase of the nursing process, and these characteristics should be integrated into the care plan. For example, a home care nurse finds out that the client being admitted to the agency has worked for 45 years on the night shift in a local factory. He has just been discharged from the hospital on a regime of insulin, 24 units of NPH every A.M. Based on the standard care plan for this client, the home care nurse would teach the client to give himself insulin at 7:30 A.M. Your initial assessment reveals that the regular sleep pattern for this client is a 3 A.M. bedtime with a 10 A.M. awakening. In this case, the home care nurse would design a personalized care plan and have the client self-administer the insulin at 11 A.M.

Agencies may use a critical path to guide the implementation of the nursing care provided and the evaluation of the outcomes of that care. A critical path details the essential interventions for each home visit for clients with specific diagnoses. It also outlines the anticipated outcomes of care based on the interventions provided. For more information about critical paths and their use in home care, refer to Chapter 8.

Documentation

Documentation of the interaction between the nurse and the client is a critical step in the nursing process. In addition to being required for reimbursement, documentation is the vehicle for communication of the client's progress to other health professionals. For a complete discussion of documentation in home care and the Medicare guidelines that govern the documentation requirements of the home care nurse, see Chapter 5.

The home care nurse uses the home visit as the mechanism for accomplishment of many of the identified strategies or interventions. The home visit is the single most important tool of the home care nurse. It is through the visit process that the nurse gains insight into the client's health and lifestyle. This information is essential in planning and implementing appropriate intervention strategies. More about the specific nature and components of the home visit is found in Chapter 3.

Evaluation

Although evaluation is one of the most significant steps in the care of clients, it is often neglected or incompletely done. Evaluation is defined as the planned, systematic comparison of the client's health status with the objectives that were identified in the planning phase. The use of the agreed-upon goals is essential to the evaluation process.

Evaluation is discussed as the final phase of the nursing process, but, in fact, some evaluation is occurring during all phases of the nursing process. The evaluation that occurs regularly throughout all phases of the nurse process is called *formative evaluation*. The home care nurse will need to evaluate the care given regularly throughout the client's interaction with the agency. For example, a home care nurse and client may mutually agree that a goal of care is "the client will be able to perform independent wound care after three teaching sessions." Following the first teaching session, the home care nurse needs to evaluate if all the planned material for that teaching session was covered. If not, perhaps the objective needs to be altered at this point rather than waiting until the three sessions are completed. Following the first teaching session, the nurse may also determine that the client had difficulty understanding the teaching that was done. Perhaps the client had difficulty performing the psychomotor skills necessary to meet the objective. It may even be that the client originally thought he or she could perform the dressing change but when required to do so, he or she felt squeamish about the procedure. Whatever the reason, the home care nurse needs to modify the objective to fit the needs and abilities of the client.

Evaluation done in the final stages of the client-nurse relationship is called *summative evaluation*. This type of evaluation occurs when the client is getting ready to be discharged from the agency. Again, the home care nurse will evaluate the client's achievement of the identified goals. At the time of discharge from the agency,

it is hoped that the client will have satisfactorily achieved the goals agreed upon in an earlier phase of the interaction. Achievement of goals is an indication that the client can be discharged from home care services.

When evaluating the effectiveness of the care plan, the home care nurse may find that there was not complete or adequate achievement of the goals. The reasons for this may not be obvious to either the nurse or the client. There are several questions the nurse can ask in the process of examining why client goals have not been achieved.

- Did I have enough information about the client and his or her problem to develop goals appropriately?
- Were the goals realistic for this client?
- Was there some factor outside the client's control (e.g., family dynamic, housing problem) that made it impossible for him or her to achieve the goals?
- Were the goals mutually agreed upon or were they developed exclusively by the nurse?
- Did the client have other priorities that prevented him or her from focusing on the identified problem and goals?
- Was the problem perceived by the client and did the client feel that resolution of the problem was a priority?
- Were the intervention strategies appropriate?
- Did the family have the resources (e.g., financial, transportation) to meet the goals?
- If other health care providers were involved in the care, was there coordination of care to facilitate the achievement of the goals?

The use of evaluation helps the home care nurse provide care that is designed to meet the needs of the client in a cost-effective and efficient manner. It also helps the nurse to modify goals and interventions as the need arises over the course of the interaction with the client. Evaluation also helps the home care nurse determine when the client can be discharged from home care services.

Discharging the Client from Services

Planning for discharge from home care should begin during the first home visit. The nurse and client should plan the care that is needed and determine how and over what period of time this care can be accomplished. The section on contracting in Chapter 8 outlines this process completely. The nurse should help the client to understand what services can realistically be offered in the home setting and with what degree of frequency. The nurse, the client, and the client's family need to set goals together. Updating these goals periodically allows everyone involved to see clearly how objectives are being accomplished and when discharge can be anticipated.

Discharge from the home care agency services is often just as stressful for clients as is discharge from the security of a hospital. In most cases, discharge means the client has progressed to self or family care and no longer requires the services of a professional nurse. At the time of discharge, families must have sufficient knowledge to cope with the day-to-day issues that arise in the client's care. They also need to know how to reach help in case of an emergency. The preparations the home care nurse makes for the discharge of the client must be clearly documented in the client's home care record. The standard criteria for discharging a client from home care are:

1. The goals for the client set out in the contract have been achieved.
2. Skilled care (nursing or therapy) is no longer required by the client.
3. The client is hospitalized and time of return to the home is unknown.
4. The client refuses further service by the agency.
5. The client moved or is moving out of the agency's service area.
6. The client expired.
7. The service now needed for the client is not available from the home health agency.
8. There is no funding available in the agency to provide the care, so the client is referred elsewhere.
9. The home situation is unsafe and intermittent care is not adequate to meet the client's needs.

In the three latter situations, agency policies should be consulted to address the issues of abandonment. Abandonment is discussed further in Chapter 10.

Although any of these situations is applicable for discharge, there are times when a client wants to continue receiving home services on a private pay basis. In this case, the nurse should consult the agency's policy manual or a supervisor (Humphrey, 1994).

Recording the discharge in the client's record simply involves clearly stating the reason for discharge and indicating how the goals were achieved. A verbal or written summary of care given, the status of the client at discharge, and the reason for discharge is the minimum of information that should be communicated to the client's physician. Individual agencies may have additional information or a form that outlines the data that is to be sent to the physician.

When a client is discharged from home care services to another agency (e.g., an extended care facility), the home care nurse can serve to ease the transition between home and nursing home by informing the staff of the way in which the client accomplished ADLs at home. Whatever information the nurse can provide to ease the transition should be communicated to the other agency personnel orally and in writing. This is often done by using an interagency communication form.

To summarize, the nursing process is a method of collecting and organizing information so that nursing care can be implemented to meet the identified needs of the client. The nursing process consists of five steps: assessment, diagnosis, planning, implementation, and evaluation. Benefits of using the nursing process in home care include enhanced communication between home care nurses, clearer justification for reimbursement for third-party payers, and the development of a care plan that is designed to meet the needs of the client.

TEST YOURSELF

1. Write your own definition of home care nursing.

2. How do home care standards relate to your practice?

3. Identify three differences between hospital and home care nursing.

4. List the six rules of developing meaningful and understandable goals.

5. Identify five ways in which you will find out about the health care resources in your community.

6. Observe a home care aide orientation or supervision visit. Identify the strategies you can use to effectively supervise home care aides in the home.

7. Mr. Powell is a 68-year-old man who has a 10-year history of emphysema. He retired 3 years ago from an upholstery company where he worked most of his adult life, and he lives with his wife and two cats in a three-room apartment on the second floor of a house. He has two grown sons who live in the area, one who works at the same upholstery company as he did. His wife does not work outside the home but spends her days doing volunteer work with her friends for the local church. Mr. Powell was recently discharged from the hospital following an acute respiratory infection. Prior to admission to the hospital, Mr. Powell was able to go up and down the stairs several times during the day and was fairly independent in his ADLs. Following this respiratory infection, Mr. Powell was discharged from the hospital in an extremely weakened state with oxygen, several medications, and orders to avoid stairs. He experiences shortness of breath after walking ten feet and this frightens him. He states, "I just don't know what to do when I get so short of breath." Home care nursing was ordered for respiratory assessment, medication teaching, and assessment of the home environment. Using the nursing care plan of your agency, develop a brief nursing care plan for the Powell family. After you have finished identifying the nursing diagnoses, write the goals, develop interventions, and identify ways to evaluate the interventions. Discuss the care plan with your supervisor.

8. Review a home care record for a client who has been discharged from service. Evaluate the client based on the list of discharge criteria in this chapter to determine the reasons for this client's discharge.

REFERENCES

American Nurses Association. (1986a). *Standards of community health nursing practice*. Washington, DC: Author.

American Nurses Association. (1986b). *Standards for home health nursing practice*. Washington, DC: Author.

Conditions of Participation, 42 C.F.R. §409, 418, 484 (1991).

Gordon, M. (1976). Nursing diagnosis and diagnostic process. *American Journal of Nursing, 76*, 1298–1300.

Humphrey, C. (1994). *Home care nursing handbook*. Gaithersburg, MD: Aspen Publishers.

Iyer, P., Taptich, B., & Bernocchi-Losey, D. (1986). *Nursing process and nursing diagnosis*. Philadelphia: Saunders.

Mundinger, M., & Jauron, G. (1975). Developing a nursing diagnosis. *Nursing Outlook, 33*, 94–98.

The Home Visit and Infection Control in Home Care

OBJECTIVES

Upon completion of this chapter, the reader will be able to identify:

1. Steps in conducting a home visit
2. Steps in bag technique
3. Caregiving and environmental issues that impact on infection control in the home
4. Measures to control the spread of communicable disease
5. Measures to prevent infection, particularly with immuno-compromised individuals
6. Measures to prevent occupational exposure to bloodborne and airborne pathogens
7. Proper handling and storage of solutions and client equipment in the home
8. Methods of hazardous waste disposal in the community
9. Infection precautions for the immuno-compromised client

KEY CONCEPTS

- **How to do a home visit**
- **Protection of home care clients from infectious disease**
- **Prevention of infection among immunocompromised home care clients**
- **Contamination potential of solutions and equipment**
- **Use of universal and respiratory precautions in home care**
- **Importance of teaching as a method of infection control**

AGENCY-SPECIFIC MATERIAL NEEDED

- Map of service area
- Nursing bag and contents
- Infection control procedures
- Medical policies that deal with infection control

- OSHA Exposure Control Plan
- CDC Guidelines for Preventing the Transmission of Tuberculosis in Health Care Settings
- MSDA sheets

INTRODUCTION: HOW TO DO A HOME VISIT

The home visit is the most important tool of the home care nurse. Home visiting requires clinical expertise combined with organization skills and common sense. This chapter begins with a discussion of how to do a home visit and includes a description of the steps involved in conducting a home visit. In order to effectively perform a home visit, the home care nurse must be knowledgeable about infection control in the home and in the community. A detailed discussion of infection control is included in this chapter.

Overall Considerations

The home visit is the most frequent way the home care nurse provides care to clients. Steps of the home visit are discussed in this section. Learning to conduct a home visit using these steps makes the implementation of the home visit easier. At first, home visiting will seem cumbersome and difficult because a great deal of planning must go into a visit so it can be completed in an efficient and effective manner. As you make more home visits, your proficiency will increase and the planning and implementation time for visits will decrease.

Home visiting is significantly different from providing care to clients in the hospital. The most obvious difference is the environment itself. In the hospital or outpatient clinic setting, the environment is controlled by the health care provider. In the home setting, the environment is controlled by the client and the family. In the home, the home care nurse does not have the immediate support of colleagues and the sophisticated structure of a hospital to assist in the provision of care. The nurse is seen as a guest in the client's home, a home that often is ill-suited to the provision of care. There may be no running water, no telephone, or the house may be in a state of disrepair. The home care nurse must recognize these values and norms and accept the client's living situation, even though it may be very different than one to which the nurse is accustomed. By working through these values, the home care nurse will be a more effective provider of care.

There are other considerations related to being a guest in the client's home. For example, be careful not to track mud or snow into the client's home as you enter. If your shoes do become dirty before you enter the home, tell the client this and ask where you may wipe them off. Always ask permission to wash your hands before starting the care for the client. These kind-nesses show respect and consideration for the client and family and set up your relationship as non-threatening.

Because the home visit provides the home care nurse with the opportunity to see the client in his or her home environment, the nurse may see the client surrounded by familiar things and be able to assess the client's cultural beliefs and traditions. Home visits also allow the nurse to observe the client/family system, which is essential for planning and implementing nursing care. During the home visit, behaviors and values, which provide insights into the family structure and function, can be observed. For example, the home care nurse may observe relationships with pets, the assignment of family roles and tasks, decor and orderliness of the home, the character of the interactions between family members (e.g., boisterous, timid, angry, or compassionate), the value placed on privacy, and many other variables that affect the client's care. This is why the home visit is seen as the single most important tool of the home care nurse.

Because the home is often not set up specifically for the care of the sick member, there may be times when you have to rearrange small pieces of furniture or items on a table. Before doing this, ask the client or family if it would be all right if, for example, you could move the trinkets on a night table so you could set up the dressing materials. Most families are more than willing to make the necessary accommodations to the home care nurse's needs. When you are finished with the procedure, always offer to replace all the rearranged items. If the procedure must be performed on a regular basis, you may want to encourage the family to find other places for the items until the area is no longer needed for the procedure. Always give the family the option of returning all items to their original position when you leave.

Personal Safety

There are certain safety factors all nurses who make home visits must take into consideration. Although it is rare that the personal safety of the nurse is compromised, the nurse's safety is a prime concern before, during, and after the home visit. If you feel there exists a potentially unsafe situation, discuss this with your supervisor before making the home visit. If you are concerned about your safety while in the home, leave and discuss this matter with your supervisor. Some agencies have an escort system, and many have specified policies and procedures concerning safety in certain agency service areas. Discuss this with your supervisor and review any policies available.

Safety Tips

There are some safety tips the home care nurse can employ during various stages of the home visit.

- Know where you are going and how to get there. Use a map for directions. There should be a section on the client's home care record indicating specific directions.
- Avoid carrying a purse or pocketbook. Have some change and your identification in your pocket. Lock your pocketbook in the trunk of your car before you leave the agency.
- Park as close to the client's home as possible. Know how you will gain access to the client's home or apartment. Lock your car doors.
- Dress appropriately and within the guidelines established by the agency. Wear comfortable shoes, ones that you can run in, if necessary.
- In the home, if you have fears about your safety, if people in the home are drunk, or there are weapons evident, do what is necessary, if you can, and then leave. If you feel you must leave immediately, do so.
- If pets are bothersome during the home visit, insist that they be put in another room. Some pets may become hostile as you being to work with a client because they may perceive that you are harming their master.
- Avoid walking down alleys or on private property to take a shortcut to or from a client's residence. Carry a flashlight for poorly lit corridors. If you are unsure about a corridor or hallway leading to a client's home, ask a family member to meet you at the entrance to the building and show you the way.
- Know the telephone numbers of your agency, the local police, and the fire department. Know the policy for emergencies at your agency.
- Keep your nursing bag within your sight. When you are not using it, keep it closed and latched. This will protect it from curious pets and children and reduce the possibility of having unwanted pests enter the bag.
- Do not attempt to break up a domestic argument. The situation can quickly turn on you.
- Never walk into a home uninvited. Always knock and be assured verbally that someone is home before entering, even when the client has left the door unlocked for you.

Home Visiting Steps

Steps of the home visit are broken down into three stages, each with activities that must be accomplished before another stage is begun. The three stages are:

1. the previsit stage
2. the visit stage
3. the postvisit stage

Each stage is described and discussed in this section. The stages of the home visit, with specific activities, are summarized in Exhibit 3–1.

The Previsit Stage

The previsit stage includes activities that prepare the home care nurse to accomplish the tasks of the home visit. The first step of this stage is to familiarize yourself with the client's chart and the purpose of your home visit. This is helpful in planning your day because some clients will require visits at specific times and some visits take longer than others. For example, if the chart indicates that the purpose of the home visit is to observe the client administer his or her morning insulin, clearly the home care nurse needs to be at the client's home early in the morning. In some cases, a home visit must be scheduled to teach a complicated procedure or observe a family member doing a return demonstration. The home care nurse will work with the family member to arrange a mutually agreeable time for the home visit. The visit may need to take place during the family member's lunch break or after working hours. In other situations, clients have sophisticated and complex procedures that need to be done. By reviewing the chart, the home care nurse can plan to spend the needed time with the client.

An important previsit activity is the telephone call to the client to confirm the visit. In most cases of follow-up visits, the home care nurse has planned with the client at the previous visit when subsequent visits will be made. Even though this may have been done previously, it is essential that the client be called to confirm that he or she is expecting a visit and that the time of the visit is convenient. This telephone call should be brief, but it is useful to ask the client how he or she is feeling and if there has been a significant change in the client's condition since the last home visit. Avoid allowing the client to go into a long description of all his or her health problems and tell him or her that you will be there shortly to discuss them. If there has been a change in the client's condition, you can plan for this visit more easily before leaving the office. Perhaps you will need to review some books to determine the proper assessment or intervention or perhaps a case conference with your supervisor is indicated.

**Exhibit 3–1
THE HOME VISITING PROCESS**

PREVISIT ACTIVITIES

- Familiarize yourself with the client's chart.
- Telephone the client to confirm visit and time.
- Conduct a thorough review of the client's chart.
- Arrange necessary equipment for the visit.
- Review the route to the client's home.
- Leave schedule for the day at the agency.

VISIT ACTIVITIES

- Conduct social phase (be brief).
- Wash hands and arrange equipment.
- Implement activities of care plan.

- Document as much of the visit as appropriate.
- Gather equipment and wash hands.
- Plan for next home visits.

POSTVISIT ACTIVITIES

- Revise care plan, if needed.
- Document the interaction.
- Communicate information to members of the health care team.
- Make referrals, if indicated.
- Care for used equipment.
- Replenish nursing bag.

Once the home visit is planned and confirmed by the telephone call, a thorough review of the chart takes place. You need to be thoroughly familiar with the client's history, medical problems, medication regime, and care plan, with special attention given to the client's specific interventions. Your supervisor or another nurse may be instrumental in filling you in on some aspects of the case, but a thorough review of the chart should provide you with the information you need. (This makes a strong case for good documentation!) From this review, you can plan the agenda of your visit. If you are unfamiliar with a medication or specific intervention, go to a nursing text. Before entering the client's home, you should have a mental picture of how the visit will unfold, but always remain flexible because priorities and clients' needs change and this affects the course of the home visit.

The next previsit activity is checking your nursing bag and arranging the necessary equipment. If your agency uses nursing bags, it is your responsibility to keep the bag well stocked and in good condition. There are certain items basic to all nursing bags, and they are listed in Exhibit 3–2. Because you have reviewed the interventions that need to be accomplished, additional necessary equipment can be easily assembled. For example, if you know that a blood sugar test is needed for Mr. Brown as part of his care plan, you must plan to do a blood test on this visit and take a glucometer with you.

Before you leave the agency, the route to the client's home should be reviewed. You should always carry a map, but if the map is reviewed in the agency and directions are written out, the chances of getting lost are

reduced. It is important that directions to the client's home be written on the record on admission. If this is done consistently, subsequent visits are easier and quicker.

You will need to leave your proposed daily schedule at the agency so you may be reached while you're out. Some agencies use a tickler system that consists of a small box and 3 × 5 cards, each with the name of a client on it. The tickler box is divided with index cards for each day of the month. As the nurse sees a client, the index card is filed behind the index card for the date of the next scheduled home visit. In this way, clients don't get lost and the scheduled visits for a specific day are easy to identify. Other agencies ask the nurses to fill out a route slip with the client's name and anticipated visit time. Many agencies use computers to assist with this function. This activity is more important than it may seem. Sometimes a client will call the agency to cancel a visit or a physician will call with new orders after a nurse has left for the day. By knowing where the nurse is, the supervisor can call the preceding client and leave that message. On a more personal note, you may need to be reached while in the field for a personal emergency, so if care is taken with your schedule the supervisor will have little difficulty reaching you.

The Visit Stage

The initial face-to-face meeting between the nurse and the client is very important because it sets the tone for the relationship to follow. The first few minutes of the home visit are generally viewed as the social phase,

Exhibit 3–2
THE CONTENTS OF THE NURSING BAG

- Soap
- Paper towels
- Forceps
- Scissors
- Thermometers (oral and rectal)
- Thermometer covers
- Cotton balls
- Tongue depressors
- Gauze (4 × 4s, 2 × 2s)
- Gloves—clean (ample supply)
- Gloves—sterile (at least one pair)
- Plastic apron
- Syringes and needles (assorted lengths and gauges)
- Tape
- Alcohol wipes
- Tape measure
- Flashlight
- Stethoscope and sphygmomanometer
- Airway

- Needle box
- Occupational Safety and Health Administration (OSHA) equipment
  - Masks
  - Protective eyewear
  - Disinfectant spray
  - Disposable gowns
- Map
- Business cards
- Copy of *Home Care Nursing Handbook,* 2nd Edition (Humphrey, 1994)

This is a list of standard equipment that is usually part of a home care nurse's bag. Your agency may have additional items that nurses are required to carry and that may need special handling orders (e.g., adrenaline). In some states, pharmacy regulations prohibit the nurse from carrying certain items such as syringes and needles. Check your agency policy for the list of specific equipment you will need.

when the client and the home care nurse may have some light conversation so that both are put at ease. After this phase, the nurse is ready to begin to implement the care plan. As discussed before, the equipment you need on the home visit will usually be carried in your nursing bag. Although "bag technique" is often thought of as an old-fashioned concept, it is an important part of asepsis in the home. Techniques for the use and care of the nursing bag are essential to reduce the spread of organisms from one client to another, from nurse to client, or from client to nurse. The steps for bag technique shown in Exhibit 3–3 should be used on every visit to maximize the efficient and effective use of the nursing bag.

As mentioned, you will begin the intervention part of the visit by using the soap in the nursing bag and washing your hands. Always wash your hands before starting the visit. Following the handwashing procedure, the implementation of the care plan begins with such activities as teaching, direct care (e.g., a wound dressing), or assessment of the client's physiological or psychosocial status. While coordinating these activities, the home care nurse is constantly observing the client, the family, and the environment to determine if some modifications need to be made in the plan of care. It is important that the home care nurse involve the client and family or the significant other at every step of the implementation process. If the primary purpose

of the visit is for the home care nurse to perform a dressing change, the nurse can describe the procedure or the wound as the care is being performed. This will help the client and family to feel like active participants in the care. Once the implementation of the care plan is complete, the nurse should gather any equipment used and wash her hands. If equipment, such as thermometers, needs to be washed or disposed of, it can be done at this time also.

If you are using a point-of-care documentation system (computer documentation done at the client's home during the visit), you will be documenting as you provide the care. Depending on when you use this equipment, you may have to wash your hands more frequently. Even if your agency is not using this system, try to accomplish as much documentation during the visit as you can. For example, if your agency uses flowsheets, as you perform, record the client assessments directly on the sheet. This will save documentation time after the visit, when you are less likely to remember the specific information.

In closing the visit, you will want to review the care the client is assuming or any aspects of the care plan that are particularly confusing. You will also set up an appointment for the next home visit and remind the client that he or she will receive a telephone call on the day of the visit to confirm the appointment. Although clients may devise their own system of remembering

Exhibit 3–3
BAG TECHNIQUE

1. Place the bag in a clean area, preferably on a wooden table. If a clean area cannot be found, the bag should always be placed on something like a newspaper to avoid contaminating the outside of the bag. Do not place your bag on stuffed furniture or at a level where an inquisitive child or pet can gain access to the bag and contaminate it or harm themselves. Always keep your bag in sight.
2. Select something that will be used to discard contaminated equipment, such as a paper or plastic bag or a bag made from newspaper.
3. Wash your hands using the soap and paper towels in your bag. It is always best to use your own soap and towels unless the client has paper towels for your use. Only use a cloth towel if the client has one for your use only. If it is not appropriate to use soap and paper towels, alcohol foam and gel can be used or rubbing your hands with an alcohol sponge with great friction can be used as a last option. Leave the equipment at the sink until the end of the visit when you will need to wash your hands again.
4. Only now, after handwashing, can the nurse enter the bag and take out the equipment needed for the visit. Place the equipment on a clean paper towel.
5. Proceed with the visit and discard dirty equipment into the paper or plastic bag. If syringes are used, you should know the agency's procedure for discarding them. Check this procedure with your supervisor before making home visits. If there is an unusually large, contaminated dressing, another bag may be needed. The family should be taught how to discard all dirty equipment safely.
6. When the visit is completed, clean the used equipment with the solution(s) recommended by your agency, as based on OSHA regulations, and wash your hands before replacing equipment in the bag. Never reenter the bag unless you have washed your hands.
7. Close the bag and leave it in a clean area until you are ready to leave.

REMEMBER

- The contents of the bag are considered clean. When items from the bag are used, they must be cleaned before they are put back in the bag (see section on infection control in this chapter). When items are taken out and used with one client, they should be either thrown away, if disposable, or cleaned before being placed back in the bag to be used on another client.
- Syringes are disposed of in a needle box labeled *biohazard*. If the client is receiving several injections, a needle box can be left in the home (see section on infection control) and disposed of when full. Remember, the needle box is considered dirty; do not keep it in your nursing bag.
- The floor is considered a dirty area—never put your bag on the floor.
- Newspaper is considered clean and can be used if other items, such as bags, are unavailable. Place handwashing supplies—soap and paper towels—at the top of the bag where they can be easily reached.
- When not in use, the bag should be kept latched. Keep the bag out of sight when traveling in the car. Bring the bag in at the end of the day because extremes in temperature can damage equipment. Avoid bringing the bag into particularly dirty homes or where a client has a communicable disease. Prepare a small bag with the specific equipment you will need. Include, in that bag, another bag in which to put back your cleaned equipment.
- Use the client's equipment as much as possible. This saves time in equipment preparation and cleanup and decreases the agency's cost per visit.

when visits are scheduled, if a client is having a particularly difficult time remembering when the home care nurse will come, marking a large calendar with the visit days is often useful.

The Postvisit Stage

The home visit is not complete at the time you leave the client's home. Many activities comprise the postvisit stage, and these need to be done before your responsibilities are fulfilled. Based on the data collected during the home visit, revisions of the care plan may be indicated. You may have identified a new problem that should be added to the problem list and documented in the record or resolved—a problem that should be noted as such. Revision of any and all aspects of the care plan is completed following the home visit.

If not already accomplished, one of the most significant activities in the postvisit stage is the documentation of the interaction. Not only does documentation allow for communication between nurses and other health care providers, it provides the basis for reimbursement. There are many ways that documentation is accomplished, and you need to be thoroughly familiar with the system used by your agency. Refer to the section on home care documentation in Chapter 5 for a detailed discussion of the documentation process.

An important postvisit activity is the communication of important information to other health care providers working with the client. It is during this stage that you may need to call the primary care provider to report the client's current condition. Case conferences with other disciplines involved (e.g., physical therapy, occupational therapy, social worker, nutritionist) may occur during this stage. Intra-agency communication is also a necessary part of this stage. If another nurse is serving as primary care nurse for the client, a brief verbal report of the visit is indicated, but the documentation on the client's chart should outline what was done on the visit and the client's status. At times, a report to the nursing supervisor is also indicated.

Referral to community agencies is also a part of postvisit activities. For example, if you determine that a client needs Meals on Wheels, you may make the referral in the client's home or wait until returning to the agency. Remember, always ask permission to use the client's telephone and make only local calls. If there is a chance that the referral source will ask for information that should not be stated in front of the client or family, make the referral at the agency.

Finally, you must care for any equipment that is to be returned to the agency and replenish your nursing bag with equipment and supplies. An ample supply of soap, paper towels, aprons, and other disposable supplies should be in your bag at all times. Agency policy will identify specific items to be carried in your bag.

The home visit is the single most important tool for a home care nurse. As a guest in the client's home, you must recognize how certain behaviors have an impact on the implementation of the client's care. There are three phases in the home visit process: previsit activities, visit activities, and postvisit activities. The effective use of the nursing bag involves a technique that is carried out in a logical way during every visit. If all the phases of the home visit process are carried out in order on every nursing visit, you will become an efficient and effective practitioner of home care nursing.

INFECTION CONTROL IN THE HOME

Recent trends in health care have resulted in increasingly ill clients being cared for at home. As hospital stays have shortened, individuals with communicable diseases and those with conditions or treatments that increase their risk of infection are being discharged home in the care of home care nurses and unskilled caregivers. In addition, clients are frequently returning home with hospital-acquired nosocomial infections, most notably urinary tract and wound infections, that may or may not have been diagnosed and treated prior to their discharge.

There are two major concerns for the home care nurse in caring for these individuals:

1. protecting the nurse, family, and community from a client who has an infectious or communicable disease
2. preventing infection in clients who may be immunocompromised by disease, age, or medical treatment

Compared to a hospital, the home is considered a safer environment for most people. Infection is less of a problem at home because of fewer numbers and types of microbes, infected individuals, and health care workers who may transmit pathogens; lower exposure potential to the serious and "exotic" infections found among hospitalized clients; greater resistance of most people to household microbes than to hospital microbes; and smaller volume of contaminated wastes handled and processed in the home. Nevertheless, a client's residence can provide special challenges for the home care nurse in preventing the spread of potentially infectious agents and protecting the client who is at risk for infection.

For example, primary caregivers, who are usually friends or family members, are frequently untrained in the direct care procedures required of them. They may know little about aseptic technique, the use and care of sterile equipment and supplies, and basic infection control practices. Additionally, a client's environment may lack the facilities, utilities, or cleanliness needed to minimize the acquisition or spread of infection. In the home, there may be little or no:

- protection from outdoor elements
- running water, flush toilets, heat, or electricity
- cooking or refrigeration units
- space or knowledge of methods for disposal of contaminated materials

Insect and rodent infestations, accumulated garbage, bed sharing, and the presence of infectious diseases among other family members also increase the risk of infection.

The unique nature of the home as a setting for care calls for the home care nurse to develop unique solutions for the problems encountered by clients, caregivers, and home health care workers. Home care agencies, licensure and certification bodies, and accrediting organizations have established policies, procedures, guidelines, and practices that address infection control, usually based on standards that have been developed nationally and are adapted from other health care settings.

INFECTION CONTROL MEASURES

Measures To Control the Spread of Communicable Disease

The presence of an individual with a communicable disease in the home need not be a health hazard to other members of the household, the home care nurse, or the community. There may be many misconceptions based on fear and lack of knowledge or understanding about the care of an individual with an infectious disease and the spread of that disease to others. Home care nurses can be instrumental in demonstrating appropriate care, instructing clients and their caregivers in infection control measures, providing answers to questions, and allaying fears. Infection control measures applied to the home setting should be based on common sense, practicality, cost effectiveness, and knowledge of disease transmission (Berg, 1988). The following suggestions provide guidance in controlling the spread of communicable disease in the home and community:

1. The most appropriate and effective method of disease prevention is handwashing. Never assume that clients or their caregivers know how and when to wash their hands. Handwashing may be the most important lesson a home care nurse can teach a client and/or caregiver to promote healthful living and to prevent the spread of disease.
2. Excessive isolation practices in the home, in addition to being impractical and inappropriate, may take time away from other care issues, compromise the quantity and quality of care, and socially isolate the client, as well as the caregivers.
3. Body fluids such as feces, urine, blood, sputum, and any irrigation returns from wound or indwelling tube care should be disposed of by flushing the material down a toilet. You should avoid pouring these fluids down a sink unless absolutely necessary. If a sink is used, clean it out well afterward and disinfect by pouring a diluted bleach solution down the drain before food or other materials are used around the sink. Body fluids from individuals with hepatitis B virus (HBV), human immunodeficiency virus (HIV), or acquired immune deficiency syndrome (AIDS) should be discarded in the same manner, as they do not require special treatment or preparation prior to private or public sewage disposal.
4. Disposable dishes are not necessary for home care clients with infectious diseases. The client's dishes and eating utensils can be washed with family dishes, in hot, soapy water or in the family dishwasher on the hot cycle.
5. The sharing of personal articles, such as combs, brushes, razors, tweezers, dental floss, water picks, and toothbrushes, and medical equipment, such as thermometers and enema kits, between an infected client and another person should be avoided.
6. Caregivers should use gloves for activities involving blood or body fluids, such as changing dressings, conducting irrigations, or changing the diapers of clients infected with enteric pathogens, and when handling contaminated or potentially contaminated materials, such as sanitary pads, dressing products, or soiled linens. The importance of handwashing before and after the use of gloves needs to be emphasized in all client and caregiver teaching.
7. Soiled dressings, used gloves, and disposable equipment or supplies should be placed in leakproof plastic bags prior to disposal in the public trash. If the material to be disposed of is not leaky, one bag should do; if it is very wet and you think it possibly will leak through the first bag, use a double bag. Always make the decision on how many bags to use based on what minimizes the risk of spreading infection. This procedure is also appropriate for discarding client care items used for or by individuals with HBV, HIV, or AIDS, unless otherwise regulated by local law.
8. Soiled linens and clothing, including those of individuals with HBV, HIV, or AIDS, can be laundered in family washers using either the hot or cold cycles and detergent. Bleach is not required for disinfecting but is advised to remove body fluid stains. Linens and clothes can be dried either outdoors, indoors, or in the family dryer on the regular cycle.
9. Blood and other body fluid spills should be wiped up with paper or cloth towels, then disinfected with a prepared household solution such as 70% alcohol, full-strength peroxide, 1:10 bleach and water solution, or Lysol or Pine-Sol, diluted as directed on the bottle. Gloves, prefer-

ably utility, should be worn to protect skin from spills and irritating disinfectants.

10. Clients with enteric infections should be discouraged from participating in food handling and preparation until the symptoms of their disease resolve or the results of two consecutive stool cultures procured at least 24 hours apart are negative. Any individual with an enteric infection should practice scrupulous handwashing at all times. If it is not possible to exclude the infected individual from food handling and preparation, such as a mother with small children, the individual must be educated to practice strict handwashing and hygiene during food preparation, serving, and cleanup.

11. Individuals with enteric infections do not require a private bathroom as long as they practice good hygiene. If the individual is unable to practice good hygiene, a private bathroom or facility should be considered. In homes where there is only one bathroom available for all family members or the individual uses a commode, bedpan, or urinal for toileting, cleaning fecal contamination immediately with household disinfectants is the best approach to infection control.

12. Clients with respiratory infections should be instructed to cover all coughs and sneezes with a tissue and discard the tissue in a designated receptacle that has been lined with a paper or plastic bag. They should also be encouraged to wash their hands after coughing or sneezing, especially if they use their hands to cover their mouths and noses.

Measures To Prevent Infection in the Home

There are numerous diseases, conditions, and treatments that predispose home care clients to infection, such as:

- impaired skin and mucous membranes, such as that caused by tubes, open wounds, reduced lubrication, and changes in pH
- impaired immune systems
- nutritional deficiencies
- tissue destruction from metastatic disease
- anemia
- extremes of age and general debilitation
- medication regimes, such as antibiotics, steroids, chemotherapy, and long-term aspirin use
- multimodal treatments, such as surgery, radiation, and chemotherapy

In addition, there are many invasive and high-tech procedures being performed in the home that increase a client's risk of microbial invasion. The client is at even greater risk when these procedures are performed by unskilled nurses or caregivers. Nurses should teach all clients and their caregivers, especially those at greatest risk, specific methods for preventing infection while being cared for at home. Areas of instruction should include:

- personal hygiene (e.g., handwashing, bathing, mouth care)
- environmental cleanliness (e.g., safe disposal of wastes)
- appropriate storage of supplies and equipment
- the types and use of disinfection agents
- modes of infectious disease transmission and prevention
- signs and symptoms of infection
- control of opportunistic infections
- importance of immunization
- skilled care procedures

Home health care nurses should also:

- be alert to infection hazards and the classic as well as unique signs and symptoms of infections in their clients
- encourage clients who exhibit signs and symptoms of infection to seek diagnosis and medical treatment
- use disposable sterile or reusable disinfected equipment and/or supplies whenever necessary
- keep cleansing and irrigating solutions as clean as possible at all times
- dispose of contaminated materials properly
- seek tuberculosis (TB) testing for themselves on a regular basis
- be adequately immunized for communicable childhood disease, hepatitis B, and influenza
- rigorously apply universal precautions
- become competent in conducting skilled procedures before performing them on clients
- practice good personal hygiene and handwashing
- avoid visiting clients when feeling ill themselves

Ancillary workers, such as home care aides, homemakers and/or companions, and volunteers, also play a role in preventing or minimizing the acquisition or spread of infection. When called upon to assume personal care, meal preparation, or home maintenance and management tasks, these support staff should:

- inform caregivers and nurses of any injuries or breaks in the skin or mucous membranes of clients for whom they are providing personal care

- be alert to signs and symptoms of infection and report any changes in a client's condition to the caregiver and home care nurse
- choose, clean, and cook food well
- wash their hands before and after food preparation, especially when working with raw food
- wash dishes and utensils in hot, soapy water
- keep kitchens, bathrooms, countertops, floors, and refrigerators clean
- keep kitchen linens, sponges, and cloths clean and dry between cleanings
- role model, demonstrate, and reinforce client and caregiver instruction
- practice good personal hygiene and hand-washing

Measures To Prevent Occupational Exposure to Infection

In December 1991, OSHA, using guidelines promulgated by the Centers for Disease Control and Prevention (CDC), established a standard for protecting individuals who are at risk for occupational exposure to bloodborne pathogens, most notably HIV and HBV (Bloodborne Pathogen Standard, 1991). All professional and ancillary staff who provide direct or indirect care because of the possibility of responding to emergency situ-ations to clients in their homes are obligated to adhere to the conditions of this standard. Components of the OSHA Bloodborne Pathogen Standard are described in Exhibit 3–4.

IMPLEMENTATION OF THE OSHA BLOODBORNE PATHOGEN STANDARD

Exposure Control Plan

Every employer whose workers are at risk for occupational exposure to bloodborne pathogens must establish a written plan called the Exposure Control Plan (ECP) to eliminate or minimize their employees' risk. These plans generally include:

- a listing of employees who are considered at risk for occupational exposure by the employer
- specific methods of compliance with the OSHA standard
- any procedures related to infection control

Exhibit 3–4
OSHA BLOODBORNE PATHOGEN STANDARD

The following is a general description of the components of the OSHA Bloodborne Pathogen Standard related to the work of home health care staff who are at risk for occupational exposure (Bloodborne Pathogen Standard, 1991).

1. Every home health care agency is required to prepare an Exposure Control Plan (ECP) that details the agency's policies and procedures in relation to the OSHA standard. This plan must be reviewed annually for appropriateness and made available to staff at all times in the event they need to refer to its contents.
2. Every agency must institute a program designed to minimize employees' risk of exposure. The program must include policies and procedures related to the application of universal precautions, the use of personal protective equipment (PPE), housekeeping and disinfection measures, the use of warning labels on contaminated or potentially contaminated articles, and the disposal of contaminated or potentially contaminated wastes, including sharps.
3. Agencies must provide the appropriate types and sizes of personal protective equipment required by their employees and training in its proper use and disposal.
4. All at-risk staff must be offered hepatitis B vaccinations free of charge, and the agency must have policies and procedures in place to ensure postexposure evaluation and medical follow up. All information and reports related to an exposure incident must be kept confidential to everyone other than the employee, the employee's physician, an appointed risk manager, and the workers' compensation carrier and be kept under lock and key for 30 years.
5. Every home health agency is required to educate its employees regarding bloodborne pathogen transmission, universal precautions, its specific work control practices, and postexposure policies prior to working in the setting and on an annual basis thereafter. Training must be offered on agency time, and the agency is required to maintain records regarding its educational efforts.

- a procedure for hepatitis B vaccination of employees
- a procedure for postexposure evaluation and medical follow up
- a procedure for communicating hazards to employees
- requirements for training and recordkeeping

Home care nurses must know the location of the ECP and review its contents during orientation and annually thereafter. Though most of the policies and procedures mandated by the standard are similar for all health care settings, practices unique to the specific home care agency and the local community, such as disposal of contaminated wastes and sharps in public trash, should be detailed in the ECP. Being familiar with the contents of the ECP is essential in providing appropriate care to home care clients and in obtaining appropriate follow up should an exposure incident occur. In addition, OSHA inspectors can and do conduct unannounced inspections, often asking staff if they are familiar with the contents and location of the ECP.

Home health care nurses are expected to comply with certain work practices that minimize their risk of exposure to bloodborne pathogens. Failure to demonstrate these work control practices can result in disciplinary action to the agency and fines levied by OSHA during an inspection or site visit. Every home health care worker at risk for occupational exposure is entitled to free postexposure follow up and medical evaluation. An agency's policies and procedures regarding this follow up should be detailed in the ECP and learned during orientation and annual bloodborne pathogen training.

The basic workplace practices included in most agencies' ECPs follow. Compare these with your specific agency policies:

- handwashing
- selecting the appropriate PPE for the situation
- maintaining universal precautions at all times
- establishing a sharps disposal system in applicable clients' homes
- disposing of contaminated materials properly and in accordance with federal, state, and local laws
- decontaminating equipment and surface areas correctly
- seeking proper follow up and treatment for an exposure incident

Handwashing is the single most effective method of infection control. Every home health care agency is required to provide handwashing products, including antiseptic towelettes and a handwashing agent that does not require running water, to its workers who are at risk for occupational exposure to bloodborne pathogens. Washing hands for 10 to 15 seconds or one refrain of "Yankee Doodle Went to Town" (Larson, 1987) is the preferred method. However, when running water is not available or when sinks are cluttered with dishes or infested with insects, antiseptic towelettes or any "dry-hand" antimicrobial skin cleanser will suffice until hands can be washed under running water.

Universal Precautions

Universal precautions refer to the treatment of all human blood and certain body fluids as if they are known to be infectious. Because neither medical history nor physical examination can reliably identify all persons infected with a bloodborne pathogen, blood and body fluid precautions must be used routinely and consistently with all clients to protect health care workers from acquiring an infectious disease.

Universal precautions apply to blood and other body fluids containing visible blood. They also apply to semen, vaginal secretions, fluids surrounding certain body organs (pleural, peritoneal, pericardial, cerebrospinal), amniotic fluid, synovial fluid, and any tissues removed from the body. Universal precautions do not apply to feces, nasal secretions, sputum, sweat, tears, urine, saliva, or vomitus (unless they contain visible blood), as these body fluids do not contain enough virus to be infectious. Human breast milk has been implicated in the perinatal transmission of HIV, but has not been found to be a mode of transmission to health care workers. Although universal precautions generally do not apply to human breast milk, gloves may be worn by health care workers who routinely handle or are exposed to breast milk, particularly in the presence of visible blood.

Although the use of gloves may not be required when dealing with such body fluids such as saliva, the home care nurse needs to use discretion in applying infection control measures to his or her practice. For example, gloves may be indicated for a digital examination of the oral mucosa, while good handwashing may be all that is necessary following exposure to drool.

Universal blood and body fluid precautions and the work practice controls described by the OSHA standard are detailed in Exhibit 3–5.

Exhibit 3–5
UNIVERSAL BLOOD AND BODY FLUID PRECAUTIONS

DO wash your hands thoroughly with soap, running water, and friction:

- before and immediately following client contact
- before applying and following removal of personal protective equipment
- between changes of personal protective equipment
- following an exposure to blood or body fluids
- after handling soiled, contaminated, or potentially contaminated materials, items, supplies, or equipment
- before and following an invasive procedure
- after sneezing, nose blowing, or coughing with a hand-to-mouth action

DO choose personal protective equipment that is the right fit.

DO wear gloves when having contact with blood or body fluids or when handling contaminated or soiled items or surfaces is anticipated. Gloves should be worn when:

- administering intramuscular (IM), intravenous (IV), or subcutaneous (SQ) medications
- handling soiled dressings or linens
- obtaining or handling laboratory specimens
- performing phlebotomies or fingersticks
- staff are experiencing minor cuts, cracks, hangnails, warts, scratches, or any skin inflammation on the hands

DO wear long-sleeve gowns or closeable long-sleeve lab coats whenever splashes, sprays, or spatters are anticipated, such as with tube or wound irrigations, enemas, or the disposal of liquids down a toilet. Gowns should also be worn when handling soiled linens or trash that could come in contact with bare arms, a uniform, or street clothes.

DO wear masks and goggles whenever splashes, sprays, spatters, or droplets are anticipated.

DO whatever is necessary to avoid needlestick or puncture injuries from sharps.

DO NOT recap, bend, break, shear, or otherwise manipulate sharps.

DO discard all disposable, soiled items (dressings, gloves, diapers, sanitary napkins, etc.) in an opaque, heavy-duty plastic bag prior to placing them in the public trash. All items with the potential to leak should be double-bagged if possible.

DO clean all blood and body fluid spills as soon as possible, wiping the spill up, then applying an EPA-approved disinfectant to the surface.

DO administer first aid following an exposure incident and contact a supervisor for follow-up instructions prior to visiting another client, if at all possible.

Personal Protective Equipment

The PPE required for universal precautions includes but is not limited to, gloves (nonsterile, sterile, and utility), long-sleeve moisture-proof gowns, face masks, glasses or goggles, and disposable mouthpieces for resuscitation purposes. Employers are responsible for supplying their staff with all of this equipment and providing the correct size or alternative PPE, such as powderless gloves, hypoallergenic gloves, or glove liners that are used when employees are allergic to the regular products provided.

Home health care nurses should maintain an ample supply of PPE in a client's home when exposure to blood or body fluids is routine or expected. Generally, home health care workers are expected to replace their supply of PPE at their discretion and to notify their supervisor of any special personal needs regarding PPE.

All disposable PPE should be used only once and properly discarded prior to leaving the client's home. Reusable glasses and utility gloves should be cleaned with a solution the agency recommends prior to leaving the client's home. If the equipment and supplies you are using are reusable, plan to leave them in the client's home for future use. Items like tourniquets and vacutainers are best cleaned at the end of the visit and left in the home. This saves the agency money and decreases the risk of contamination on future visits.

OSHA requires home health care agencies, not the staff themselves, to clean, launder, repair, replace, or dispose of any damaged personal protective equipment. If the home care employee has damaged personal or agency equipment, everything should be placed in a Ziploc bag and returned to the agency. OSHA requires that all contaminated material be transported back to the agency in a puncture-proof container.

Specimen Collection

Any specimens collected for laboratory analysis, such as blood, sputum, throat cultures, or urine, should be placed in a puncture-resistant, leak-proof, and clearly labeled container prior to transportation or shipping to a laboratory. Home care nurses should check with local laboratories regarding their requirements for receiving specimens, as many now request that specimens be placed in the laboratory's own plastic bag or a Ziploc bag prior to handling by their personnel.

Housekeeping and Disinfection Measures

All surfaces and equipment contaminated with blood or body fluids should be cleaned of organic material first, then cleaned with an effective Environmental Protection Agency (EPA)–approved disinfectant. Whenever possible, home health care workers should use the cleaning/disinfecting products that clients have in their homes or instruct them to purchase the correct disinfectant. Approved disinfectants most commonly found are: 70% alcohol; 1 to 10 bleach to water solution; 3% peroxide; boiling water; diluted phenolics such as Lysol or Pine Sol; or a 1 to 3 white vinegar to water mixture (Rutala, 1990). If blood glucose monitors with removable strip platforms or doors, such as Lifescan's One Touch I and II machines, are being used between clients, these platforms or doors must be replaced following each client use. The procedure for these machines allows blood to seep under and dry beneath the platforms or doors, thereby increasing home care nurses' and other clients' risk of exposure to bloodborne pathogens. If replacing these platforms or doors between clients is not possible, they must be disinfected with an EPA-approved product and procedure prior to using the machine with another client.

Care of Solutions and Client Equipment

Sterile solutions, equipment, and supplies used in the care of home care clients can be easily contaminated, even though these items are generally used for only one client. Any sterile solution that is poured from one container to another for the purposes of cleaning, packing, or irrigating provides an excellent medium for bacterial growth. Though commercially prepared irrigating solutions (e.g., sterile water, normal saline, acetic acid) are labeled for single use only because they do not contain a preservative, home care nurses often leave containers of solutions in clients' homes for extended periods of time. Studies have shown, however, that

these solutions are readily contaminated within a very short period of time (Brown, Skylis, Sulisz, Friedman, & Richter, 1985; Kaczmarck, Sula, & Hutchinson, 1982), suggesting that they should be replaced on a frequent, routine basis. To minimize the risk of contamination of solutions, home care nurses and/or caregivers should:

1. Purchase or prepare small volumes of solutions (250 mL or less) to reduce the storage interval (Brown et al., 1985).
2. Inspect all solutions for clarity, particulate matter, and turbidity prior to use.
3. Prepare small volumes of mixtures (peroxide and normal saline) at the time they are needed and for single use only.
4. Date bottles when opened and discard solutions within a reasonable period of time (three to seven days for normal saline and sterile water) or according to the manufacturer's suggestions (Brown et al., 1985).
5. Refrigerate normal saline and any solutions prepared with normal saline to retard bacterial growth (Barrett & Coleman, 1993). Be careful, however, not to put a cold solution directly on a wound; allow it to warm up first. If this is not feasible, then leave the solution set out all the time and prepare new solution more frequently.
6. Whenever feasible, consider purchasing or preparing normal saline, sterile water, or other wound-cleansing products in spray bottles, as the likelihood of contamination is lessened when the cap or lid is rarely removed and replaced.
7. Pour sterile solutions into sterile containers.
8. Pour off a small volume of solution (5 mL) in a sink, toilet, or container prior to use to minimize the flow of microbes from around the neck of the bottle into the solution as it is poured into another container.
9. Use sterile equipment to withdraw sterile products from sterile containers.
10. Never leave solutions in irrigation containers at the bedside as bacteria can grow rapidly in moist, static environments.
11. Suggest that your agency or organization establish and implement a policy to discard solutions within a reasonable time following their opening or preparation.

Home care nurses must keep themselves abreast of current practice and exercise thoughtfulness in the use of sterile fluids, equipment, and supplies when providing direct care to clients in their homes. Although maintaining sterility is required for IV therapy, catheter insertions, injections, some tube irrigations, and some wound care, using a clean technique is often sufficient when conducting a procedure in the home. For example, insulin-dependent diabetics are now being encouraged to reuse their syringes until blunt as insulin contains an antimicrobial preservative, and research has shown that diabetics do not suffer skin infections from repeated use of needles. However, in other circumstances where injections are administered for medications that do not contain preservatives, such as B12 or Calcimar, nurses should not reuse syringes unless they are resterilized.

Direct care procedures, whether performed by nurses or caregivers, should always be conducted with the cleanest solutions, equipment, and supplies available. Home care nurses need to be aware of and sensitive to a client's ability to purchase and prepare sterile equipment and supplies and to offer as many alternatives as possible to minimize the financial and work burden on the family unit. For example, if the sterile items required to conduct a procedure are not available or adequately prepared, any available equipment can be quickly and adequately disinfected as directed here. Although disinfecting does not ensure sterility of equipment, in the home situation disinfecting supplies is often sufficient for most procedures.

The quickest and most effective methods for disinfecting reusable equipment in the home are as follows. When choosing the method to be used, consider the characteristics of the specific equipment:

- boiling in a covered pan for 15 to 20 minutes (boiling promotes the formation of rust on metal objects and can melt plastic items)
- cleaning items of all organic matter with soap and water, then submerging them in a 1-part bleach to 10-parts water solution for a few minutes (this dilution of bleach and water is corrosive and will deteriorate rubber, is unstable within a few hours, and is inactivated by organic matter)
- soaking objects for 10 minutes in a 3% to 6% hydrogen peroxide *or* an acetic acid solution (1 part white vinegar to 3 parts water), then rinsing with sterile water (Simmons, Trusler, Roccaforte, Smith, & Scott, 1990)
- cleaning metal items with a pressure cooker: cover items with a small amount of water, heat the cooker to 121°F with the gauge in place that measures up to 15 pounds of pressure per square inch, and cook the items for 10 minutes at this level of pressure (Barrett & Coleman, 1993)
- microwaving hard plastic items (e.g., self-catheters) in a closeable (Ziploc) plastic bag with moisture (wet paper towel) on high for 10 to 12 minutes (Doughty, 1991).

It is important for home care nurses to use sterilized or adequately disinfected equipment *every time* a sterile or clean procedure is performed, as many of the microbes present on individuals and in all households can be potentially infectious to immunocompromised clients. Whenever there is a question regarding the sterility of solutions, equipment, or supplies, it is best to forgo the use of the items, choosing to use other items or an alternative method of providing care to ensure the level of cleanliness required of the procedure and by the client's condition.

Contaminated Material

Contaminated materials provide a means of transmission of bloodborne pathogens. Though the AIDS virus is thought to be inactivated when dried, the hepatitis B virus can survive on surfaces, dried and at room temperature, for a least one week (Bond et al., 1981). The types of contaminated materials encountered in the delivery of home care include:

- items that could release liquid or semiliquid blood if compressed, such as soaked dressings, IV tubing, catheters, suction equipment, etc.
- items caked with dried blood or body fluids containing blood that could be released during handling, such as soiled dressings
- pathological and/or microbial wastes, such as body tissues and specimens containing blood or body fluids containing blood

Contaminated materials, particularly those involving liquid or semiliquid products, should be double bagged to prevent leakage and exposure to others. The unsterile glove used to remove small dressings or wipe spills can be used as the primary container when removed from the hand inside out, while plastic bags, such as the ones obtained with grocery purchases, can serve as the secondary container.

Whenever possible, contaminated or potentially contaminated materials should be placed immediately in outdoor trash receptacles to prevent the accidental exposure of caregivers or other health workers providing care in the home. However, if clients resist the removal of these materials, home care nurses should use discretion in working with the family. You can label the indoor trash container with a biohazard sticker or dispose of the materials in a red plastic bag to warn others in the home of their exposure potential. This material should also be kept in a secluded area of the home, away from view. Home health care workers and caregivers should always wear PPE when handling soiled materials. Teaching clients and caregivers universal precautions and disposal of biohazardous waste is a critical aspect of every home care nursing visit.

Hazardous Waste Disposal

Most hazardous waste generated during the provision of home care can be discarded in sewer or public trash disposal systems. Home health care nurses should take the time to identify and understand local laws regarding waste and trash disposal, as they assume precedence over state and federal regulations. Staff of a local health department or any local environmental program should know the community's regulations regarding waste disposal, and the agency will include this information through its hazardous waste disposal policy in the orientation program.

Disposal of Sharps

To minimize the risk of needlesticks or puncture wounds, a sharps disposal system should be established in clients' homes where:

- clients are self-injecting medications
- clients are using lancets to monitor specific blood values via fingerstick
- nurses are injecting clients with IM, IV, or SQ medications
- nurses are using lancets, needles, or vacutainers to obtain and/or monitor blood values
- nurses are utilizing disposable sharps, such as scissors, forceps, or tweezers, to conduct specific procedures

OSHA requires that a sharps disposal system be established and maintained in a client's home, whenever appropriate, as long as home health care workers are providing care. Sharps containers must be puncture-resistant, leak-proof, labeled with a biohazard sticker or other warning, opaque, and with a twist-on or securely fastened cap or lid. Plastic detergent or bleach containers fit these criteria. Any container is preferable to disposing of unprotected sharps in the trash. The sharps container should be easily accessible to personnel; located as close as possible to the area where sharps are used; replaced routinely, preferably when ¾ full; and stored out of the sight and reach of confused individuals, children, and pets. A good place to store the container is on top of the refrigerator, in a closet, or behind a closed, secure door.

Home health care nurses should always be prepared to dispose of a needle or lancet without recapping, bending, breaking, shearing, or otherwise manipulat-

ing it. Nurses are frequently called upon to administer a single dose of injectable medication or to perform a one-time-only venipuncture or fingerstick for assessment purposes. If self-sheathing syringes, fully enclosed lancet tips, or needleless systems are not available to conduct these procedures, home health care nurses should have a backup plan to dispose of sharps. Some nurses carry red sharps containers or other containers, such as baby bottles or small plastic containers, in their nursing bags or automobiles. Placing an uncapped sharp in a container, whether it be glass, metal, or plastic, is preferable to attempting to recap. Any sharp transported in a bag or container from one location to another places the health care worker and others at risk for exposure, particularly in the presence of a curious individual or animal or in the event of an accident.

Sharps containers, usually red, provided by a vendor or agency must be returned to the provider for medical waste disposal, usually when ¾ full or when care or treatment is discontinued. These red boxes must be permanently closed, secured, and placed in a secondary container prior to transporting from a client's home to the vendor or agency. Once in the vendor's store, agency's office, or hospital, all red boxes containing sharps should be placed in a labeled, red-plastic, covered container in a locked storage area until a waste removal company disposes of them according to local laws.

Though private citizens are not required by most state and local laws to dispose of their sharps in any particular fashion, the EPA recommends that all sharps users dispose of their needles, syringes, lancets, and other sharp objects in a hard plastic or metal container with a screw-on or tightly secured lid (Environmental Protection Agency, 1990) prior to their disposal in public trash. Some communities urge residents to dispose of their sharps in designated medical waste areas, such as an incinerator in a hospital, while others discourage the use of coffee cans as they can rust, are often recyclable, and do not have screw-on or tightly secured lids.

For clients or individuals disposing of their sharps containers in the public trash, nurses should instruct them to:

- discard containers when they are ¾ full or before needles begin to penetrate the walls of hard plastic bottles
- tape down the lids of full containers prior to disposal in the trash
- bury containers deeply in an opaque trash bag (black, green, or white plastic bag or brown paper bag) prior to curbside pickup

• protect sharps-containing trash from human or animal scavengers and excessive or unusual outdoor elements

Disposal of Contaminated Materials

The EPA recommends discarding disposable materials and products soiled with blood or body fluids, such as dressings, diapers, sanitary napkins, paper towels, and PPE, in opaque, heavy-duty, leak-proof plastic bags secured tightly with a tie or string. Saturated items with the capacity to leak should be double bagged, if possible, for added protection against exposure. All contaminated materials should be removed from the client's residence as soon as possible and discarded in a tamper-resistant receptacle for public trash removal. This is considered a safe practice; if red trash bags are used in the client's home, trash haulers will not pick them up in regular trash.

Blood, body fluids (urine, drainage from indwelling catheters), semisolid excreta (vomit, sputum, feces), irrigants (wound, enema, catheter irrigations), and solutions removed from the body (peritoneal dialysis solutions) should be flushed down the toilet with as little splashing, spattering, and spillage as possible. Sinks, drains, or outdoor irrigation/runoff systems should not be used for the disposal of these liquids.

Nurses need to inform and reassure their clients that it is not necessary to label hazardous waste or inform the people who remove or handle trash of its potentially infectious nature, if the waste is correctly prepared to protect others and the environment prior to placement in the public trash system. They should also be assured that properly functioning public sewage systems process waste adequately to prevent the spread of diseases that could result from the disposal of potentially contaminated liquids in their toilets.

PROTECTION FROM EXPOSURE TO TUBERCULOSIS

In response to the recent rise in tuberculosis (TB), the appearance of drug-resistant strains of TB, and the increase in health care workers infected with TB following workplace exposure, OSHA is enforcing the guidelines established by the CDC in 1990 for the prevention of the transmission of tuberculosis in health care settings (Centers for Disease Control and Prevention, 1990b). All employers of health workers providing direct care to clients in their homes are obligated to adhere to the conditions set forth by OSHA's Enforcement Directive (U.S. Department of Labor, 1993), the most important of which are outlined in Exhibit 3–6.

The two most common routes of transmission of airborne pathogens are droplets and direct contact. To prevent or reduce the likelihood of the spread of infectious respiratory diseases, especially TB, home health care nurses should:

Exhibit 3–6
OSHA ENFORCEMENT DIRECTIVE

The following is a general description of the components of the OSHA Enforcement Directive for the protection of health care workers at risk for occupational exposure to TB (U.S. Department of Labor, 1993):

1. Health care agencies are required to institute work controls designed to prevent the spread of TB and to reduce the concentration of infectious droplet nuclei.
2. Health care agencies are required to establish policies and procedures related to the use, selection, inspection, cleaning, maintenance, and storage of respirators.
3. Health care workers must be trained regarding the proper use, application, and care of personal respirators.
4. Employees must be individually tested to ensure the proper fitting of their personal respirators, including the medical evaluation of those who could suffer ill effects while wearing a respirator (individuals with cardiac or respiratory conditions).
5. Employers are required to establish TB surveillance protocols for their workers and procedures for recording, follow up, counseling and/or treatment of positive test results, symptoms of TB, or diagnosed infection.
6. All TB exposure incidents must be recorded, evaluated, and treated according to established protocols.
7. Employees must be trained in the hazards of TB transmission, its signs and symptoms, medical surveillance and therapy, and agency-specific protocols and procedures related to respiratory pathogens.

- Cover their own noses and mouths (with their hands, tissues, or a mask) whenever they experience a respiratory illness.
- Instruct clients and family members to cover their noses and mouths (with their hands, tissues, or a mask) when coughing or sneezing, particularly in the presence of purulent sputum or hemoptysis.
- Instruct clients and caregivers to discard used tissues in a container and to wash their hands well, particularly after handling soiled tissues.
- Wear OSHA-approved respiratory protection (respirator) when working with a client or family member who has an undiagnosed cough, untreated TB, suspected TB, or a cough- or sputum-producing treatment or who fails to take his or her anti-TB medications as ordered. The respirator should be donned as soon as possible upon entering the home and prior to close client contact.
- Conduct cough- or sputum-inducing procedures in well-ventilated areas away from other household members and following the donning of a respirator.
- Encourage clients or their family members to seek evaluation and treatment for any undiagnosed pulmonary symptoms.
- Be aware of clinical situations, such as the client's nonadherence to TB medication regime, the presence of drug-resistant TB, and individuals at risk for acquiring TB infection; environmental conditions (e.g., unsanitary conditions, confined living spaces, transient individuals in the home); and procedures (e.g., endotracheal suctioning or the administration of aerosolized medications that produce coughing) that put a caregiver or family member at risk for respiratory infections.
- Assist in the relocation of immunosuppressed persons as well as children under age five from the homes of clients with infectious TB.
- Participate in any employer-sponsored TB screening and prevention programs.
- Support and encourage clients with TB to understand their prescriptions, follow their doctor's orders, be compliant, remain positive while on long-term medication therapy, and verbalize any concerns that interfere with the treatment regime or plan of care.

It is important to keep in mind that OSHA's Enforcement Directive to protect workers from exposure to TB is different from OSHA's Bloodborne Pathogen Standard. Universal precautions require that *all* individuals be treated as if they are infected with bloodborne pathogens, whereas only those individuals suspected of or diagnosed as having tuberculosis require the imple-

mentation of respiratory precautions (National Association for Home Care, 1994). Respiratory precautions can be discontinued when the client has improved clinically; when a cough has diminished in severity, frequency, and/or sputum production; when cough- or sputum-producing procedures are discontinued; and/or when the number of organisms in a client's sputum smears has declined to an acceptable level following treatment (CDC, 1990b).

PRECAUTIONS FOR THE IMMUNOCOMPROMISED CLIENT

Immunocompromised clients are frequently seen in the home care setting. The inability of an individual to resist infection can be the result of many conditions: malignant or chronic diseases (e.g., AIDS, cancer), treatments (e.g., chemotherapy, radiation, multimodal treatments); medications (e.g., long-term steroids, antibiotics), transplantation, and extremes of age, all of which pose unique challenges to the home care nurse. For the client who is immunocompromised, there are special precautions that must be taken to avoid exposure to potentially infectious agents. Immunocompromised clients should be taught to:

- Avoid crowds and contact with family members or visitors who have a contagious or potentially contagious condition or disease, such as boils, cold sores, fever blisters, shingles, the common cold, flu, chickenpox, or measles (Berg, 1988; Humphrey, 1994).
- Avoid raw or unpasteurized dairy products (eggs, milk), raw seafood, undercooked meats and/or foods prepared with mayonnaise (tuna fish or egg salad), or raw eggs (fresh Caesar salad dressing).
- Use precautions when caring for pets as they frequently carry microbes that can cause opportunistic infections. Avoid emptying litter boxes and cleaning turtle bowls, fish aquariums, small animal environs, and birdcages. Birds and turtles should not be handled without gloves unless they have been examined for the diseases of psittacosis and salmonella by a veterinarian (CDC, 1990a). If no one but the client is available to clean pet cages and litter boxes, gloves should be worn at all times during the cleaning procedure and hands should be washed immediately afterward (San Francisco AIDS Foundation, 1989). Cat litter boxes should be emptied and cleaned, not just sifted, every day.
- Wear gardening gloves and masks when tending to dirt, gardens, and brush outdoors, as many de-

caying fungi and microbes can cause diseases, such as aspergillosis, in immunocompromised individuals although these are normally not harmful to healthy individuals (San Francisco AIDS Foundation, 1989).

- Empty and replace the water in cut flower vases frequently to prevent the growth of potentially harmful microbes in standing water (Humphrey, 1994).
- Use small containers for food and use the contents completely at one serving to prevent bacterial growth in leftovers (Humphrey, 1994).
- Avoid agitating linens when removing them from a bed to prevent excessive airborne activity.
- Eat a well-balanced diet and drink plenty of fluids.
- Maintain good, overall hygiene—bathe regularly, check for cracks in the skin, wash hands frequently and with a mild soap; apply lotion when skin is dry to prevent cracks and breaks; and take good care of the mouth, teeth, and gums.
- Avoid stress and get plenty of rest.
- Wash children's toys frequently; toss soiled books, magazines, and newspapers as they cannot be adequately cleaned; and separate soiled from clean items.
- Keep kitchens and bathrooms clean because common microbes can be dangerous to immunocompromised clients. Clean counters and floors frequently; separate sponges for cleaning the bathroom and kitchen and for cleaning dishes, floors, toilets, and countertops; clean the refrigerator regularly to prevent mold; and keep garbage in covered trash cans.
- Avoid organically grown fruits and vegetables or make sure they are peeled and/or cooked before eating.
- Consider immunizations, particularly the influenza vaccine.
- Change air conditioning and heating filters and clean vaporizers and humidifiers on a regular basis.
- Avoid unnecessary invasive medical and nursing procedures (Humphrey, 1994).

CONCLUSION

Prevention of infection and spread of communicable disease can be accomplished when clients, caregivers, and home care nurses fully understand the principles of infection control and commit themselves to following recommended practices and procedures. Safe, effective, and humanistic care can be offered and provided to home care clients experiencing immunosuppression or a communicable disease without unduly compromising the health, welfare, or lifestyle of the client or other members of the household. In addition, caring for a client with an infectious disease at home need not be a danger to caregivers, home health care workers, or the community in which the client resides.

TEST YOURSELF

1. Discuss how you feel about making home visits.

2. You are going on a home visit to a client with an extremely unclean house. What are the most important aspects of bag technique in this situation?

3. List five caregiving and environmental factors that increase an individual's risk of infection while he or she recuperates from a health problem at home.

4. Identify five things a caregiver could do to protect his or her family from acquiring the communicable disease of one of its members.

5. Home care nurses can be very instrumental in preventing infections among their immunocompromised clientele. Describe five personal or client-related interventions nurses can implement to protect their clients from infection.

6. What type(s) of personal protective equipment (PPE) would a nurse wear in order to conduct wound care that included irrigation, packing, and dressing? How would the nurse dispose of the packing and dressings removed from the wound and the PPE used to provide care?

7. Name three circumstances in which a nurse would don a respirator to provide care to a client.

8. List four things a nurse or caregiver can do to ensure the sterility of solutions used for cleaning or irrigation purposes.

9. Describe the recommended method for disposal of sharps in the public trash system. Include three characteristics of a sharps container and how and when the container should be discarded in order to protect trash handlers and the environment.

10. Describe six measures an immunocompromised client can take to protect himself or herself from infection.

REFERENCES

Berg, R. (1988). *The APIC curriculum for infection control practice.* Dubuque, IA: Kendall/Hunt Publishers.

Bloodborne Pathogen Standard, 29 C.F.R. §1910.1030 (1991).

Bond, W.W., Favero, M.S., Peterson, N.J., Gravell, C.R., Ebert, J.W., & Maynard, J.E. (1981). Survival of hepatitis B virus after drying and storage for one week. *Lancet, 2,* 550–551.

Brown, D., Skylis, T., Sulisz, C., Friedman, C., & Richter, D. (1985). Sterile water and saline solution: Potential reservoirs of nosocomial infection. *American Journal of Infection Control, 13,* 35–39.

Centers for Disease Control and Prevention. (1990a). *Caring for someone with AIDS.* Atlanta: Author.

Centers for Disease Control and Prevention. (1990b). Guidelines for preventing the transmission of tuberculosis in health-care settings, with special focus on HIV-related issues. *Morbidity and Mortality Weekly Report, 39,* December 7.

Doughty, D. (1991). *Urinary and fecal incontinence.* St. Louis: Mosby.

Environmental Protection Agency, Office of Solid Waste. (1990). *Disposal tips for home health care.* Washington, DC: U.S. Government Printing Office.

Humphrey, C. (1994). *Home care nursing handbook* (2nd ed.). Gaithersburg, MD: Aspen Publishers.

Kaczmarck, E., Sula, J., & Hutchinson, R. (1982). Sterility of partially used irrigating solutions. *American Journal of Hospital Pharmacy, 39,* 1534–1536.

Larson, E. (1987). Handwashing: It's essential even when you use gloves. *American Journal of Nursing, 89,* 934–941.

National Association for Home Care. (1994). *Home care employer's guide to OSHA tuberculosis requirements.* Washington, DC: Author.

Rutala, W. (1990). APIC guideline for selection and use of disinfectants. *American Journal of Infection Control, 18,* 24A–38A.

San Francisco AIDS Foundation. (1989). *Infection precautions for people with AIDS: Household guidelines.* San Francisco: Author.

Simmons, B., Trusler, M., Roccaforte, J., Smith, P., & Scott, R. (1990). Infection control for home health. *Infection Control and Hospital Epidemiology, 11,* 362–370.

U.S. Department of Labor. (1993, October 8). Memorandum for Regional Administrators from Roger A. Clark, Director, regarding the Enforcement Policy and Procedures for Occupational Exposure to Tuberculosis.

The Medicare Home Care Benefit

OBJECTIVES

Upon completion of this chapter, the reader will be able to identify:

1. Why knowledge of Medicare is important to the home care nurse
2. The regulatory impact of the Medicare Conditions of Participation
3. Medicare home health coverage criteria
4. Categories of skilled nursing services
5. Strategies for determining frequency and duration of nursing services
6. Medicare coverage criteria for other health care disciplines

KEY CONCEPTS

- **General Medicare information essential to the home care nurse's practice**
- **Medicare home health coverage criteria**
- **Types of skilled nursing activities**
- **Medicare coverage for other disciplines**

AGENCY-SPECIFIC MATERIAL NEEDED

- HIM-11 Medicare Manual—Transmittal 222 (Appendix O)
- Medicare Conditions of Participation
- Home care licensing and accreditation information relative to agency
- Fiscal intermediary (FI) coverage manual
- Agency student nurse policy
- Home care aide assignment/plan of care form
- Case conference form

INTRODUCTION

Medicare is currently the largest payment source for home care in the United States. With this in mind, it is important that the home care nurse learn all the aspects of the Medicare home care benefit as a foundation for learning home care. This chapter outlines the Medicare home care benefit, first discussing why the nurse should thoroughly understand the benefit and then going into the general principles governing its administration. The importance of learning the application of skilled services, how to determine frequency and duration, and the Medicare coverage guidelines for other home care disciplines are also covered.

As the nurse reads this chapter and the following one on home care documentation, she should refer to the agency-specific materials outlined above as well as Transmittal 222 (Appendix O) and the Medicare Glossary (Appendix M). The information found in Transmittal 222 is very specific and can expand on the terms and concepts presented in this chapter.

WHY KNOWLEDGE OF MEDICARE IS IMPORTANT TO THE HOME CARE NURSE

Home care nursing is a unique profession that has become more visible since the inception of Medicare in 1965. The Medicare program offers a national insurance plan for the elderly and disabled population of the United States that includes a home health benefit. Initially, the home health benefit was allowed only after the patient had been in the hospital and was limited to 100 visits in a calendar year. In the 1970s, Congress lifted these provisions, recognizing that home care services were as valuable a choice for patients as other health care services, regardless of hospitalization.

Also in the 1970s, private health insurance policies began to add home health coverage for their members, expanding the benefit to those under the age of 65, which increased the variety of patients seen by the home care industry. Private insurance companies generally structure their home care benefits similar to Medicare's rules, as do some state Medicaid programs. Differences are found usually with acute care versus long-term care coverage, and this has provided an opportunity for insurance companies to offer long-term care policies. Consequently, no matter what age patients are, if they have insurance that includes home care coverage, that provision was modeled after the Medicare home health benefit, or developed to supplement it.

It is important, therefore, that the home care nurse understand the basic provisions of the Medicare home health benefit no matter what type of home health agency she is employed in. It is essential that she have a thorough knowledge of how to apply these principles when providing service to Medicare clients. The home health agency that participates in the Medicare program is responsible for seeing that each nurse is well educated on the coverage criteria that affects all areas of home care services so each client has equal access to care as Congress intended. It is also important that the nurse understand Medicare coverage for care to the frail, disabled, and the elderly as much as for other areas of specialized, high-technology clinical practice.

Because Medicare is the largest payer of home health care benefits, the nurse should consider Medicare guidelines that influence coverage by other payers for home care benefits. Even as the health care environment changes, the Medicare home health care coverage guidelines will remain important as determinants of coverage. For example, Medicare uses terms such as *homebound*, meaning those patients who require skilled nursing care on an intermittent basis and as long as it is medically reasonable and necessary. Medicare uses general terms and concepts that most home health care insurance providers use in their policies and so, if the nurse understands Medicare, it is easier to understand the various coverage guidelines that national insurance companies use. Even in light of the changes occurring in managed care, the terms and concepts used in the Medicare program are important to comprehend.

The nurse's judgment, based on her first home visit evaluation and review of the physician's orders, determines whether the client's requirements are covered by Medicare. Additionally, the nurse's initial and ongoing documentation is continually scrutinized by the agency to ensure that the client's needs are being assessed and met and if the services are reimbursable.

For services that a home health agency provides to patients who self-pay or are paid out-of-pocket by family members or significant others, the client or payer usually dictates the rules by which payment is authorized, especially in regard to frequency and duration. The services of private duty nursing and paraprofessionals (home care aides) are the main services paid for in this manner, and it is important for the nurse to understand the differences between Medicare coverage and other coverage for type of services delivered so that she can educate the patient and family in these areas.

Additionally, for the nurse who has a desire for upward mobility in home care, especially in the areas of management, administration, case management, or other opportunities, knowledge of Medicare is essential. In the future, more nurses will be involved in all community-based services for both the acutely ill and the long-term care needs of all clients in addition to the ill. In this way, understanding coverage criteria is foundational to implementing and evaluating these services.

MEDICARE AND HOME HEALTH

Medicare is a federal insurance program for people age 65 or over, for the disabled, and for persons with chronic renal disorders. The people who receive Medicare benefits are called beneficiaries. There are two parts to Medicare Insurance, Part A and Part B. Part A is automatically available at no cost when a beneficiary has been contributing to the Social Security program. Part A covers hospitalizations, related inpatient services, and home care. Part B covers outpatient services, including physician visits, lab work, covered home medical equipment (at 80%), and certain supplies. Part B is an optional insurance coverage and subject to monthly premiums that are deducted from the beneficiary's monthly Social Security check.

Each client who has Medicare is issued a Medicare card, which is red, white, and blue. The card indicates the client's identification number, which is often identical to the client's Social Security number, with an added initial to indicate the origin of benefits. The card indicates if the client has Part A and/or Part B and is always checked upon admission and at other times indicated by agency policy by the home care nurse.

Medicare is governed by the Health Care Financing Administration (HCFA). The federal government has divided the country into ten regions with different insurance companies responsible for administering the Medicare home care benefit. These insurance companies are called fiscal intermediaries (FIs) and are responsible for seeing that the Medicare regulations are carried out appropriately in the areas of billing, financial audit, and service delivery that deals with clinical practice issues.

The criteria for Medicare coverage are explained in detail in the Medicare Home Health Agency Health Insurance Manual-11 (HIM-11), revised by HCFA (HCFA, 1989). All home health agencies should have a copy of this manual, and the nurse should read sections 203–206. The home health agency may have additional material that will help the nurse understand the manual. Some FIs have developed Medicare training manuals that contain HIM-11 sections 203–206.7 and have additional, clarifying information regarding

documentation and coverage issues. The National Association for Home Care (NAHC) has video tapes and sample test questions to further educate the home care staff on important elements to know when performing home care and documenting it.

On December 22, 1994, the government issued through the *Federal Register* a notice that took the home care principles within HIM-11 and placed them into law, giving the instructions a stronger regulatory authority, and making it even more important that the home care nurse understand the coverage guidelines. The significance for home care nursing in this action is that home health care is now recognized by the government as a formal, specialized field of nursing practice. This action complements the actions taken by the American Nurses Association (ANA), when home care was recognized as a specialty area of nursing practice, which is discussed in Chapter 2. Now the national Medicare program clearly defines home health nursing as a skill that includes nursing functions such as management and evaluation, teaching, assessment, and direct (hands-on) care. Also, this definition of skilled nursing is shared in other Medicare settings, such as hospitals, to provide a consistent application of the law for nursing among the different settings in which Medicare beneficiaries receive health care.

AN OVERVIEW OF MEDICARE RULES

General Medicare Rules

The Medicare eligibility and coverage rules, which are discussed later in this chapter, along with the survey and certification rules form the basic primer of Medicare information about how to implement the home care benefit. These rules determine access, payment, and the criteria for home care agency licensure with which agencies must comply. Other Medicare rules do not relate to the direct home care visit as much as the ones mentioned here, but they are discussed in other sections of this work and are important in understanding Medicare home care coverage.

The legal rules regarding fraud and abuse, especially in the area of obtaining referrals, are covered in Chapter 10. Other Medicare rules apply to the accounting aspects that determine the agency's cost and charges for services. These rules are commonly referred to as audit and reimbursement rules. Agency administrative and financial personnel work with auditors from the Medicare program, usually through the FI, to monitor and adjust reimbursement rates based on agency costs and the geographic area they serve, that is, urban or rural.

Thirty-nine states have their own home health licensure laws separate and distinct from Medicare. These vary significantly from state to state. Most home care agencies must also follow some universal rules for issues that are regulated by the Environmental Protection Agency (EPA), Food and Drug Administration (FDA), and the Occupational Safety and Health Administration (OSHA). Many of these apply to employer/employee relationships and offer protection, such as infection control standards and communicable disease precautions that are discussed in other chapters. With all the regulations and rules, home health agencies and their staffs must have up-to-date information and usually use in-services, newsletters, periodicals, and conferences to stay ahead of this regulated environment.

Medicare Conditions of Participation

The Medicare Conditions of Participation (COPs) are rules that agencies must comply with to participate in the Medicare program. The COPs set expectations for the registered nurse and other disciplines to follow relative to clinical issues and, additionally, set administrative and operational expectations for the agency. Adherence to these rules is measured annually by a survey and certification process that is implemented by the state surveyor(s), or the home care agency may have an accrediting organization, such as the Joint Commission on Accreditation of Healthcare Organizations (Joint Commission) or Community Health Accreditation Program (CHAP), perform the Medicare Certification Survey. Whichever is chosen, the agency is reviewed on an annual basis for compliance with the COPs and can be reviewed more often if complaints or deficiencies are found throughout the year.

It is important for the nurse to understand the COPs because surveyors determine the agency's quality of care issues, which give an impression of the quality of nursing care provided. Additionally, they measure overall agency compliance with the COPs. Compliance with the regulations is determined by observing home visits, reading client records, and reviewing agency policies and procedures. The surveyor interviews the nurses, other staff, and clients to determine if the conditions have been met.

Medicare Coverage Criteria

Clients must meet five criteria to have home care services reimbursed by Medicare. They must be homebound, have services provided under a plan of care (POC), have only reasonable and necessary serv-

ices reimbursed, require skilled service, and require service only on a part-time or intermittent basis. It is important that the home care nurse realize how much her judgment is relied upon for determining these factors.

Homebound

Clients must be confined to the home (HIM-11, Section 204). A client is considered homebound by Medicare, if:

- leaving the home requires a considerable and taxing effort
- absences from the home for nonmedical reasons are infrequent and are for a short period of time
- absences from home care are for the purpose of receiving medical treatment (regardless of the frequency)
- the client attends adult day care for the purpose of receiving medical care

Most often confusion is found with regard to occasional absences from the home for nonmedical purposes. For example, an occasional trip to the barber, a walk around the block, or a short ride or visit would not negate that the client is homebound. The nurse's judgment, based on objective review of the client's functional status, would greatly affect what is or is not a "taxing effort." Because there are no guidelines on how to determine what is meant by infrequent or short duration, then the taxing effort becomes a key documentation issue and important decision-making concept (HIM-11, Section 204.1).

Services Provided under a Plan of Care

Services must be provided under a POC established and approved by a physician (HIM-11, Section 204.2). There must be a verbal authorization and written physician's order for all care provided. The POC that is found on the HCFA Form 485 contains pertinent client information and all ordered services signed by the physician. The POC must be updated and reviewed by the physician every 60 to 62 days and any changes to the POC between review dates require supplemental physician orders.

Reasonable and Necessary

The terms *reasonable* and *necessary* also require the nurse's judgment because the guidelines are minimal (HIM-11, Section 203.1). The services must be consistent with the nature and severity of the individual's illness or injury, his or her particular medical needs, and accepted standards of medical practice. Services related to the *prevention* of an illness or injury unrelated to the restoration potential are not covered under Medicare.

A finding that care is not reasonable and necessary must be based on information in the POC and in the medical record with respect to the unique medical condition of the individual. That means that a denial of coverage may not be made solely on the reviewer's general inferences about clients with similar diagnoses or on data related to utilization generally, but must be based upon objective clinical evidence regarding the client's individual need for care. This is another of the many reasons why the nurse's documentation is so important.

Skilled Service

The client must have a need for skilled nursing (SN) care on an intermittent, part-time basis, or physical therapy (PT), speech therapy (ST), or a continued need for occupational therapy (OT) (HIM-11, Sections 204.4–205).

A *skilled nursing service* is a service that must be provided by a registered nurse, or by a licensed practical nurse (LPN) or licensed vocational nurse (LVN) under the supervision of a registered nurse to be safe and effective. In determining whether a service requires the skills of a nurse, consider both the inherent complexity of the service, the condition of the client, and accepted standards of medical and nursing practice (HIM-11, Section 205.1 A1).

Categories of skilled nursing reimbursable by Medicare include observation and evaluation, treatments and procedures, teaching and training, and management and evaluation of the client's plan of care. These are discussed in a later section of this chapter. The assessment and evaluation of various aspects of a client's care (medications, physical assessment, performance of procedures) are skilled because it takes the education and training of the nurse to implement them. For example, assessing the effect of medications on a client and observing for side effects of medications (a skill), determining the condition of a client with an acute episode of congestive heart failure (a skill), or monitoring the condition of a wound (a skill) are all considered skilled services.

A skilled procedure or treatment can be taught to a nonmedically trained person by a nurse and still be considered a skilled service because it takes the nurse's training to teach the client and caregiver the complex procedure or treatment. An example of teaching as a skill is found when working with a client who is receiving a sterile wound care procedure three times a day. The procedure (sterile wound care) can be taught to the client's caregiver who, as part of the teaching process, is observed by the nurse several times before being allowed to perform it independently. Teaching this procedure has been a skilled service, and although the nurse may no longer visit to change the dressing, she still may visit the client at a frequency and duration determined in consultation with the physician to observe the wound healing (another skill). Teaching and training are covered Medicare services and are just as important in home care as the provision of direct, hands-on care.

SN, PT, and ST are called *primary disciplines*. One of these services is needed to open a home care case. Once a primary discipline is involved, *secondary disciplines* (medical social services, OT, and home care aide services) are then reimbursable. Except for the OT, secondary disciplines are unable to continue service without the involvement of at least one primary discipline. Occupational therapists may only stay on a case once the patient has been discharged from the primary discipline to complete the OT goals outlined in the care plan. Auxiliary services, such as respiratory therapy and registered dietitians, are not allowed as *direct* reimbursement, but can be incorporated into the agency's administrative costs. Unfortunately, there is great disincentive to using these and other auxiliary services because of this reimbursement issue.

Part-Time and Intermittent

Part-time means skilled nursing and aide services combined may not exceed 8 hours per day or 35 hours per week. However, documentation justifying the need for additional care may be determined by the agency to be covered, knowing that the FI will later review the record and reimbursement on a case-by-case basis.

Intermittent means an individual must have a medically predictable, recurring need for skilled services (SN, PT, ST) every 60 to 90 days. One-time nursing visits are not allowable unless, after the first visit, a situation arises that makes the preauthorized additional visits unreasonable (e.g., client is institutionalized, expires, or refuses further treatment).

CATEGORIES OF SKILLED NURSING SERVICES

The nurse should be familiar with the requirements for access to services, but must be knowledgeable of the criteria for skilled nursing services. The detailed guidelines for other home care disciplines can be found later in this chapter. Skilled nursing services encompass four major areas:

1. observation and assessment
2. teaching and training
3. performance of skilled treatments and procedures, also known as direct, hands-on care
4. management and evaluation of a client care plan

Observation and Assessment

Observation and assessment are reasonable and necessary when the *likelihood of change* in a client's condition requires skilled nursing to identify and evaluate the client's need for possible modification of treatment or initiation of additional medical procedures related to a specific *medical event*. A medical event may be defined as a change in a client's condition, such as a medication change or a sign of a serious complication (a symptom), a hospitalization, an emergency department visit, *or* other alteration in the client's medical condition and/or plan of treatment. These changes are found or anticipated by the nurse, which is what makes that professional assessment a skill. In other words, a layperson, such as the client or the caregiver, would be unable to assess or anticipate this event. Often these signals are such that it is likely that skilled observation and assessment by a licensed nurse will result in changes to the treatment of the client and then the services would be covered. At other times, reporting these signals to the physician remains important but does not necessitate a change in the plan.

In nursing terms, this category is equivalent to the nurse looking for side effects, not only from medication reactions, but from positional changes, activity level fluctuations, and basically the healing process with a critical eye for the signs and symptoms of impending medical problems. Some examples would be signs of infection, excessive shortness of breath after activity, and unusual edema considering the client's condition and circumstance.

Observation is one part, while assessment adds to the complex skilled process in which the nurse relies on training, education, and experience to formulate the necessary action to resolve or minimize the impact of the recognized symptoms. Documenting observed and assessed complications or side effects is crucial to the reimbursement of such important skilled services.

Teaching and Training

Skilled nursing visits for teaching and training of either a client or caregiver in various aspects of client care and disease management would be reasonable and necessary if what is being taught requires the knowledge and expertise of a skilled nurse, the teaching is new and not reinforcement of previous learning, and it is related to the client's main diagnosis and condition. Examples of skilled teaching and training are, but are not limited to, injections, prescribed diet instruction, medication instruction, ostomy care, catheter care, and dressing change procedures.

Teaching is a complex process that requires the expert skill of a home care nurse not only to teach but to evaluate the effectiveness of the teaching. The steps of the teaching process are outlined in Chapter 7. Often, teaching may be the only skilled service that a client needs, but as stated earlier, any of these skilled services can be provided as the sole reason for visiting. Home care nurses should always assess the client's need for teaching and realize that it is as valuable a service and as important as the hands-on, technical care that is rendered. With effective teaching the client can prevent future exacerbations and complications or, if they occur, understand what to do.

Performance of Skilled Treatments and Procedures

Certain treatments and procedures are reimbursable under Medicare if they are reasonable and necessary to the care of the client's illness or injury and require the skill of a licensed nurse. Examples of this skill include B12 injections for pernicious anemia, administration of intravenous therapy, insulin injections, wound care, venipuncture when the test is necessary to the diagnosis or treatment of the illness, and Foley catheter maintenance. Noncovered treatments include administration of eye drops and most oral medications. Wound care provided by a skilled nurse at a frequency of five times a week or more (e.g., daily) or for greater than 21 consecutive days' duration may be denied if the documentation is not sufficient to support the need. It is also essential that the home care nurse provide an anticipated end date for any daily nursing visits to Medicare clients. This date may change during the client's time on service based on his or her progress or lack of progress but, if expanded, needs to also have a projected end date.

Management and Evaluation of a Care Plan

Management and evaluation (M&E) of a client care plan is a covered Medicare home care service when the need is clear from the assessment or visiting note and is ordered on the care plan. The client's recovery and safety cannot be ensured unless the total care, skilled or not, is planned and managed by a registered nurse (RN). The focus of the nurse's skill in M&E is on the professional nurse's supervision of the delivery of care (either unskilled or mixed services) by multiple caregivers. M&E of the care plan is usually found with overlapping medical conditions as indicated by numerous diagnoses, and care provided is of such complexity that the client's medical condition would be jeopardized if it is not managed by a skilled nurse.

In order for M&E to be a skill, there must be a conglomerate of care needs and integration of caregivers who need to be managed in a strategic manner. This skill differs from observation and evaluation. The nurse is not primarily assessing the client as much as evaluating the care being rendered and managing it to eradicate medical complications often resulting from an unorganized care plan. This oversight by the nurse would indicate needed modifications to the care plan. The goal of M&E is then *not* to teach new material but to evaluate the interrelationships of the care given to see that complications or exacerbations are prevented and ensure the medical safety of the client. Home care agencies may have policies that give the nurse more direction in applying this coverage criterion to clients. It is a skill that requires the leadership concept of problem solving inherent to the profession.

An analogy that may illustrate M&E when the nurse assesses that the multiple caregivers (formal and informal, or both) are engaged in separate activities is that of a train with various cars going in different directions. Unless the engineer coordinates the cars and steers them in the same direction, harm may result when the cars go onto separate tracks. The care plan (the train map) must be developed and constantly revised by the nurse (the engineer) to demonstrate the newly coordinated plan to which each car (caregiver) agrees.

Additional Skilled Coverage Issues

Skilled nursing visits conducted by student nurses when a home health agency participates in clinical training programs with a school of nursing are covered visits through Medicare. Procedures for the use of student nurses in home care vary based on agency policy and state regulations. You should consult your agency's individual procedures in this area. Psychiatric nursing visits are also reimbursed if the nurse is a trained psychiatric nurse.

Although nursing visits to supervise the activities of a home care aide are required by Medicare to be conducted either every 14 days or every 60 days for nonmedical care, they are not reimbursable as a covered service. If the client needs the nurse to perform a skilled

service at the same visit that she is performing supervisory activities, the visit would be covered if the skill is clear on the record. The nurse always needs to use the visit time efficiently when multiple skills are to be performed in one visit. The nurse should remember that each skill is unique and should be documented as such.

DETERMINING FREQUENCY AND DURATION

On the initial visit, as well as on subsequent visits, the nurse must decide, in conjunction with the client's physician and the client and family, how often each week a client needs to be seen (frequency) and the length of time (duration) the client will be on service. Many insurers, as well as Medicare, develop unpublished screens to process claims as internal guidelines regarding frequency and duration. Medicare is used as an example in this section. The unique needs of each client should always be considered along with any internal agency guidelines.

Duration is usually the certification period determined by the client's reimbursement source. For Medicare, it is 62 days; other payment sources may differ. The Medicare certification must be reviewed to determine if the client needs another period of time (62 days) to accomplish the home care goals. A progress report, developed by the nurse, for the first 62 days is sent to the physician who, after review, develops the care plan for the next 62 days with the nurse's input and signs the plan authorizing the care. The renewal of orders for a new certification period is called a recertification, or recert.

The frequency of visits is based on the client's diagnosis, acuteness of the condition, client or family's ability to learn, presence of a person to teach, physician orders, and nurse's judgment of the condition and needs of the client, as well as applicable state, federal, or agency rules and policies. Historically, frequency has generally been planned with higher frequency beginning the first week of care and tapering down as the severity of the client's condition improves. HCFA Form 485, Home Health Certification and Plan of Care (see Appendix D) requires specific frequency and duration entries in Field 21 for each discipline involved in the care of the client.

When planning frequency, know your agency's treatment week; Medicare's is usually Sunday through Saturday. It is helpful to use a calendar with that week as your guide for completing the frequency and duration part of your admission paperwork.

Format for Writing Frequency and Duration

Frequency and duration are always written for the 62 days (nine weeks) of the certification period unless an earlier discharge is anticipated. For example, if the agency's week was Sunday through Saturday and a client was admitted Wednesday for observation and assessment and teaching, which required visits Wednesday, Thursday, and Friday the first week, the visit frequency for the first week of the certification period would be:

3 wk 1 (for week 1 of service) = 3 visits for first week of service
or
1 da 3 (for week 1 of service) = daily visits for 3 days

If the client's condition and the teaching needs warranted visits three times a week, tapering down to two times a week, and then possibly discharge at the end of the certification period, the remaining frequency (for that certification period) would be:

3 wk 5 = 3 visits a week for 5 weeks (service weeks 2–6)
2 wk 2 = 2 visits a week for 2 weeks (service weeks 7–8)
1 wk 1 = 1 visit a week for 1 week (service week 9)

Some agencies range their visit frequency; for example, using the preceding situation, weeks two to six of service might be written 2–3 wk5 or 1–2 wk2. Check with your agency if you range visits or use the preceding example. When additional pro re nata (prn, which means "as necessary") visits are necessary, the projected frequency of the prn visits should be added to the initial frequency on HCFA Form 485 and should *always* be quantified and qualified. An example would be SN prn × 2 for occlusion or displacement of the Foley catheter. If a client requires more visits than planned, the physician should be contacted for an order. Keep in mind that frequency is always found in the physician's order. The nurse can decrease the frequency at any time based on the client's needs through communication with the client and physician and documentation of why the visits were decreased in the client record.

Certification, recertification, and interim orders for changes (verbal orders) must all be followed by the physician's signed confirmation in a timely manner. The nurse needs to be well informed of the agency's rules regarding timely processing because the agency billing and licensure are both at stake if not done according to the regulatory guidelines.

Determining Visit Frequency

All aspects of the client's situation must be assessed to determine frequency of visits. This will re-

quire the nurse to evaluate the factors and guidelines presented in Exhibit 4–1.

PROFESSIONAL AND PARAPROFESSIONAL HOME CARE PROVIDERS

This section identifies the roles and functions of the other professionals who provide care to clients in their homes. In addition, the Medicare guidelines that influence the reimbursement for the specific type of care are detailed in this section. The role and functions of the home care nurse are not included in this section; they are described in Chapter 2.

Role of the Home Care Nurse in Working with Other Disciplines

Many professionals and paraprofessionals are involved in delivering home care. The needs of the client dictate the type of provider(s) that will be involved in the plan of care. If the home care nurse is involved in the care of the client, she is responsible for the case coordination. This means that the nurse will organize the development of the plan of care in collaboration with the other home care providers. The nurse will then assess the client's progress toward preestablished goals. In some cases, skilled nursing is not involved in the plan of care. In those situations, another professional assumes the case coordination function.

Through periodic case conferences, all providers and increasingly clients and family members are involved in planning future care and have the opportunity to discuss the client's response to the current plan of care. This can occur using a variety of high-technology telecommunication systems. Medicare and other third-party payers require that the case conferences be documented and where these are kept is up to the home care agency. Some accrediting agencies also require that notes from case conferences be kept in a notebook designated for that purpose. Modifications to the plan of care must be documented in the clinical record. Third-party payers often require that they be informed of substantive changes in the plan of care either verbally or in writing. Supervisory visits also need to be recorded and filed in the client's home care record.

As the case coordinator, the home care nurse is responsible for ensuring that the POC is designed and implemented to meet the short- and long-term goals of the client, and includes all disciplines that are involved with the client's care. The nurse should be sure that the services provided by nursing and the home care aide

Exhibit 4–1
FACTORS AND GUIDELINES THAT AFFECT FREQUENCY OF VISITS

FACTORS THAT AFFECT FREQUENCY OF VISITS

- The *current status* of the disease process, injury, or situation that necessitates home health care.
- Identification of *actual versus potential problems*. Visits may be needed more frequently to accomplish immediate goals and then readjusted to meet longer-term goals.
- The *prognosis* of the case and the likelihood of complications arising that are related to nursing care frequency.
- The *goals* agreed upon, time frames established, and contract expectations understood by the client, family, and agency staff.
- The ongoing need for *nursing assessment, monitoring,* and *evaluation* of progress toward goals.
- The *patient teaching* that needs to be accomplished and the need for appropriate follow up.
- The type and complexity of *direct nursing care* that must be given to meet short- and long-term goals.
- The client's *current mental status* and the nurse's understanding of the client's situation and current knowledge of the disease, injury, or condition. One goal of home health intervention, consistent with the community health standards of practice, is to increase the client's or responsible person's knowledge and understanding, so this factor will be a dynamic, changing factor in determination of future visit frequency.
- The client's or responsible person's *willingness* to provide needed care.
- The client's *environment*.
- The client's and caregiver's overall capabilities for *compliance with instruction*.

The nurse makes a professional evaluation of all the preceding factors to determine visit frequency. As the situation changes over time, these factors must be constantly reassessed so that new physician orders can be obtained to maintain appropriate visit frequency. It is not possible to develop a "cookbook" system to determine visit frequency because no two client situations are alike and the ability to determine frequency requires the skill of a professional nurse.

GUIDELINES FOR DETERMINING VISIT FREQUENCY

Some general guidelines can be used in assisting the nurse in determining visit frequency. If a client requests more service than the physician or nurse feels is needed, agency policy and procedures should be consulted.

Clients Who Need To Be Seen the Next Day or More than Once a Day

Any of the following seven factors can apply to these clients:

1. The client's condition is unstable, and a serious change in the client's condition could potentially occur within 24 hours.
2. The care plan involves a complex procedure, such as dressing changes or wound care, that requires a nurse to complete, teach about, or oversee completion of the procedure. Examples of procedures that might require daily or more frequent visits include injections, intravenous (IV) therapy, tube feeds, and catheter irrigations.
3. Members of the support system in the home are having difficulty understanding or coping with the client's condition or care needs and require the direction and supervision of the nurse.
4. The nurse has an incomplete database on which to make a judgment and because of a reported and unexpected symptom or issue, more data need to be obtained the next day in order to manage the client properly.
5. The immediate acute teaching need or subject matter of teaching is so complex that it must be divided into smaller segments; for example, the client who has had numerous medication changes.
6. A caregiver is being sought who can be taught procedures, such as insulin injections or dressing changes.
7. The physician orders need to be specifically followed.

Note: For all visits that are daily, a projected end point is required for nursing, but should also be considered for other disciplines.

Next Visit—Two to Three Days

In the majority of cases, there should be *no more than* two or three days between the initial and subsequent visits, for health and safety reasons. Remember, if the client was just discharged from the hospital, the first day at home (the initial visit) provides the baseline data at the client's "best." To determine the client's actual condition after hospitalization, daily visits for two or three days in a row give a more accurate picture of the client's overall situation and needs so an appropriate care plan can be developed. The types of situations where the client should be seen within two to three days are:

continues

Exhibit 4–1 continued

1. The client's condition needs intermittent visits rather than daily; for example, to continue teaching and/or monitoring.
2. The caregiver is providing skilled interventions that need to be monitored by the nurse.
3. The nurse is evaluating the effectiveness of teaching that has been done. The nurse is continuing to evaluate past teaching and implement new teaching from the care plan.
4. The nurse continues to provide ordered skilled interventions that only a nurse can do.
5. The nurse is evaluating the effectiveness of the care plan (e.g., medications, procedures, teaching, compliance with diet, caregiver and other support systems).

Weekly Visits

The following factors can apply:

1. The client is more stable and, as such, more independent.
2. The care plan requires a skilled nurse for ordered interventions in this time frame, such as injections, application of treatments or dressings, laboratory testing, and, in some cases, the prefilling of insulin syringes (refer to your agency's Medicare training manual).
3. The skills of observation and assessment are almost exhausted. Although still reasonable and necessary, visits are not required more frequently than once a week for a couple of weeks. The nurse must be careful if this situation applies, because some FIs do not consider observation and assessment less often than two times per week as reasonable and necessary.
4. The client's or caregiver's compliance with teaching has progressed but must be evaluated.

Monthly or Longer

The following factors can apply:

1. *Specific orders* are given for treatments, such as injections, blood draws, or Foley catheter changes.
2. The care plan involves a skilled need at this frequency (e.g., laboratory work).
3. The visit is required to fulfill regulations or compliance with reimbursement guidelines, such as supervisor visits for state Medicaid programs, which may be considered administrative, versus direct skilled nursing care.
4. The nurse must evaluate the entire client/family/environment situation to determine continued safe conditions and continued use of adequate and appropriate care and services to ensure that discharge is appropriate.

Remember, at any time throughout the certification period, the frequency of visits might need to be increased or decreased to meet the client's needs and to be considered reasonable and necessary. Such changes as hospitalization, onset, exacerbation, or worsening of a condition, and/or the introduction of new medications indicates that visits need to be increased. If visits are not increased when these factors are present, documentation should indicate why they were not.

When there is no change in the care plan and the client's condition is unchanged, it is usually time to decrease visits and plan for discharge. As always, the nurse must evaluate the client's progression toward the goals of the care plan and have an anticipated discharge date that is constantly reviewed throughout the episode for the client to be well prepared and clear on the expectations for self-care learning.

Source: Adapted from Carolyn Humphrey, *Home Care Nursing Handbook*, ed 2, pp. 23–26, Aspen Publishers, Inc., © 1994.

are coordinated with the services provided by other disciplines involved with the client (PT, ST, OT, medical social worker [MSW]). Also, the nurse needs to ensure that documentation reflects why the client's condition requires that other disciplines be involved in the care.

The COPs further emphasize that agencies have a responsibility to coordinate care. The nurse generally acts as liaison for all parties interested and participating in the care. Additionally, with increased quality management activities using both internal and exter-

nal review, the coordination of all disciplines becomes a key element for monitoring quality. Efficient and effective information sharing can enhance outcome achievement and client satisfaction.

Medicare Coverage for Other Providers

Physical Therapy

Home care patients of all ages and with a wide variety of diagnoses may require PT services. The patient's need for PT is based on documentation of a deficit in self-care, mobility, safety, range of motion, or strength. Medical diagnosis alone does not establish the need for PT. The presence of a functional limitation is the most significant factor in determining if PT services are needed. The two main roles of the physical therapist in the home are to provide skilled intervention to improve the patient's level of functioning (LOF) in one of the previously mentioned areas and to establish a safe and effective maintenance program.

PT is one of the three *primary* skilled home health services covered by Medicare; SN and ST are the others. Insurance companies with a home health benefit often cover PT services as does workers' compensation, health maintenance organizations (HMOs), and Medicaid. The determination of whether the services will be covered is dependent on the skilled need of the patient and the cost-effectiveness of providing the PT in the home.

Examples of therapy services include assessment of needs and development of a therapy program for the beneficiary. The physical therapist functions also include:

- therapeutic exercises
- gait training
- active range of motion exercises
- ultrasound
- shortwave and microwave diathermy treatments
- hot packs, infrared treatments
- paraffin
- whirlpool baths

All PT services must be consistent with the nature and severity of the patient's illness or injury to be considered reasonable and necessary. Once the beneficiary has attained optimal functioning with no further evidence of improvement, the service would no longer be considered reasonable and necessary care. If a beneficiary had a cardiovascular accident (CVA) one year ago with therapy and has progressed to a maximum level of functioning, services would not be reimbursable. Similarly, a patient who has had abdominal surgery and is discharged home complaining of general weakness could be expected to recover with time, and PT would not be considered reasonable and necessary for the nature of the illness. The beneficiary would need a musculoskeletal or neuromuscular diagnosis to qualify for services under Medicare.

Coverage Guidelines for PT. For PT services to be covered by Medicare, the following seven requirements must be met:

1. The services must relate directly and specifically to an active written POC established by the physician after any needed consultation with the physical therapist. This POC requires the documentation of functional limitations and safety measures to protect against injury. These measures are critical in order to justify the need for skilled rehabilitation. Documentation of the patient's functional limitations in activities of daily living (ADLs) and mobility as well as safety factors requiring skilled intervention is essential.

The development, implementation, management, and evaluation of a patient care plan based on the physician's orders calls for skilled PT services when, because of the patient's condition, those activities require the involvement of a skilled physical therapist to meet the patient's needs, promote recovery, and ensure medical safety. When the skills of a therapist are needed to manage and periodically reevaluate the appropriateness of a maintenance program or an identified danger to the patient, these services would be covered, even if the skills of a physical therapist are not needed to carry out the activities performed as part of the maintenance program.

2. The PT services must be reasonable and necessary to the treatment of the patient's illness or injury or to the restoration of maintenance of function. It is necessary to determine whether individual therapy services are skilled and whether, in view of the patient's overall condition, skilled management of the services provided is needed. (Skilled management might be needed even if many or all of the specific services needed to treat the illness or injury do not require the skills of a therapist.) Skilled management involves a finding that the patient's recovery or safety cannot be ensured unless the total care, skilled or not, is planned and managed by skilled rehabilitation personnel. The therapist should document the necessary precautions and the medical complications and safety factors that warrant skilled management. If the skills of a therapist are needed to establish a reasonable and necessary maintenance program until it can be safely and effectively carried out by nonskilled individuals, this would be considered coverable by Medicare. Also, if a danger to the patient's safety is identified and there is a need to reevaluate periodically the appropriateness of the care furnished, the services may be covered because the program is not yet fully established for safety and effectiveness.

"A service that is ordinarily considered non-skilled could be considered a skilled therapy service in cases in which there is clear documentation that, because of special medical complications, skilled rehabilitation personnel are required to perform or supervise the service or to observe the beneficiary. However, the importance of a particular service to a beneficiary or the frequency with which it must be performed does not, by itself, make a nonskilled service into a skilled service" (HIM-11, Section 205.2).

3. The PT services must constitute a specific and effective treatment for the patient's unique medical condition.
4. The PT services must be consistent with the nature and severity of the illness or injury, and the amount, frequency, and duration of services must be reasonable given the patient's particular medical needs.
5. The PT services must be of such a level of complexity and sophistication (or the patient's condition must be so severe) that only a qualified physical therapist or a PT assistant (PTA), under a therapist's supervision, can safely or effectively perform the necessary treatment.
6. There must be an expectation, based on the assessment made by the physician of the patient's rehabilitation potential, either that the condition of the patient will improve materially in a reasonable and generally predictable period of time or that the services are necessary to the establishment of a safe and effective maintenance program. "If there is not a reasonable expectation of improvement in a patient's condition, there may still be a need for skilled PT services to establish a maintenance program. A special medical complication might also necessitate skilled PT services to perform exercises or treatments that are normally considered nonskilled, even when no rehabilitation potential is present (e.g., for a terminally ill patient or a patient with pathological fractures)" (HIM-11, Section 205.2). In this situation, it is important to document the reasons for PT and provide documentation that is clear and specific.
7. The services must be considered reasonable under accepted standards of medical practice and must also be considered specific and effective treatment for the patient's condition.

Reimbursement Criteria for PT Services. A patient must meet all the criteria listed below to have PT in the home covered by Medicare:

1. The functional limitations must render the patient homebound.
2. There must be signed physician orders for PT services.
3. The patient must have a fair to good rehabilitation potential. There must be evidence that the patient's condition will improve in a reasonable period of time.
4. There must be a comprehensive assessment documented in the clinical record.
5. There must be a realistic POC identified in the clinical record.
6. The interventions must be designed to help patients meet the goals of improved functional ability and require the skill of a physical therapist.
7. Progress notes and reevaluations must reflect movement toward a goal.

Physical Therapy Assistants. When the needs of the patient are not complex, some PT services may be provided by a PTA. A PTA is someone who is trained to perform specific therapy activities under the direction and supervision of a licensed physical therapist. States have practice acts that govern the scope of practice for a PTA. This practice usually involves:

- performing active and passive range of motion
- performing therapeutic massage, and heat and cold applications to patients with stable conditions
- motivating and assisting patients to improve their functional ability
- observing and recording patient condition and reporting changes to the physical therapist
- participating in case conferences as appropriate
- documenting patient progress in the home care record

The PTA cannot be responsible for evaluation of the patient's condition, teaching, supervision, assessment of gait, and, establishment of, or revision to the POC. The physical therapist should provide on-site supervision of the PTA every two weeks or after four to six visits are made to the patient by the assistant. Supervisory visits are essential for Medicare reimbursement; however, it is important to remember that if the PT is providing exclusively supervision, it is not a reimbursable visit under Medicare. Specific treatments or skilled intervention must be given if the PT visit is to be reimbursable under Medicare.

Speech Therapy

ST services are provided to patients of all ages who have speech and language problems, including difficulties or delays in language development. Problems with speech and language may be either expressive or receptive. In addition, ST services are also helpful with patients who are experiencing dysphagia (difficulty swallowing). The speech therapist works with patients to improve their ability to carry out independently ADLs related to communication or swallowing. For example, the types of activities the therapist engages in may relate to talking on the telephone, eating, or managing oral secretions.

Examples of diagnoses seen when ST is provided under Medicare include, but are not limited to: new diagnosis of a CVA, Parkinson's disease, amyotrophic lateral sclerosis (ALS), multiple sclerosis (MS), dysphasia, and dysphagia.

ST is one of the three *primary skilled* services covered by Medicare. Because communication disorders or swallowing difficulties would not necessarily restrict a patient's ability to leave the home, it is necessary to identify the patient's functional limitations that support the patient's homebound status especially if ST is the only skilled service being provided. Other third-party payers may not require that the patient be homebound to receive reimbursable ST visits.

Coverage Guidelines for ST. Medicare will reimburse for ST services that are designed to meet the specific goals of the patient. These services include:

- assessment
- diagnostic testing and evaluation
- maintenance therapy
- therapeutic services
- aural rehabilitation
- teaching and training

Assessments are done to ascertain the type, causal factors, severity, and prognosis of the specific disorder. Reevaluation is necessary for patients whose condition had previously contraindicated ST and now these services are needed. Maintenance ST services are designed to maintain the patient's current level of function in the face of a debilitating illness (e.g., MS). Therapeutic services are designed to restore patients to their previous level of function following a medical problem. Aural rehabilitation focuses on procedures or treatments for patients with communication problems related to impaired hearing acuity. Teaching and training of the patient, family, or caregiver is a covered service under Medicare if all other conditions are met.

Specific ST services that are *not* covered under Medicare are:

- nondiagnostic and nontherapeutic routine
- repetitive and reinforcing procedures
- assessment related to specific work skills or work settings

For ST to be covered by Medicare, the following conditions must be met:

1. The patient must be homebound.
2. The services must be directed toward specific speech, language, or voice production or dysphagia treatment.
3. The services must be provided by a speech/language pathologist, and it must be reasonable to expect that the interventions will improve the patient's ability to function independently in the communication and swallowing areas in which there is a deficit.
4. It must be demonstrated that the patient has a reasonable probability that the ST service will result in improvement of the patient's condition in a reasonable and predictable period of time. This is done through the collaboration of the physician with the speech/language pathologist.
5. The therapy must be reasonable and necessary to meet the specified therapeutic goals which are part of the written POC (HIM-11, Section 205.2C).

Reimbursement Criteria for ST Services. In order for ST services to be covered, all the following criteria must be met:

1. The homebound status must be clearly documented including the functional limitations that render the patient homebound.
2. The patient must have a medical diagnosis that suggests a language disorder or swallowing problem.
3. The written POC must include goals that can be accomplished only by a speech/language pathologist.
4. Specific treatment procedures to be conducted by the speech/language pathologist are included in the written POC.
5. There must be signed physician orders for ST services.
6. There must be evidence that there will be improvement in the patient's condition in a reasonable period of time.
7. Documentation should reflect a measurable progress toward a goal.
8. There must be evidence of teaching the maintenance program to a family member or significant other following discharge from ST services.

Occupational Therapy

Patients of all age groups may require the assistance of the occupational therapist. This therapist helps the patient acquire the skills necessary to accomplish ADLs. Occupational therapists focus their interventions on the patient's upper extremities and on the fine muscle skills needed to perform functional activities, such as eating or dressing. In addition to assisting patients to develop self-care skills, the occupational therapist is involved in assessing the patient's home for safety and suggesting modifications to improve the patient's ability to function independently. These modifications may include the installation of grab bars in the bathtub or the modification of the kitchen to make meal preparation possible.

Skilled OT services include assessment and development of a therapy program that may include:

- Selecting and teaching task-oriented therapeutic activities designed to restore physical function (e.g., use of specific activities to restore upper body strength for a recent CVA).
- Planning, implementing, and supervising therapeutic tasks and activities designed to restore sensory integrative function.
- Planning, implementing, and supervising of individualized therapeutic programs as part of an overall "active treatment" program for a patient diagnosed with a psychiatric illness (e.g., use of craft activities requiring a patient to follow directions/patterns to reduce confusion and for reality orientation for the schizophrenic client).
- Teaching ADLs and instrumental ADLs (IADLs) (e.g., to promote or restore independence to the CVA patient).
- Designing, fabricating, and fitting orthotic and self-help devices (e.g., for patients with rheumatoid arthritis and amputees).

Medicare reimbursement for OT services is more limited than for PT or ST. OT services are considered one of the secondary home health care services under Medicare. This means that one of the skilled services as defined by Medicare (SN, PT, or ST) must be needed and is being provided in order for OT services to be reimbursed. There is an exception to this rule. If a skilled service is being provided in addition to OT and the skilled service is no longer needed, the occupational therapist can continue to provide reimbursed home care visits until the OT goals established on the written plan of care are met or until the patient no longer meets the criteria for Medicare home care services. Other third-party payers also reimburse for OT services on a more limited basis than PT.

Coverage Guidelines for OT. Medicare will cover OT services that are designed to restore or improve the level of functioning of the patient. These services include:

- assessing and evaluating the patient's condition, needs, goals planned, and treatment potential
- using therapeutic activities to restore physical or sensory integrative function
- planning, implementing, and supervising individualized therapeutic activity programs as part of an overall treatment program for patients with a diagnosed psychiatric illness
- teaching clients how to improve their ability to be independent in their ADLs through energy conservation and work simplification
- designing, fabricating, and fitting self-help devices
- assessing the need of and training patients in vocational and prevocational activities designed to restore function in ADLs (HIM-11, Section 205.2)

OT services that are *not* covered by Medicare include:

- implementation of an activity program to maintain function at a level to which it has been restored
- therapy provided to patients with a temporary loss of function that would reasonably be expected to return spontaneously without therapy
- services related specifically to employment or work skills

Guidelines for Medicare Reimbursement for OT. In order for OT services to be covered, all the following criteria must be met:

1. A primary service must have been initiated prior to occupational therapy.
2. The patient must be homebound.
3. The OT must relate to the primary or secondary diagnosis.
4. The rehabilitation potential must be fair to good.
5. The level of complexity of the POC must require a qualified occupational therapist.
6. There must be documentation that the patient is making progress toward a goal.
7. The therapy must be provided for a recent illness or injury that has resulted in a loss of function.
8. The therapy must be reasonable and necessary and not a duplication of the physical therapy services.
9. There must be periodic reevaluations of the patient's functional status and progress.

OT Assistants. A certified OT assistant (OTA) may provide services to a patient in the home under the direction of a qualified occupational therapist if there is an OTA practice act in the state. The occupational therapist consults with the physician and determines the POC. The OTA may provide selected services to the patient as identified in the POC. The occupational therapist must be available by telephone to the assistant at all times when care is being given. Supervisory visits must be done periodically and clearly documented in the clinical record. Lack of supervision can be a reason for denial of payment from Medicare and other third-party payers.

The OTA can perform the following activities:

- conduct noncomplex active and passive therapeutic exercises
- assist patients in learning therapeutic tasks and functional ADLs
- observe, record, and report to the occupational therapist the patient's response to the POC
- confer with members of the health care team for planning, modifying, and coordinating the treatment plan
- document the patient's response to care in the clinical record

Medical Social Worker

A MSW is involved in the psychosocial problems of both adults and children. Although MSWs focus on psychosocial problems, their interventions must contribute significantly to the patient's medical condition. The social problems the patient experiences must impede the progress or stability of the patient's medical condition.

Medical social services (MSS) must be provided by a qualified MSW. The MSW must have a master's degree from a school of social work accredited by the Council on Social Work Education and one year of social work experience in a health setting. Medical social work is one of the most difficult services to get reimbursed. As with any type of care, reimbursement is based on patient needs, specific criteria for reimbursement, and effective documentation. Medicaid does not provide any reimbursement for medical social work services because Medicaid recipients are assigned a case worker when they enroll in Medicaid. Medicare considers MSS a secondary service, which means that it can be initiated only when at least one of the primary services of SN, PT, or ST is also being provided.

Coverage Guidelines for Medical Social Work. Medicare will pay for medical social work services that contribute significantly to the patient's medical condition. These services are:

1. *Psychosocial assessments.* Skilled assessments of the social and emotional factors related to the patient's illness, need for care, response to treatment, and adjustment to care (followed by collaboration with the physician and nurse or therapist to develop the care plan) are coverable upon admission, at least once every two months, and upon discharge.
2. *Financial–environmental assessment.* An assessment of the relationship of the patient's medical, nursing, and therapy requirements to the home situation and the patient's financial resources, as well as the availability of community resources, is coverable.
3. *Counseling.* Counseling services required by the patient to cope with his or her medical condition and response to treatment are coverable. Remember, counseling a patient's family is covered only if this service is incidental to other covered MSS being provided to the patient and it is reasonable and necessary to the treatment of the patient's illness or injury. A recent ruling by HCFA will allow MSW visits to a client's family if the documentation validates that the intervention impacts positively on the client's POC.
4. *Short-term therapy.* Goal-oriented interventions directed toward management of terminal illness, reaction and adjustments to an illness, strengthening the family's support, and resolving conflicts related to the chronicity of an illness are examples of short-term therapy. *Note:* When skilled assessment is involved in counseling services, specifically identify the assessment services for Medicare patients.
5. *Community resource planning.* Establishing the need for and making referrals to community resources, such as supplemental health care, Meals on Wheels, food stamps, advocacy, and linkage, are covered. *Note:* Medicare does not cover the services of a MSW to complete or assist in the completion of an application for Medicaid, because federal regulations require the state to provide assistance in completing the application to anyone who chooses to apply for Medicaid. Also, if the only documented service provided is telephoning Meals on Wheels, this would not be a covered MSW visit, because the call could be placed by any individual.

6. *Long-range planning.* Assessment of a patient's needs for long-term care is covered, including evaluating the home and family situation, helping the patient and family to develop an in-home care plan, and arranging for placement (HIM-11, Section 206.3).

Reimbursement Guidelines for Medical Social Work. In order for medical social work to be covered by Medicare, all the following criteria must be met:

1. The patient must be homebound and receiving at least one primary service (SN, PT, or ST).
2. The medical social work services must be prescribed by a physician and written in the physician's POC.
3. The POC must indicate why the required services necessitate the skills of a qualified MSW. There must be documentation that there is a clear and specific link between the social and emotional needs of the patient and the patient's medical condition and rate of recovery.
4. The services must be delivered to resolve or manage a problem that is an impediment to the patient's medical recovery.
5. The services must be reasonable and necessary to the treatment of the patient's illness or injury.
6. The services must be provided to the patient or the patient and family but not only to the family.

Social Work Assistants. The social work assistant (SWA) provides psychosocial care to patients under the direction of a qualified MSW. The MSW must provide periodic supervision to the assistant in the form of case conferences or joint visits or both, depending on the needs of the patient and the skills of the assistant. Each supervisory visit must be clearly documented in the patient's clinical record.

Home Care Aide

The home care aide (HCA) is a paraprofessional involved in a range of services that extend from basic housekeeping to complex personal care. Services that are performed by the HCA typically include ensuring a clean, healthy home environment, shopping and meal preparation, grooming, bathing, and other personal care services for the patient. Three levels of HCA have been identified, each with its own focus.

Home Care Aide I. The HCA I assists with environmental services such as housekeeping and homemaking to preserve a safe, sanitary, and healthy home. The HCA I is not involved in providing any personal care to patients (National Association for Home Care, 1992). In many agencies, the HCA I is referred to as a homemaker.

Home Care Aide II. The HCA II can perform nonmedically directed personal care in addition to all the duties of the HCA I. The HCA II is not to be assigned duties related to medication administration and wound care (NAHC, 1992).

Home Care Aide III. The HCA III can perform all the duties performed by the HCA I and II. Additionally, the HCA III works under a medically supervised POC to assist the patient and family with household management and personal care. The HCA III activities that may be part of the medically supervised POC include nonsterile wound care, assistance with self-administered medications, and rehabilitation services (NAHC, 1992). A HCA III may be certified or uncertified. To be certified, a HCA III must attend a course of study that includes instruction on the personal care of clients and household management skills. Medicare will reimburse the home care agency only for care provided by a certified HCA III. In many agencies, the HCA III is called a home health aide.

It is the responsibility of the RN to determine the specific personal care and health-related services to be provided by the HCA. Although this evaluation is usually conducted at the time of the admission visit, HCA services can be initiated later if the patient's physical condition deteriorates, the family can no longer manage the care of the patient without assistance, or there are other factors that make placement of a HCA necessary. The RN cannot assign duties to the HCA that he or she has not been evaluated as competent to perform.

Medicare-certified home care agencies must have a plan in place to determine the competency of all HCAs and provide training if necessary. In addition to yearly evaluations of competency, HCAs must receive 12 hours of inservice education every calendar year. These programs must be provided by qualified RNs and can be either in the home care agency or in some other type of educational setting (community college, vocational school, etc.)

Supervision of paraprofessionals, such as HCAs, in the home is the responsibility of the home care nurse. A detailed description of the home care nurse's responsibility for supervision of HCAs appears in Chapter 2. If the home care nurse is not directly involved in the patient's care by providing a skilled service, the home care nurse can delegate the responsibility to other professionals, such as the physical therapist or the speech therapist. Medicare mandates that the HCA III be supervised every two weeks. This means that the home care nurse makes a visit to the patient's home either when the HCA is present to observe the aide providing care or when the HCA is absent to assess the relationship between the HCA and the patient (HIM-11, Section 206.2). For those patients not under Medicare,

6667666666

licensure requirements vary from state to state regarding frequency of HCA supervision, and agency policies outline supervision of paraprofessionals. Medicare considers a HCA service to be a secondary service, which means that it can only be initiated when one of the primary services of SN, PT, or ST is being provided to the patient. When the skilled service is no longer necessary, the HCA must also be discontinued.

Medicare Guidelines for Coverage of a HCA. Medicare will pay for HCA services for patients who are unable to meet their personal care needs without assistance. In addition, HCAs can be involved in household duties that are incidental and do not significantly contribute to the time spent by the HCA. The covered services are:

1. Personal care duties, including:
   - assisting the patent with bathing and skin care
   - assisting the patient to transfer into and out of bed
   - caring for the patient's hair and teeth
   - assisting with exercises, ambulation, and range of motion as directed by skilled personnel
   - assisting with medications that are specifically ordered by a physician and that are ordinarily self-administered (e.g., the HCA can give the patient the pill container and water or can prefill insulin syringes if permitted by state law; check with your state's nurse practice act; Illinois and Michigan are among many states that do not permit HCAs to prefill insulin syringes)
   - retraining the patient in necessary self-help skills
   - assisting in feeding the patient and promoting adequate fluid intake
   - assisting with catheter site care or irrigations under nursing supervision
2. Household duties, including:
   - changing the bed
   - light cleaning
   - making arrangements to ensure safety and enable the patient to reach necessary supplies or medications
   - laundering, as necessary, for the patient's comfort and cleanliness
   - promoting the proper nutrition for the patient by purchasing the necessary food
   - assisting in the preparation of meals
   - washing the dishes and utensils during the visit

Health-related services must be the primary reason for any HCA visit. A commonly used guideline is that household tasks should not take up more than 25% of the HCA's home visit time.

Reimbursement Guidelines for HCAs. In order for HCA services to be covered, all the following criteria must be met:

1. The patient must be homebound and receiving a primary service (SN, PT, or ST).
2. The HCA services must be prescribed by a physician and written in the physician's POC.
3. The HCA must be able to perform hands-on personal care for the patient. If the family is providing the personal care services, HCA services would not be considered reasonable and necessary.
4. An RN must determine the specific personal care services to be provided to the patient.
5. The HCA must be supervised every 14 days, and that supervision must be documented in the clinical record. If the HCA is assigned to assist with therapeutic exercises, the therapist should periodically supervise the HCA and document the supervision in the clinical record.
6. HCA services must be provided on a part-time, intermittent basis. HCA services are usually provided one to two hours a day, several days a week. When extensive personal care is required, combined SN and HCA services are allowed 8 hours a day and up to 35 hours per week. More hours can be allowed under exceptional circumstances. An example of an exceptional circumstance would be the care of a patient in the final stages of a terminal illness. In this situation, the provision of a HCA beyond 35 hours a week may be permitted because the care is needed for a finite and predictable period of time.

Other General Providers

Nutritionist. A home care nutritionist is involved in assisting patients in the management of their therapeutic diets. The nutritionist can either provide direct nutritional counseling to patients or provide consultation and direction to the home care nurse. If an agency has this service available, it is usually on a contractual basis. Nutritional services are not usually a reimbursable service from third-party payers.

Nurse Practitioner/Clinical Nurse Specialist. This nurse may provide total patient care, supervise others in difficult cases related to their specialty, or direct a special program. For example, a pediatric nurse practitioner may not only deliver direct care to the agency's pediatric patients but may act as a consultant to staff RNs to develop a care plan for their pediatric patients.

Enterostomal Therapist (ET). An agency may have an ET on staff who will provide direct care to patients or act as a consultant to staff members whose patients have bowel or bladder problems or wound management problems.

Respiratory Therapist (RT). Some home health agencies work on a contractual basis with RTs for patients who have a diagnosis related to their respiratory function. This relationship is especially important with patients who are on ventilator support. Often the RT works with the durable medical equipment (DME) in providing not only the technical products and services (e.g., ventilator, oxygen) but the professional treatment as well.

TEST YOURSELF

1. Identify the regulatory agency that administers the Medicare home health care benefit and the document that describes the regulations.

2. Identify the five criteria that a client must meet to be eligible for home care services under Medicare. Define each in your own words.

3. List the three primary disciplines identified by Medicare. List two secondary disciplines.

4. Identify the four areas of nursing practice that are described by Medicare. Describe a clinical situation that is an example of each one.

5. Describe a clinical situation in which a client would need a visit the day after admission, two days after admission, and once a week or once a month.

6. Identify two roles and responsibilities of the home care nurse in working with other professionals and paraprofessionals.

7. Identify three criteria that make a patient eligible for Medicare covered home care for:
   - physical therapy
   - occupational therapy
   - speech therapy
   - home care aide services
   - medical social worker services.

REFERENCES

Health Care Financing Administration (April 1989). *Medicare home health agency health insurance manual pub. 11.* Washington, DC: Author.

National Association for Home Care. (1992). *National uniformity for paraprofessional title, qualifications, and supervision position paper.* Washington, DC: Author.

Documentation in Home Care

OBJECTIVES

Upon completion of this chapter, the reader will be able to identify:

1. How home care nursing standards and the scope of home care practice influence documentation
2. How the Medicare Conditions of Participation and the Medicare coverage criteria affect documentation
3. Standards and principles of documentation common to all types of nursing practice
4. Strategies to document sensitive areas of practice
5. Various parts of a home care record and their purposes
6. Critical elements to document on HCFA Forms 485, 486, and 487
7. The fiscal intermediary audit process and the agency's denial/appeal process

KEY CONCEPTS

- **Effects of the home care standards and scope of practice on home care documentation**
- **Standards and guidelines of documentation**
- **How to complete HCFA Forms 485, 486, 487, and 488**
- **Documenting to satisfy clinical practice standards and Medicare regulations**

AGENCY-SPECIFIC MATERIAL NEEDED

- HIM-11 manual and supportive materials
- Transmittal 222 (see Appendix O)
- HCFA Forms 485, 486, 487, and Fiscal Intermediary Request Form (488)
- Any videotapes available on documenting for Medicare
- A blank copy of the agency's clinical record
- Agency procedure for certification and recertification
- Copies of the ANA publications *Standards for Home Health Nursing Practice* and *A Statement on the Scope of Home Health Nursing Practice*
- MIS manual, if agency is computerized

INTRODUCTION

The previous chapter discusses the Medicare home care benefit and the coverage criteria for nursing and other disciplines. This chapter covers the effects the American Nurses Association (ANA) publications *Standards for Home Health Nursing Practice* (ANA, 1986) and *A Statement on the Scope of Home Health Nursing Practice* (ANA, 1991) have on documentation, general principles of home care documentation from a practical and legal perspective, the components of the home care client record, and descriptions of how to complete the Medicare forms used in home care.

Numerous examples and suggestions will enable readers to apply these concepts to their own specific agency materials and forms. Now that you have begun to understand the coverage criteria for Medicare, this chapter will help you understand how to document effectively as you care for your clients. It is important to note that the home care nurse documents in the client record not only to ensure Medicare coverage but to reflect the needs of the client and family, the physician orders, the nursing care plan, and the progress toward the mutually agreed-upon goals.

The traditional nursing care provided and documented in an institutional setting was focused on medical and surgical procedures and was mandated by physician's orders and protocols based on the medical model of health delivery. As the nursing profession progresses, documentation now includes nursing protocols based on research and established standards of practice. Today, the nursing care plan created in any health care environment should provide documentation that builds on both the nursing care needed by the client and the individualized physician's orders.

When Medicare was enacted in 1965, specific documentation requirements for home care were part of the law and regulations. Although many of these requirements have been slightly modified, the Medicare documentation requirements that exist today are the same ones that were begun 30 years ago. As health care reform moves forward, home care and home care nursing will be in demand. Crucial to the ability to provide nursing services in the home is nursing's ability to justify what the client's needs are, what the nurse does in the home, and why she does it. Nothing can replace the significance of home care documentation data when health care is revamping its agenda and nursing is increasing in its importance. Documenting the care given to a home care client is just as important as the quality of care provided. Home care nursing is provided in the client's place of residence and the nurse has an incredible amount of independence. With this autonomy, the nurse has a professional responsibility to be accurate and comprehensive in her documentation of client care and to rely on her professional integrity to see that the care is provided with high standards. From the individual client home visit to the agency's quality improvement program to state and national issues, accurate and timely documentation of home care services is used to validate that needed services were provided to the Medicare beneficiary. These data are also used for health policy decisions, to document and project the costs of services, and to determine what will be covered in the future.

HOME CARE DOCUMENTATION

Documentation and the Standards for Home Health Nursing Practice

Home care nursing is considered a specialty nursing profession as acknowledged by the ANA. Two publications by the ANA, *Standards for Home Health Nursing Practice* (ANA, 1986) and *A Statement on the Scope of Home Health Nursing Practice* (ANA, 1991), identify the profession as a specialty with two basic categories, generalists and specialists within home care. This led to the development of a certification exam that is administered by the credentialing center of the ANA and is discussed in Chapter 2.

Most state nurse practice acts rarely differentiate home care nursing from other types of nursing. Consider the *Standards for Home Health Nursing Practice* as national guidelines for the profession to apply in daily practice. These guidelines include organization, nursing theory, data collection, diagnosis, planning, intervention, evaluation, continuity of care, interdisciplinary collaboration, professional development, research, and ethics. Each section of the *Standards* elaborates on the necessary functions and processes associated with home care nursing. Throughout the entire document, the need to document in a standardized, systematic, and concise form is stated.

The importance of documentation is found in the basics of nursing practice and reinforced in *A Statement on the Scope of Home Health Nursing Practice*. This document clearly delineates several distinguishing characteristics that make home care nursing a specialty within the nursing community. The specific language of the document addresses the nurse applying a holistic approach to clients' health and illness that emphasizes the use of a client-focused nursing care plan with goal attainment. These two documents indicate a clear relationship between the importance of documentation and the professional factors affecting this nursing specialty.

How the home care nurse documents varies from agency to agency and payer to payer. Although formats for documentation are always changing, as seen in the development of critical pathways, the constant in home care documentation is that detail is necessary and that the importance of accuracy and comprehensiveness will remain paramount. Documentation is important from an external perspective as well as an internal one. In addition to internal agency audits and reviews, Medicare surveyors, the Joint Commission on Accreditation of Healthcare Organizations (Joint Commission), the Community Health Association for Programs (CHAP), and others focus on documentation to retrospectively decide if the care provided was adequate and appropriate.

General Documentation Issues

The home health care record is a written account of the client's history, status, and progress and usually contains a physician's plan of treatment (doctor's orders), client care forms, and business and financial data. The record is the database for planning individualized care for the client and serves to communicate information to all health professionals involved in the client's care. It also serves an important legal function; it documents evidence for the client's Medicare, workers' compensation, insurance, or litigation-related claims. It is, therefore, paramount that the home health nurse recognize the importance of quality documentation and value it as much as hands-on care for clients. Not only is proper documentation necessary to justify reimbursement for third-party payers, it is also the key to the nurse's and agency's protection from liability. The phrase "if it wasn't charted, it wasn't done" reminds us that the best evidence of an event is usually what is in writing. Because most malpractice claims occur long after the events take place, when recollection can be unclear, the written record is given great significance. The written record can be the best indicator of what actually happened because it was written at the time of the event.

Using the following guidelines will help ensure that the home care nurse meets the practice standards required by the legal duty to communicate:

1. *The record must be accurate in all respects.* Poor documentation can lead to errors in the care of the client. For example, doctor's orders must always be up to date. Persons who care for the client on weekends or intermittent caregivers, such as student nurses, must be able to rely on the accuracy of orders for medication and treatment.

2. *The actual content of the record should contain measurable and objective information rather than subjective statements.* A statement made by a client can be recorded in quotation marks to indicate the source of the data. In general, conclusions should be avoided and the actual data recorded. For example, instead of recording that a client is "not eating enough" (conclusion), measurable objective data, such as amount of weight loss, daily intake, or statements from family members should be noted. Such phrases as "client appears comfortable" are not helpful because no observations are recorded to support this conclusion.

3. *Initial and ongoing assessments and nursing interventions must be documented in the record.* The nurse should record who was notified of changes in the client's status, including times and dates and any other follow-up care. There is a clear legal duty to communicate essential findings to those who need to know (e.g., the client's physician).

In a suit that involved documentation in the recovery room, a plaintiff won his case, in part, because of inadequate recording on his chart (*Wagner v. Kaiser Foundation Hospitals*, 1979). After surgery to correct a tear duct obstruction, the patient eventually sustained neurological damage as a result of the anesthesia and a period of subsequent hypoxia after surgery. During the approximately two hours he was in the recovery room, the nurses' notes showed the recording of his blood pressure and pulse at 15-minute intervals, but with no record of his respirations. The written nursing note entries stated the patient was "doing well" and that there were "no apparent complications." The defendant's expert witnesses stated that it was standard policy to observe and count respirations and that the information was not charted unless there was something unusual. The court concluded, however, that failure to monitor the patient's respirations properly led to his problem not being discovered. Because the respirations were not recorded, the jury was allowed to conclude that they were not assessed. Thus, even routine nursing care should be recorded, and one should not rely on the claim that "we always do it." This type of evidence would not be persuasive in the courtroom.

In another malpractice case against a hospital for negligent treatment, the plaintiff presented evidence of failure to document. He indicated that observations of circulation to his toes were not made (*Collins v. Westlake*, 1974). There was a written doctor's order to "watch condition of toes," even though the doctor testified that it was usually routine in such injuries for the nurses to check the circulation in the foot without a physician order. The nurse who was on duty part of the evening stated that normally a nurse does not chart each observation every time the patient is checked and that usually only abnormal findings are recorded.

The only entries on the nurse's notes the night in question were as follows:

> 12:30 Unable to sleep. Milk given.
> 1:30 Awakened for pain.
> 6:00 A good night—states he feels better. Left foot is cold—color is dusky—appears to have no feeling on foot. Dr. Hubbard notified. (*Collins v. Westlake*, 1974).

On appeal, the court concluded that there was no evidence in the record of the case that the circulation in the plaintiff's foot was observed by the nurse on duty at any time between 11:00 P.M. and 6:00 A.M. on the days in question. Therefore, the nurse's failure to recognize the condition led to the dangerous impairment of circulation that resulted in the amputation of the patient's foot.

4. *In the home care situation, it is important not only to document direct observations, but also to indicate what was taught to family members and the client, and what their response to instructions was, in order to ensure proper monitoring of the client's condition.* Client education documentation, including instruction to family members, needs to be an ongoing part of the record. In some cases, written instructions provided to the client and his or her family can be persuasive evidence that such instructions were given. In an emergency room case where a mother claimed that she was not instructed to observe her son for complications of a head injury after he was discharged, one of the issues was verbal versus written instructions (*Crawford v. Earl Long Memorial Hospital*, 1983). A dispute arose between the nurse, who testified that she gave these instructions verbally, and the mother of the plaintiff. If the instructions had been in writing, it would have helped substantiate the claim that the client received the information. Written instructions should not replace verbal explanations and discussion but should be used as a supplement to them. It is also recommended that the nurse document evaluative statements related to the client's understanding of the instruction. For example, "Client correctly drew up 40 U of NPH insulin and administered it in left thigh." In cases when detailed or complex instructions are needed, standard written instructions should be given. An example might be written instructions for tracheostomy care in the home. Some computer companies have teaching instructions that can be generated and given to clients, whereas other agencies use preprinted instruction sheets. These instructions should be reviewed and updated periodically by home care nurses and administrators at the agency.

In order to improve documentation of side effects from medications, one home health agency devised a system of peel-off medication labels for each drug to be placed in the client's record (Plastaras, 1987). On the client's drug profile sheet was listed each drug with a corresponding preprinted label listing side effects. By having the information in a quick and usable form, documentation was easier and the nurses could instruct clients more efficiently. This system is an example of an improved way to recognize complications of drug therapy and drug interactions. This system also helps the nurse and the agency protect themselves against potential liability.

Basic Principles of Effective Documentation

It is important to keep in mind some of the basic principles of good documentation, including how to correct errors and ensure proper timing of entries. Errors should remain legible by drawing a single line through the incorrect material and initialing above the error. If a large amount of information is charted on the wrong record, a line should appear through it, with the statement "charted in error," or "charted on wrong record." One should *not* use correction fluid or erase on the chart. In no case should records be destroyed or substituted at a later date. Doing so can give the impression that there was an error made or that there was an attempt to cover up for a mistake. In a Connecticut case, a large verdict was entered in the plaintiff's favor after a finding of negligence on the part of the hospital staff (*Pisel v. Stamford Hospital*, 1980). Part of the evidence presented at trial was that the director of nursing had ordered the staff to destroy the original notes and to rewrite the nursing notes surrounding the incident of the patient's injury. In upholding the lower court's judgment, the appeals court stated that the falsified record could be considered evidence of the hospital's awareness of its negligence.

Entries must also be made in a timely manner, because other caregivers may need to rely on the information and the clinical record is the major means of communicating client data. Also, by documenting immediately, the information is more likely to be accurate. If one remembers additional data not recorded at the time of a previous note, they should be included later as an addendum. The addendum should be dated the day it is written and titled "late entry."

The nurse should avoid contradictions or inconsistencies in the chart. Likewise, negative or derogatory comments about clients or other providers should not be made in the report. The nurse should also make sure that reports for scheduled tests are documented and included in the chart. These reports should be stamped or initialed with the date and time received so there is no question as to when they became a part of the record. If reports are faxed from the agency to the physician or vice versa, the agency should have a policy and procedure for documenting the time and date this occurred and where to file them in the home care record. Proxy charting, or signing for care given by someone else, is not a good practice. Countersigning, for example, a registered nurse (RN) signing with a home health aide, or a clinical instructor with a student nurse, would be proper if the RN is responsible for the case through proper delegation of tasks to the other caregiver. It should be clear who actually delivered the care.

Other charting pointers include:

- Always use standard abbreviations that are approved by the agency; unapproved ones can be misinterpreted.
- All phone conversations with the client, physician, or home care providers should be documented in the record.
- Any instructions to the client to make an appointment or follow up with his or her physician should be noted. The client's failure to keep appointments with the home care nurse or others can provide evidence of the client's failure to comply with the recommended plan of treatment. This could later be used to help the agency establish the client's contributory negligence for an alleged injury and in some states could negate his or her claim or reduce the liability of others.

Documentation of Sensitive Areas of Practice

Questions arise as to what should be documented in situations that involve potentially sensitive areas of practice. One example might include when the nurse questions whether care by another health professional is inappropriate or substandard. Both case law and professional standards impose a duty on the nurse to report questionable care and, in some instances, to take further action beyond documentation to protect the client from harm.

The ANA *Code for Nurses with Interpretive Statements* (1985) offers suggestions about how to handle questionable practice by another member of the health team. The first approach would be for the nurse to discuss her concerns about the care and the possible harm it may cause to the client with the person carrying out the questionable practice. If this does not yield any positive results, the findings should be reported to the appropriate authority within the agency or institution, following established formal channels. Every agency or practice setting should have a process for handling concerns of this type without fear of reprisal on the part of any employee who makes such a complaint. Written documentation of dates, times, observations, and events that validate the nurse's concerns should be recorded. In some cases, part of the documentation could be in a client's record, such as failure of a physician to return calls made on certain dates.

Once there is legitimate concern raised or a detrimental pattern established on the part of another caregiver, separate documentation should be completed in the form of incident reports or a log. All documentation should indicate clearly who was notified and what action, if any, was taken. This information should then be shared with the immediate supervisor who needs to have notice of any serious or immediate threat to the health care of the client.

If the problem is not corrected within the employment setting and continues to jeopardize the client's welfare and safety, other authorities may need to be contacted. An example would be a practice committee or state licensing board for specific categories of health care workers or professionals. Some nurses think, mistakenly, that if they document substandard or questionable care in the client's record, that alone will meet the duty owed to the client. In fact, when nurses knew or should have known that medical care was substandard, courts have imposed a duty upon them to act beyond mere documentation. This point is illustrated by the case of *Utter v. United Hospital Center* (1977), a successful malpractice case against both a hospital and physician. The patient presented persuasive evidence that the nurses did not take proper steps to ensure his safety. Three days after the plaintiff had a cast put on in the emergency room, he showed signs of deteriorating. The nurses noted some of the abnormal findings in the record, but not others. The charge nurse testified that she called the physician and informed him of the patient's symptoms, but he did nothing further. A hospital policy manual stated that in such cases the supervisor and department chairperson should request consultation. Even if the data were properly documented in the patient's record, the court stated that the nurses had an obligation to use positive action even beyond documentation. Thus, even if the agency does not have a policy regarding what to do in this situation, the nurse has an obligation to act in circumstances where harm is likely to come to a patient. The steps that the nurse takes to meet this obligation should be carefully and objectively documented in the client's record.

Another case illustrates that nurses' complaints and action taken by review committees will be supported when proper steps are taken. In *Scappatura v. Baptist Hospital* (1978), the chief of staff of a hospital temporarily suspended a physician's privileges, acting on information from nurses that the postoperative measures taken by the physician were "extreme, unusual, and perhaps unsafe." The nurses informed their supervisor of the situation. The supervisor initiated the steps for suspension through a written memorandum of the incident to the medical director. The court upheld the emergency suspension, pending a later thorough investigation, even though a formal due process hearing was not held.

A more difficult situation arises when the questionable practice that may have a detrimental effect on the client is by someone in the client's home who is not licensed or employed by an agency. For example, a home care nurse may question the activities of a person employed by the client as a homemaker or helper. The nurse's responsibility to the client in this situation will depend on a number of factors. The same general steps should be followed as outlined previously, with some modification, depending on the circumstances. For example, the home care nurse would first need to determine that the concern stems from the potential detrimental effect to the client's health, because this is the basis of the nurse-client relationship. Personal concerns of the client, such as how he or she chooses to spend money or leisure time, need to be separated from genuine health concerns.

Although the nurse is not responsible for the quality of care provided by private employees of the client, she does have a duty to the client at least to inform him or her of the concern and the basis for it. A proper notation of this conversation should be made in the client's record. If the client is fully competent, he or she has a right to take or withhold any action desired. If, however, the situation affects the care plan or the quality of care provided by the agency, there should be a mutu-

ally satisfactory resolution of the problem. An example would be if the nurse is teaching the client a sterile technique dressing change, but the homemaker follows a nonsterile procedure when the nurse is not there. If the nurse notices this, she must act on the situation, because the agency is responsible for the 24-hour care of the client with regard to the specified plan of care.

A different course of action may be required if the client is not competent. The nurse should then inform the client's family of the concern and let them make any decisions in the client's best interest. If no family member is available, state or local protective agencies may need to be informed. In an emergency situation, police or local authorities should be contacted, especially if illegal or unethical conduct is suspected. An example would be if the nurse has grounds to suspect that someone is taking advantage of the client by unauthorized use of his or her money or possessions.

Documentation of Abuse

Another sensitive area of documentation arises when the nurse suspects that an abuse or neglect situation exists in the home. This situation is reportable by statute to Children's Protective Services (CPS) if a child is involved or to Adult Protective Services (APS) if an adult is the client. Civil or criminal liability can occur if the nurse or other person who suspects the abuse does not report it to the proper authorities and further abuse or neglect occurs. Suspected abuse or neglect presents a challenging situation because documentation and testimony by the home care nurse will likely be part of the evidence if a formal complaint is filed against an individual (see guidelines for testifying as a witness, Chapter 10).

The nurse's primary role as the helper of the client and family may seem to be in direct opposition to her role as an investigator, gathering data that could have a negative or punitive effect on an individual. The welfare and safety of the client must be at the core of the nurse's actions, but at the same time she must provide support and guidance for the client and family. Documentation in potentially abusive situations must contain precise and ongoing evaluation of the home environment, family interaction, and physical and emotional status of the client. The principles underlying documentation are the same whether the client is a child or an adult. The nurse should check with her supervisor regarding the regulations and procedures in her state and agency. Vague terms such as *seems* and *appears* should not be used because they indicate uncertainty. Some guidelines for assessing for abuse are as follows:

If the client is an adult or child:

- Any abnormal findings, such as bruises or cuts, need to be precisely located and measured. Also, any changes in physical assessment from the previous visit that cannot be linked to the diagnosis or progression of the disease should be noted.
- The nurse should obtain a diet history and compare this to daily food and caloric requirements for the client.
- Food supplies should be checked to see if appropriate types and amounts of foods are available in the home and the client should verbalize a 24-hour recall of the previous day's meals.
- The nurse can direct other care providers, such as the home care aide, to observe for such things as sufficient food provision (e.g., whether food is left out for the client who will be alone for long periods of time), safety of the home, overall condition of the client upon arrival of the care provider, and verbal comments from the client and family that need to be evaluated.
- The caregiver's understanding of the client's functional limitations and cognitive abilities should be thoroughly evaluated because frustration and abuse may be occurring because unrealistic goals are being placed on the client.
- The home environment in general needs to be considered and documented in the record and conditions (e.g., appropriate temperature, cleanliness, sanitation, presence or absence of water and sleeping space) should be noted.
- Safety considerations, such as open stairways, access to hazardous substances, or no access to emergency assistance, should be noted.
- Physical condition of the living quarters should be noted, as this is often considered in a decision to remove a child or an adult from his or her home.
- A detailed family history should be obtained, as it will often help clarify other stresses in the environment and may reveal ways that the family relieves stress.

Additional guidelines if the client is a child:

- With a child, growth charts should be used and the child's specific data recorded on them. Developmental data should be included using such standard measurement tools as the Denver Developmental Screening Test (DDST) (Frankenburg & Dodds, 1969).
- Parent-child interaction can be documented by recording whether the child is comforted by the parent and the parent's response to situations requiring discipline or safety measures.
- It is also important to determine the parent's perception of the parenting role and whether expectations for the child are developmentally appropriate. Abusive parents sometimes have unrealistic expectations for the child, expecting behavior appropriate for an older child.

The child's emotional health and environment may be difficult to assess and document. That type of assessment should be based on observations of parent-child interaction, presence of toys or other stimulation in the environment, and the child's overall behavior. Emotional abuse of the child, although difficult to prove, may be evidenced by extreme perfectionism by the parent or constant belittling of the child's efforts to perform tasks. Any such behavior should be objectively noted in the record.

Helberg (1983) suggests that a community health nurse may be aided in balancing conflicting roles with the abusive family by contracting with them for mutually agreed-upon services. The nurse can list broad teaching goals relating to the child's developmental level and behavior, improving the coping behavior and responses of the parent and assisting in advocacy for better conditions for the family related to housing and finances. The parents could agree to work with the nurse to help alter the conditions that initiate the abusive behavior. Any failure of the parents to keep appointments or refuse services should be documented, because this serves as important evidence in any subsequent court proceeding.

THE HOME CARE RECORD

The home care chart is used by the agency to document client needs and services provided and serves as a legal record of all client activities performed by the agency. Documentation from the chart may be submitted to third-party payers, including Medicare, to justify payment for the services provided. The content of the chart varies from agency to agency, and the specific information included in the chart is dictated by agency policies and state and federal regulations. To ensure compliance with the various requirements, specific forms are used so information can be easily documented and reviewed. Standardized care plans, such as the one shown in Appendix B, may be used frequently in home care charts. The increasing use of critical paths, discussed in Chapter 8, is another way of standardizing the documentation of care.

Agencies may use skilled notes, in-home logs, or preprinted flowsheets for charting and communicating to other health team members client data, such as vital signs, assessments, treatments, procedures, and changes in the plan of care. Often these forms are printed on special paper with noncarbon copies so copies can be distributed to the appropriate departments based on agency policy. An example of an in-home log is found in Appendix C. Although there are variations in records and forms in all home health agencies, all home care records include the components listed in this chapter. As each chart component is discussed, the new nurse should have a copy of the agency's record available so that easy comparison can be made.

COMMON FORMS AND THEIR PURPOSES

Intake Form

The intake form contains the initial client information received by the agency when the client is referred for service. These data may be given by telephone to the person in the agency responsible for taking referral information. The form includes basic demographic information, a brief history of the client's illness and past problems, preliminary physician's orders, current medications, specific services ordered, and payer sources.

Patient Consent, Advance Directive, and Other Admission Forms

It is important that at the start of the initial home visit, consent be obtained from the patient or responsible party for treatment prior to providing treatment. Upon admission, according to the Omnibus Budget Reconciliation Act (OBRA) of 1990, the home health agency is required to notify patients of the following:

- patient bill of rights
- patient responsibilities
- any ordered home care services
- their consent to treatment by the agency
- certification for Medicare (Title XVIII of Social Security) and Medicaid (Title XIX), if applicable
- any applicable charges for services and how billing will be handled
- assignment of benefits for private insurance cases
- their need to have an advance medical directive and the agency's provision of assistance to do so

- frequency of visits
- duration of visits
- date of next visit
- the agency's complaint policy and the Medicare comment line toll free phone number
- how to reach the agency 24 hours a day

Initial Evaluation Form

This database includes findings from the initial nursing assessment, including the client's past medical problems, mobility, and safety concerns. It also includes information about the client's lifestyle before the current illness, available support systems, emotional factors related to the client's current problems, and concerns about adequacy of housing, food, and other economic and social issues that affect the home care plan.

Agencies have numerous ways of capturing this important information and may use physical databases, psychosocial, and socioeconomic data collection tools; or they may use computers with integrated screens that collect this information to be printed out in various formats. It is important to understand that, regardless of what format the initial evaluation is in, the nurse's assessment should be comprehensive, including all aspects of client, family, physical, psychosocial, cultural, and economic information that are relative to determining and justifying the care the client needs. Also at the initial visit, verification of payer sources is completed, including sources of payment for home care services, client's income and expenses, and any other forms and information the agency might require for financial records.

Medication Record

The medication record includes information about all client medications, both over-the-counter and prescription drugs. Any new or changed dosages of medications are noted on this form. Special care should be given to ensure that all medications, dosages, and times of administration the patient has been given are consistent with the information on the physician's order form. If they are not, the nurse should confirm the medication orders with the client's physician. Medicare's Conditions of Participation (1991) require that, in addition to being taught the dose and time, the patient be taught about side effects and contraindications of his or her medications. On this form or on other agency forms, this information is either printed out or the nurse is asked to write it down to leave with the client. Documentation must show that the nurse as well as the client are aware of side effects and contraindications.

Nursing Care Plan

The nursing care plan details the client's individual problem list and outlines the nursing diagnoses and interventions developed by the nurse in collaboration with the client, family, physician, and other members of the health team. Some home health agencies use the North American Nursing Diagnosis Association (NANDA)–approved nursing diagnoses in the care plan. A list of NANDA diagnoses can be found in Appendix A. Included in the client's care plan are the individualized long- and short-term goals of care that are used to evaluate the client's progress toward expected outcomes and indicate when the client has reached these goals and is ready for discharge. Some agencies use the Health Care Financing Administration (HCFA) Form 485 as the care plan for the client, while others use the HCFA Form 485 and a separate nursing care plan. Either way is acceptable to licensure and accrediting bodies. The HCFA Form 485 is discussed later in this chapter.

Nurse's Note and Narrative

The nurse's note section often includes a checklist for the physical assessment of the client and a narrative portion that may include specific treatments, procedures, patient teaching, additional documentation of patient status, and evaluation of teaching, as well as the measurement of the client's progress toward goals. The use of a prescribed format for collecting nursing information on each visit not only makes it easier for the nurse to do the paperwork but also ensures consistency between visits. The narrative needs to be as clear, concise, and brief as possible without losing meaningful content. It is important to document comments made by the client and caregiver that are relevant to the care as well as the nurse's direct observations on the narrative, but not to repeat information already recorded on other areas of the note and the checklist.

The narrative may be used as the specific place to pull together a brief summary of nursing observations and interventions to present a total picture of the client's condition. For instance, a client has congestive heart failure (CHF). On this visit, the nurse observes pitting edema of the feet and rales, which represent changes in the client's condition since the previous visit. The nurse would record clearly in the narrative the symptoms that indicate that the client may be going into CHF, her plans to consult with the physician regarding medication or diet changes, and the need for

increased frequency of nursing visits to evaluate the client's response to the changes in the plan of care. This use of the narrative results in accurate, effective documentation that indicates that the skill of the nurse was necessary to assess and develop such effective interventions.

Home Care Aide Assignment Sheet

Home care aides are required to work under the direct supervision of a RN. At the initial client evaluation, the RN develops an assignment of personal care and light housekeeping tasks for the home care aide to perform that is individualized for each client. This plan should include any special client needs and specific personal care goals that have been shared with the client and family. One copy of this written plan is kept in the client's home, one is given to the aide, and one is placed on the client's agency record. The assignment sheet should be reviewed and updated with each subsequent recertification period and as the client's condition warrants.

Supervisory Visit Forms

The Medicare Conditions of Participation (1991) require that home care aides be closely supervised to ensure their competence in providing care. During the supervisory visit, the nurse should assess the relationship between the aide and the client and determine if the goals are being met. Some agencies use a separate supervisory note for this function, while others integrate the information into the nursing visit note. Whichever format is used, simply checking a box on a visit note that says "aide supervised" is not enough. The nurse's goal must be to document in a way that shows the agency is in compliance not only with the frequency of the supervision but also with its intent.

The documentation of every aide supervisory visit should include the following information:

1. *Date of Visit.* The Conditions of Participation have specific frequency requirements that differ depending on whether the client is under a skilled plan of care or is receiving nonskilled care only.
2. *Assessment of Client-Aide Relationship.* Documentation should include subjective comments from the client about the relationship and/or the nurse's objective comments based on observation of the aide–client relationship.
3. *Progress toward Goals.* Note the client's comments or objective observations reflecting progress to-

ward goals involving the home care aide services, such as bathing, ambulation, etc.

If the aide is present during the visit, include the aide's name, observation comments regarding the aide's performance of assigned duties and any nursing instructions, and a review of the aide assignment sheet or education provided. Be sure to follow up on any questions or issues raised during the supervisory visit. Perhaps the client reports that the day aide is always 20 minutes late. The nurse should bring this concern to the aide supervisor, document it in the aide's personnel file, and if appropriate, also document it in the client's home care record and report back to the client. A prompt, attentive response can defuse further problems with the aide and prevent the client from having a complaint against the agency.

If a client is receiving only therapy services, the therapist can make the supervisory visit. The same documentation guidelines apply if the therapist supervises the aide. However, it is good practice to let a RN review and initial the supervisory notes completed by the therapist. This is a good way to demonstrate coordination of services. Further discussion on aide supervision is found in Chapter 2.

Other Health Team Members' Notes

Client notes of any other home care disciplines involved in the client's care, including noncovered services or contracted disciplines, should be located in the client's permanent record. It is important that the nurse become familiar with these forms and their content to ensure that coordination of services takes place. At patient care conferences and at other times when discussion between service providers occurs, the nurse needs to be familiar with the interventions toward the goals other disciplines and service providers have made. These can be found on their assessment and visit notes or in a separate note often set aside specific to that discipline.

Physician's Orders—Plan of Treatment

This section of the record contains all medical orders for the client, including the initial certification, any recertification, and all supplemental orders. The physician's order sheet that orders home health services for a defined period of time is called the plan of treatment (POT). Most agencies choose to use the required Medicare HCFA Form 485 as the POT for all home care clients (Appendix D) although there may be a separate form for the initial physician's orders, which is completed at the time the client is referred or admitted to the agency.

The period of time covered by the orders should be spelled out on the form, and although the time period is usually based on agency policy, government regulation, or both, two months (62 days) is common. The POT includes such information as diagnoses, medications, diet, allergies, prognoses, activity limitations, and specific home health services ordered (e.g., nursing, therapy, home care aide). The home care nurse, using information from the intake sheet, which includes the initial physician's orders, the initial evaluation form(s), and the client and family's perception of need, completes the POT, including the nursing interventions and the frequency and duration of services. This initial POT is then forwarded to the physician who verifies the orders, signs the form, and returns it to the agency. If additional services or skills are identified after the initial assessment, or, because of a change in the client's condition the frequency and duration of home care needs to be changed, supplemental physician's orders must be obtained.

Some insurance companies may require specific statements or information to be placed on the physician's orders. For example, the words *medically necessary* might be needed in the orders if home care aide services are required. The nurse should be aware of the client's individual policy requirements before writing the physician's orders; this is usually done in collaboration with the agency's billing department.

Communication Notes

Communication notes are used by many agencies and should be created when there is needed documentation that does not occur during the course of a client visit and does not require a verbal physician's order. Such notes include phone calls to physicians, family members, other health care team members involved in the client's care, and any other communication regarding the client that is important to be noted in the client's permanent record. Many agencies use these forms especially to communicate information from the home care aide to the client's primary nurse. The note is given to the nurse and then when action is taken on the identified issue, the nurse or aide supervisor returns the note to the aide so the aide is assured the communication was acted upon. This document can and should become part of the client's record because it is an excellent way to show that coordination of all services was done.

Conference Summary

Many agencies use a form for documenting the interdisciplinary conferences held to discuss the client's current or prospective plan of care. The conference may be a regularly scheduled one that must be held at least every recertification period (62 days) or one that occurs as the need arises to ensure coordination of client services. The conference summary form may contain identified patient problems, interventions toward expected outcomes, plans for discharge, or psychosocial factors affecting the client's progress toward goals.

Discharge Summary

The agency may have a specific form that is used when a client is discharged from service. This form is used as a checkoff sheet to ensure that each discipline in the case is discharged appropriately and at a certain time. Additionally, a summary of the client's condition at discharge, reason for discharge, and progress toward goals is also included in this record. Some agencies use the discharge summary form as a communication tool with the client's physician and/or referral source when the discharge is complete. Some states require that a copy be sent to the physician; check your agency's policy.

MEDICARE FORMS IN HOME CARE

The Medicare forms used in home care are the HCFA Forms 485, 486, and 487. The HCFA Form 485, as previously referred, is also known as the POT. The HCFA Form 486 is an optional form that may be used to substantiate need for services provided and to assist the fiscal intermediary (FI) in making coverage determinations. The HCFA Form 487 is simply an addendum to the plan of care/medical update and patient information and may be used to provide additional documentation of any elements of the HCFA Forms 485 and 486.

HCFA has produced a workbook and videotape that describe in detail how to fill out Forms 485, 486, and 487. These tools can be helpful. If the home health agency does not have these available, the nurse can check the written guidelines in this text or developed by the agency to guide her through the completion of these forms.

HCFA Form 485

HCFA Form 485 (Appendix D) is the POT for the physician(s) who is caring for the patient and requires the attending physician's signature. The HCFA Form 485 must be reviewed at least every 60 days and is completed with each certification and recertification. The form should include both Medicare covered and noncovered services. When completing the HCFA Form 485 (as well as 486), no field may be left blank. There are some fields where N/A is applicable—Fields 4, 10, 12, 13, 14, and 15.

This section outlines guidelines on completing the HCFA Form 485.

Field 1: Patient's Health Insurance Claim (HIC) Number

Enter the patient's complete Medicare number or payer source identification, which can be obtained from the patient's health insurance card.

Field 2: Start of Care Date

The start of care (SOC) date is the six-digit number that reflects the date of the first Medicare billable service. This date remains unchanged on subsequent POTs or recertifications until the patient is discharged (e.g., 020595).

Field 3: Certification Period

This identifies the period covered by each physician's POT. Enter the six-digit month, day, and year. On the initial certification, the *From* date must match the SOC date. The *To* date can be up to, but never exceeding, two calendar months and mathematically never exceeding 62 days. Always repeat the *To* date on subsequent recertification as the next sequential *From* date. *To* in this situation means up to, but not including. Services delivered in the *To* date are covered in the next certification period (e.g., initial certification from 020595 to 040595 covers visits made on 2/5 through 4/4, not visits made on 4/5; recertification from 040595 to 060595 covers visits made on or through 6/4).

Field 4: Medical Record Number

This optional field may be used by the agency to assign a patient number that is unique to the agency. If the agency does not use such a number, N/A must be entered.

Field 5: Provider Number

In this field, enter the agency's six-digit number issued by Medicare. It contains two digits, a hyphen, and four digits (e.g., 74-1234).

Field 6: Patient's Name and Address

Enter the patient's last name, first name, and middle initial as they appear on his or her health insurance card, which has been checked on the initial visit. This is followed by the patient's address. The telephone number is optional.

Field 7: Provider's Name, Address, and Telephone Number

Enter the provider's name and address. The telephone number is optional.

Field 8: Date of Birth

Enter the patient's birth date utilizing the six-digit number. If the patient was born prior to 1900, the complete year must be included. (e.g., 070664 or 10241898).

Field 9: Patient's Sex

Check the appropriate box.

Field 10: Medications: Dose/Frequency/Route

Enter physician's orders for all medications including dose, frequency, and route of administration for each. The HCFA Form 487, which is an addendum sheet, may be used for drugs that cannot be listed on the HCFA Form 485. Denote a (N) for any medications that are new within the last 30 days and a (C) for any changes of current medications within the past 60 days including dose, frequency, and route. All medications, including over-the-counter (OTC) medications, must also be listed here. If the patient has no medications, you must enter N/A. Oxygen should also be listed in Field 10, if applicable.

Field 11: ICD-9-CM Code, Principal Diagnosis, and Onset/Exacerbation Date

The *International Classification of Diseases, 9th Revision, Clinical Modification (ICD-9-CM)* is the code book used by all health care providers when coding a patient's disease and procedures for billing purposes. (If your agency requires the nurse to complete the ICD-9-CM code in the HCFA Form 485, you will receive more in-depth instructions during your orientation.) Using the ICD-9-CM code book, enter the code appropriate for the principal diagnosis in the space provided. Also in Field 11, enter the principal diagnosis itself. The principal diagnosis is the diagnosis that is most related to the current POT, represents the most acute condition, and requires the most intense services. For each diagnosis listed, identify the most current onset or exacerbation date that best justifies the need for covered services (e.g., 428.0 CHF (E) 020595). Be as specific as possible. A general, nonspecific diagnosis does not carry the weight of a specific diagnosis. Also, be aware that some reimbursements are diagnosis specific and require a specific diagnosis for coverage (e.g., Vit B12 or Calcimar injections).

Field 12: ICD-9-CM Code, Surgical Procedure, and Date

Enter the surgical procedures relevant to the care rendered, if applicable. For example, if the patient's principal diagnosis is a fracture of the left hip, then the relevant surgical procedure may be ORIF of the L hip. If no surgical procedures are applicable, enter N/A in this field. Do not include surgical ICD-9-CM codes if they are not relevant to the skilled care being provided.

Field 13: ICD-9-CM Codes, Other Pertinent Diagnoses, and Onset/Exacerbation Dates

Enter all pertinent ICD-9-CM codes and diagnoses relevant to the care rendered. Other diagnoses affecting the patient's condition are listed in order to reflect the seriousness of the patient's condition and the services being provided. Again, the HCFA Form 487 may be utilized to provide additional documentation. If no secondary diagnoses are applicable, denote N/A in this field. Exclude diagnoses that relate to an earlier episode that has no bearing on the current POT. The priority of diagnosis and onset/exacerbation date should be evaluated with each recertification to reflect changes in the patient's condition and the POT during the previous two months. Remember to draw a picture of the patient with the use of specific codes and descriptors.

Field 14: Durable Medical Equipment (DME) and Supplies

This is the area to enter all *nonroutine* supplies that are being billed to Medicare. Enter N/A if no supplies or DME is billed. If the supply is inherent to the service, it does not need to be itemized (or necessarily listed) in order to bill (e.g., if the order is for a Foley cathether change, indicated in Field 21, then the supply "Foley catheter" does not need to be repeated in Field 14).

Field 15: Safety Measures

Enter any safety measures ordered by the physician or identified by the agency for the patient. Enter N/A if no safety measures are applicable.

Field 16: Nutritional Requirements

Enter the prescribed diet, including any therapeutic diets, fluid restrictions, dietary requirements, enteral feedings, and nutritional supplements (e.g., Ensure tid).

Field 17: Allergies

Enter medications to which the patient is allergic and any other allergies the patient reports or experiences. The abbreviation NKA (No Known Allergies) may be used here, if applicable.

Completing Fields 18A and 18B

Both Fields 18A and 18B are extremely important in supporting the patient's homebound status. Be sure to use measurable descriptors in order to support the patient's limitations. To help establish homebound status, the nurse must be specific regarding physical or psychological limitations, such as "patient can only walk 20 feet before becoming severely dyspneic" or "patient refuses to use stairs for fear of falling." In describing prior functional status, the greater the gap between abilities before the patient became ill and the present, the better. This is especially true for patients who need physical therapy services. For example, most patients are weak following major abdominal surgery for cancer with creation of a colostomy. If the patient was totally independent, however, and drove and played golf before surgery and now requires the assistance of one person to transfer or ambulate with a walker, then physical therapy could be justified for muscle strengthening and assisting the patient with progressive ambulation.

Field 18A: Functional Limitations

Check all items that the physician and/or the agency have assessed as current limitations for the patient. If *Other* is checked, the limitation must be described in detail.

Field 18B: Activities Permitted

Check the activities allowed by the physician's orders. If *Other* is checked, describe the additional activities.

Field 19: Mental Status

Check the blocks most appropriate to the patient's status. If *Other* is checked, describe the condition in detail.

Field 20: Prognosis

Check the box which specifies the most appropriate prognosis for the patient: Poor, Guarded, Fair, Good, or Excellent.

Field 21: Orders for Discipline and Treatments

As previously stressed, Medicare considers skilled care to be assessing, observing, teaching, performing skilled procedures, and evaluating. The nurse should be sure to include the terms *assessing, observing, teaching,* and *evaluating* in the physician's orders in this section. This will help to avoid the use of words denoting minimal skill, such as *reinforce* or *encourage*. For example, for a patient with a new colostomy who also had an exacerbation of chronic obstructive pulmonary disease (COPD) and CHF postoperatively, the nurse might write: Skilled nursing (SN) to assess cardiorespiratory status and response to new medications, bowel status, and skin integrity around stoma. Teach colostomy care, bowel regime, to help normalize stool and diet. Also teach correct medication use and the effects and side effects of meds, pacing of activity, COPD, CHF disease processes, and symptoms for the patient to observe and report.

For the patient with a coronary artery bypass graft (CABG) who developed arrhythmias and cardiac arrest and then urinary retention postoperatively, the nurse might write: SN to assess cardiac status, particularly rate, rhythm, and response to new medications, healing of incisions, intake and output, and amount of residual urine. Teach the patient medications and symptoms of wound complications to observe and report. Teach self-catheterization using clean technique and a #16 Foley straight catheter.

When writing direct care skills in orders, be sure to note the specific procedure you will be performing. For example, the directions could be phrased as "SN to pack wound bid with a wet to moist saline dressing," or "SN to insert a #18 Foley catheter with 5 cc balloon 1mo2 and 4 prn for Foley dysfunction."

In this section, the amount, frequency, and duration of visits must be detailed. The key is to estimate the number of visits that will cover any unexpected visits if a new problem has developed or the patient is learning more slowly than expected. It is essential to anticipate a few as-needed visits in some patient situations or estimate visit ranges to adjust for changes in the patient's condition. If you do write for as-needed visits, you must quantify them (how many you are requesting) and qualify them (what specifically you are anticipating happening that will indicate a need for an as-needed visit). For example, for a CHF patient with new medications, diet, and little understanding of the disease, the nurse might write this section in two ways:

1. "SN to visit 4wk1, 3wk1, 2wk1, 1wk3, and 3 prn if problems arise with patient's condition or teaching progresses slowly." This approach allows for a six-week parameter of coverage. If the patient's condition warrants additional visits beyond those initially requested, a physician's order to cover the change would be indicated.
2. "SN: 4-5wk1, 2-3wk4, 1-2wk4." This approach develops a nine-week parameter of care that will cover nursing visits until the next certification period (60 days). By doing this, you will have orders for the entire certification period and not need to send additional, interim orders unless the visits needed go beyond those in the original order. The home care nurse can discuss these two approaches with the supervisor and orientation coordinator and further explore the agency's policies regarding this.

Field 22: Goals/Rehabilitation Potential/Discharge Plans

Enter realistic, achievable goals as identified by the physician, agency, and the patient. These goals should be measurable and individualized for the patient. Goals need to be updated with each recertification to reflect the resolution, continuation, or the identification of any new problems. Check your agency's nursing and patient record policies regarding goal setting. The following are examples of realistic, measurable goals:

- Patient will be knowledgeable about all new medications within two weeks.
- Patient/caregiver will be independent in IV administration in two visits.
- Dressing changes will be decreased from daily visits within three weeks.
- Patient will be independent in preparation and insulin administration within one week.

Rehabilitation potential addresses the patient's ability to attain the goals and an estimate of the time needed to achieve them. The words *fair* or *poor* alone are not very useful. An example of a rehabilitation potential for a patient being seen post-operatively for a repair of a fractured hip would be "Rehab potential good for patient to ambulate independently with walker by 4-10-95."

Discharge plans include a statement of where or how the patient will be cared for once home health services are not provided.

Field 23: Nurse's Signature and Date of Verbal SOC

This field verifies for surveyors, HCFA representatives, and intermediaries that a nurse spoke to the attending physician and has received verbal authorization to visit the patient.

Field 24: Physician's Name and Address

Enter the attending physician who has established the POT and certifies/recertifies the medical necessity of the visits and/or services.

Field 25: Date Home Health Agency Received Signed POT

Enter the date the agency receives the signed copy of the HCFA Form 485 from the physician. The field can be left blank if the physician dated his or her signature (Field 27). Usually agencies use a dated "Received" stamp on all chart correspondence.

Field 26: Physician Certification

Indicate for initial certification or recertification.

Field 27: Attending Physician's Signature and Date Signed

The attending physician signs and dates the POT. Rubber signature stamps are not acceptable. The form may be signed by another physician who is authorized by the attending physician. If the signature is not dated, the agency must complete Field 25.

The Importance of Completing HCFA Form 485 Correctly

Every FI hires nurse reviewers who, by looking at various parts of selected clients' home care records, determine if the client and home care services meet the coverage criteria for the Medicare home care benefit. The Intermediary Medical Information Request is a form utilized by FIs to request additional information from the agency to justify billed services. Some FIs use their own form, a HCFA Form 488, or simply send a letter to request further information before making or possibly denying payment.

If the documentation sent clearly indicates that the client's condition and the care provided meet the Medicare criteria for reimbursement, the bill is paid. If the FI does not find the documentation to be clear regarding its criteria for reimbursement, it will send a request for more information (HCFA Form 488) to the agency.

When the agency receives this request or other communication, it usually involves copying portions of the client's nursing and/or other discipline record to provide the requested information.

When the agency responds to the FI's request for further information, client documentation on HCFA Forms 485 and 487 is usually submitted to the FI along with other relevant materials (most likely at least nursing visit notes for the time period in question) for a process called medical review. Information on these forms must be supported by information in the client's home care record. It is important that the home care nurse understand how to document not only on the HCFA Forms 485 and 487 but in the clinical record as well to ensure that the materials sent for medical review are comprehensive and paint a picture of the care given to the client.

HCFA Form 486

HCFA Form 486 (see Appendix E) encompasses the summary data needed by FIs to make coverage determinations on home health claims. HCFA Form 486 may be submitted for response to a FI's request for further information, but the agency does not need to complete one on each patient routinely, unless it chooses to do so for its own internal needs. The form, which is completed by the agency and signed by a nurse or therapist, reflects orders from all physicians contributing to the patient's POT and provides a brief description of the type of services rendered during the billing period, as well as a description of the patient's current health status.

Agencies can choose to use the HCFA Form 486 as a multipurpose tool by routinely completing it for quality management activities. Someone assigned in the agency can review each case periodically to evaluate how care is progressing and if services are covered, using the form to collect such data. HCFA Form 486 can be sent to the physician periodically to fulfill the agency's requirement for reporting to the physician regarding the patient's progress and summary of care.

Because the top section of HCFA Form 486 is similar to HCFA Form 485 and is self-explanatory, the following discussion identifies only those fields that need special clarification as to content.

Field 15: Updated Information: New Orders/ Treatments/Clinical Facts/Summary from Each Discipline

It is important in this field to list not only vital signs and other factual data, but to tell the story of the patient's situation in a concise way. This will show the intermediary that the services provided were needed. It is important that objective data and problem areas be stressed. Document teaching that needs to be accomplished and stress any current or ongoing knowledge deficits the patient and family may still have.

The home care nurse must describe ways the patient is at high risk for developing potential problems and include any relevant information from the patient's hospital stay indicating complications or other problems that developed prior to or during the hospitalization. Note the following examples of clinical data that could be included in this section. Both discuss the same patient at the same point of recovery, but which really justifies the services requested?

Patient Situation: The patient has just been discharged from an acute hospital with a below-the-knee amputation of the right leg.

Example 1

SN: Right stump, incision had 3×1 cm separation on admission with serous, pink drainage saturating 2 4×4s. Now wound size 1×0.5 cm. Redness has decreased, serous drainage only. Able to ambulate well. Having difficulty breathing. Taking pain medication as required. PT in to visit yesterday.

Example 2

SN: Wife has learned correct dressing change technique. Occasional cough, bi-basilar rales. LLE 2 + edema. Exertional dyspnea. Blood glucose 100. On admission, required pain medication q 4 hr. By 02/21/95, required medication only upon awakening and again at bedtime. Wound on right stump had 3×1 cm separation on admission with serous, pink drainage saturating 2 4×4s. Now wound size 1×0.5 cm, redness has decreased, serous drainage only.

PT: 20 degree flexion contracture right knee. Improved to 10 degree by 02/21/95. Required assist of one to transfer on admission and able to ambulate 30 feet. Now able to ambulate 50 feet with standby assist but requires assist of one to transfer. On 02/13/95, increased repetitions of Theraband exercises to right hip flexors and extensors. As of 02/21/95 strength in right hip and quads remains F+. Cannot navigate stairs, inclines, or unlevel surfaces or get from floor to chair unassisted.

AIDE: Continues to require standby assist to ambulate. Requires assist to transfer. Has progressed from needing complete assistance with bathing to requiring assist only on his back, left lower extremity, and hair shampoo.

The second example certainly gives the reviewer clear reasons why assessing, observing, and teaching skills were needed and would justify the increased visit frequency.

Field 16: Functional Limitations—Reason Homebound/Prior Functional Status

This section expands on the checklist on functional limitations of HCFA Form 485. As in all documentation on HCFA Forms 485, 486, and 487, the nurse must be sure that the patient's total home care record will substantiate anything written on any of the three forms. In completing all of the forms, the nurse must remember that functional limitations include not only physical limitations, such as ambulation difficulties or activities of daily living (ADLs), but also things such as slowness to grasp new concepts, illiteracy, visual limitations, and anxiety.

Field 18: Unusual Home/Social Environment

In filling out this section, information about the actual home or social environment should be included. For example, a lack of electricity, running water, or needed DME could be the rationale for continued service because it makes the care given more complex than with patients who do have the appropriate setting and supplies. Another example would be the patient's spouse who might be very anxious about the patient's condition and therefore slow to learn his or her care. These areas are important to note for they show the impact of these issues on the type of care needed and show the frequency and duration variances of delivering that care. Additionally, this exemplifies the importance of practicing home care nursing with a family and community focus.

If the home health agency does not use the HCFA Form 486 routinely, the nurse must review the information discussed here to be sure documentation regarding these areas is clear in the visit notes. The nurse has to be vigilant in documenting the patient's homebound status and the ongoing assessment information that indicates the patient's status is changing and that he or she is not stable or chronic. Reviewing this information can be done easily by summarizing the information in the notes and the patient's progress toward goals either formally or informally during the recertification process and patient care conference.

FI REQUEST FOR FURTHER INFORMATION

FIs send requests for further client information, sometimes called a query, to agencies periodically. There are several names for the form, based on the individual FI. The purpose of this section is to explain the concept and process involved in the FI's request and the nurse's role.

The FI request for information form will indicate the dates of service in question and the time the agency has to respond to the inquiry, which is usually a short period of time, around 30 days. The agency will send the FI the additional information, which will likely include the HCFA Forms 485, 486, and 487 and/or skilled notes and any other pertinent information requested that enables the FI to see the picture of the client situation the nurse described in the documentation. After reviewing the additional documentation, the FI may choose to pay the claim or to deny all or any part of the billed services that the FI considers noncovered services or that do not comply with the criteria of the home health benefit.

WHEN THE AGENCY RECEIVES A DENIAL FROM THE FI

Dealing with Medicare and the FIs can be frustrating and time consuming when coverage for a client who was thought to be qualified is denied or when HCFA changes a procedure or a way of interpreting a set of criteria. Even the best organized system of tracking this internal information and the changes that occur in the regulations and interpretations is time consuming for the agency and the nurse.

If the agency receives a denial for services, it has recourse through the Medicare program to appeal denials of covered services and ask for reconsideration of the claim(s). This process is complex and beyond the scope of a beginning nurse's orientation. It will be important, however, once you are feeling comfortable with the day-to-day operations and expectations of your role in working with Medicare clients that you learn how FI requests are handled at your agency, the reconsideration and appeal process, and the process that can take the agency's appeal to the highest level, that of the federal court, where the case can be heard by an administrative law judge (ALJ).

The client will receive written notice when a denial of a home care claim for service provided to him or her has been made by the FI to the agency. Significant frustration can be felt by the agency, the home care nurse, and the client and family when this happens. Additionally, the client and family may be confused regarding whether the services provided were necessary, and they may question if the agency is knowledgeable about the Medicare program. When the home care nurse understands the criteria and the processes outlined in the preceding sections, she can explain to the client these Medicare requirements and limitations. This will enable the client to understand the cause of the denials and thereby cast a more positive light on the agency.

When this happens, the client, family, and agency can work together to appeal the denial, if necessary, and the agency then acts as a client advocate to ensure that the beneficiary is receiving the care to which he or she is entitled.

DOCUMENTATION HINTS

Documentation in the client's Medicare home care record should use language found in the HIM-11 manual under the criteria for skilled services. This holds true for documentation on HCFA Forms 485, 486, and 487 as well. Although the following guidelines are essential for Medicare clients, they also address sound clinical practice, are descriptive, and therefore can be used for all home care clients, regardless of payment source, to document clearly the skilled level of care provided.

The following documentation hints are meant to be a guide to assist the nurse in accurately documenting in the client's record what the status *actually* is. They should by no means be interpreted as a way to obtain coverage if the client is not experiencing the documented problems or instability. Documentation decisions are up to the nurse as she assesses the client from visit to visit and should be taken very seriously to substantiate the reasons the client needs home care. If the nurse is struggling to define a skill and is having difficulty in documenting the care using these hints, then the client indeed may be ready for discharge from home care.

- Use words such as:
  - –observation/assessment
  - –management/evaluation
  - –teaching/instruction
  - –performance of skilled procedures
  - –acute (rather than chronic)
  - –specific observations (rather than general weakness)
- Support the reasonable potential for complications or ineffective healing.
- Rarely use the words *stable, plateau, independence,* or *maintenance* unless these are used in the context of explaining the remaining unstable aspects of the client's condition. The word *stable* should be used only when the client is ready for discharge.
- Support the client's inability to perform a procedure (such as administer insulin) and the nonavailability of an able or willing caregiver. When there is a caregiver in the home, the documentation should indicate that the caregiver is unable or unwilling to perform specific procedures, if that is the situation.

- When the teaching constitutes reinstruction, indicate the specific changes in the client's environment and condition that necessitated modifications or reinstruction.
- Document that the skills of a nurse are required based on the inherent complexity of the service, condition of the patient, and accepted standards of practice.
- Answer these key documentation questions:
  - –Can the services be furnished safely and effectively without the skills of a nurse?
  - –Is the care consistent with the client's medical condition and accepted standards of practice?
- Document briefly the factors resulting in a high likelihood of complication or factors ensuring that essential skilled services are achieving the purpose of promoting the client's recovery and safety.
- Document the reasons that the client's condition could change and lead to a subsequent acute episode or medical complication.
- Document why skilled observation and assessment are needed to determine if treatment should be changed.
- Always document any modifications made to the treatment or any additional medical procedures initiated as a result of the nurse's assessments.
- When documenting wound care, be specific regarding:
  - –nature of drainage
  - –amount of drainage
  - –procedure performed
  - –amount and type of irrigation solution
  - –any edema, pain, or heat
  - –length and width of packing
  - –number and size of dressings applied
  - –condition of surrounding area
  - –name of any topical ointments, creams, or other medications applied
  - –measurement and description of wound dimensions and condition
- When documenting other skilled procedures, follow the same principles as in documenting for wound care. *Be specific and use details.*
- Document facts, not opinions. Be objective, not subjective.
- Use complete and accurate documentation, and reflect the care actually given at each visit.
- Be as brief and concise as possible.
- Document the true, accurate clinical findings. If the client is improving but still is unstable and needs more care, indicate that the client remains unstable and needs further care, not just that the client is improving. For example, a statement

might read, "client's wound measures 3 inches long, ½ inch wide, and 1 inch deep. Last week it was 3½ inches long, ½ inch wide, and 1¼ inches deep," instead of only recording "wound healing nicely."

- Include in each note:
  - –type of visit—routine or as needed
  - –why the visit is necessary
  - –specific observations to substantiate why the visit is necessary—remember, observation is a skill
  - –skilled care given
  - –client's response
- Relate documented care to the client's diagnosis and the care plan.
- Use quantifiable, measurable terms.
- Be technical, mathematical and scientific.
- When teaching, document client and family progress or lack of progress toward the goals.
- Elaborate on factors affecting the lack of progress.
- Evaluate progress in the context of client goals.
- Write clinical notes so they can stand alone.

DOCUMENTING HOMEBOUND STATUS

Initial and periodic documentation that the patient's functional limitations meet the Medicare homebound criteria is very important and is an area that is especially reviewed by the FI. At least monthly, documentation should indicate and reinforce that the patient is homebound. Exhibit 5–1 shows examples of patient situations indicating homebound status that can assist you in better documenting the client's actual status.

The information presented in this section will help the nurse new to home care understand the important aspects of documentation. Documentation should always reflect the progress toward established goals. Without justification of the need for skilled nursing care, reimbursement from any payer source is unlikely. It is important to remember that the nurse may be the only agency employee to see the client and that all reviewers will look at the home care record to support the medical necessity of all services provided by the agency. Remember to be clear and concise and to professionally paint a picture of the client, and your documentation will be effective.

Exhibit 5–1
TIPS FOR DOCUMENTING HOMEBOUND STATUS

- Always explain why trips outside the home are taken. The client usually leaves the home only for activities related to therapy or physician's appointments. Clients may leave the home for church, beauty shop, or barber visits with a "considerable and taxing effort."
- Specify the client's needed level of assistance when possible (e.g., moderate, maximum one person, two people).
- Specify gait devices and/or equipment, such as Hoyer lifts or wheelchairs, when possible.
- Note precautions, such as cardiac or orthopedic restrictions.
- Note pain with activities.
- Note increases in blood pressure, pulse, and swelling, as appropriate.
- Note absence of rails for stairs, uneven surfaces that must be navigated, or any other obstacle to leaving the home.
- Remember, there is no magic distance that qualifies or disqualifies the client from being considered homebound.

Source: Adapted from Carolyn J. Humphrey, *Home Care Nursing Handbook*, ed 2, Aspen Publishers, Inc., © 1994.

TEST YOURSELF

1. Identify four documentation principles that must be kept in mind when recording in a home care record.

2. Complete HCFA Form 485 for one of your first observational visits. Review it with your supervisor or the orientation coordinator.

3. Once the client's HCFA Form 485 has been signed by the physician and returned to the agency, can you write additional information on it?

4. Using the form your agency uses to document a home care aide supervisory visit and using the record of a client who currently has a home care aide, document a supervisory visit as if you were the nurse conducting it and the aide was present.

5. When you make an incorrect entry on a client's record, what should you do?

6. Mrs. Doe, an 83-year-old woman, is seen by the agency for COPD and hypertensive episodes. She lives with her son and daughter-in-law in a three-bedroom house and is able to ambulate only with assistance and the use of a walker. On your most recent visit, you noticed several bruises on Mrs. Doe's arms and legs as well as a three-pound weight loss since your previous visit, one week ago. Although Mrs. Doe denies any problems, you notice that she is left alone all day while her family works, and there is no indication there has been any food or water left for her while she is alone. What would you do?

7. The agency receives a referral on April 4 for Mr. White, who is to have physical therapy only visits after his release from a local rehabilitation center on April 5. The nurse conducts an evaluation visit to Mr. White on April 6 and finds no nursing needs. The home care aide visits Mr. White on April 7, and the physical therapist makes her first visit on April 8.

   • What is Mr. White's SOC date for Field 2 of HCFA Form 485?
   • What is the verbal SOC date and where on HCFA Form 485 do you enter that?
   • What violation of Medicare regulations occurred in Mr. White's scenario?

REFERENCES

American Nurses Association. (1985). *Code for nurses with interpretative statements.* Washington, DC: Author.

American Nurses Association. (1986). *Standards for home health nursing practice.* Kansas City, MO: Author.

American Nurses Association. (1991). *A statement on the scope of home health nursing practice.* Washington, DC: Author.

Collins v. Westlake, 57 Ill 2d 388, 312 N.E. 614 (1974).

Conditions of Participation, 42 C.F.R. § 409, 418, 484 (1991).

Crawford v. Earl Long Memorial Hospital, et al., La App 1 Cir (1983), 431 So. 2d. 70 (1983).

Frankenburg, W.K., & Dodds, J.B. (1969). *Denver developmental screening test* (DDST). Denver, CO: University of Colorado Medical Center.

Helberg, J. (1983). Documentation in child abuse. *American Journal of Nursing, 83,* 223–239.

Pisel v. Stamford Hospital, 180 Conn. 314, 430 A. 2d (1980).

Plastaras, C. (1987). Documentation of the side effects of medication. *Home Health Care Nurse, 5,* 36–38.

Scappatura v. Baptist Hospital, 120 Ariz. 204, 584 P. 2d 1195 (1978).

Utter v. United Hospital Center, 236 S.E. 2d 213 (W. Va. 1977).

Wagner v. Kaiser Foundation Hospitals, 185 Or. 81, 589 P. 2d 1106 (1979).

Quality Management in Home Care

OBJECTIVES

Upon completion of the chapter, the reader will be able to identify:

1. Essential components of an integrated quality management program
2. Aspects of a quality assessment program and the measures commonly used to evaluate each aspect
3. The significance of the inter-relationship between structure, process, and outcome
4. The role of performance improvement within a home care agency
5. Basic concepts of performance improvement
6. Roles of the board and leaders in performance improvement
7. The role of the home care nurse in performance improvment
8. Joint Commission standards relative to performance improvement

KEY CONCEPTS

- **Quality assessment/quality improvement**
- **Structure, process, outcome**
- **Performance improvement**
- **Program evaluation**
- **Joint Commission standards relative to performance improvement**

AGENCY-SPECIFIC MATERIAL NEEDED

- Agency mission or philosophy
- Agency objectives
- Organizational chart
- Staff nurse job description
- Agency's quality management program
- Outcome evaluation instrument
- Process evaluation instrument (record audit tool)
- Joint Commission's *Accreditation Manual for Home Care*, if agency is accredited

INTRODUCTION

Historically, quality was assumed in health care. The 1990s mark a new era of focused interest on health care quality and cost. Quality measurement is new to health care, whereas business and industry have employed sophisticated methods of quality control for many years. Nurses are the primary managers of care in most health care settings. It is nursing that is cited so often in consumer satisfaction surveys as the indicator of quality. The nurse must practice both the art of professional nursing; that of communication, compassion, and interpersonal skills; as well as the science, the technical skills for care delivery.

This focus on quality and the cost of care, as well as changes in payment methodology and payer attitude, has shifted the provision of care to community-based settings and away from institutions. This has resulted in the growth of home health care as a means of providing care in a more cost-effective manner. The growth of home care and the emphasis on the nursing role in home care place the home care nurse in a critical position, not only in the direct provision of care but also as an active participant in the implementation of quality programs that demonstrate excellence.

HISTORY OF TOTAL QUALITY CONTROL

Several have tried to define quality in the service area of health care. Avedis Donabedian (1966) believed almost 20 years ago that all systems include inputs, processes, and outputs but called them *structure, process,* and *outcomes.* He further defined health care systems in terms of efficiency and achieving a desired goal at minimum expense. The effectiveness links the system to outcomes with the goals of improved or maintained health.

A leader in the quality arena in the recent past is Dr. W.E. Deming, best known for his work in Japan after World War II. His work assisted many U.S. companies in improving quality. Deming proposed that there must be dedication to improvement of quality and productivity for an organization to be in a competitive position and that decreased quality means decreased productivity (Deming, 1982).

J.M. Juran, another leader in the field of quality, first recognized that product quality does not happen by accident but is a result of careful planning. Juran created the Juran trilogy, which states that there are three basic managerial processes in a successful organization. They are (1) quality planning, (2) quality control, and (3) quality improvement (Juran, 1988).

The first quality review in health care, developed by the American College of Surgeons and Dr. E.A. Codman in 1918, required peer review of hospitals and physicians. In 1980, the then-named Joint Commission on Accreditation of Hospitals (JCAH) introduced the first quality assurance standard. This standard focused only on "the problems," with each department in an institution required to perform a number of chart audits. In 1986, the JCAH agenda for change introduced the final draft of 12 key principles that characterize a quality health care organization as follows:

1. mission
2. culture
3. strategic planning and resources programs
4. organizational change
5. role of governing body, management, and clinical leadership
6. leadership qualification, development, and assessment
7. resources
8. clinical competence of practitioners
9. recruitment, development, evaluation, and retention policies and practices
10. evaluation and improvement in client care
11. organization, integration, and coordination
12. continuity and comprehensiveness of care

Historically, health providers assessed and monitored performance through quality assurance to determine if performance conformed to standards. The limitation of this traditional quality approach was that it was of a static nature and settled for a given level of performance and nothing beyond. Traditional quality assurance focused primarily on individual performance and clinical aspects and was often punitive. The quality assurance activities were delegated to a few who were responsible for monitoring quality. In 1992, the Joint Commission on the Accreditation of Healthcare Organizations (Joint Commission) changed *quality assurance* to *quality assessment,* stating that quality could not be assured, but rather assessed and improved.

This chapter gives the new home care nurse an overview of the definition of many terms used in quality assessment and methods used by most home health agencies in evaluating and improving the services they provide. Because the concept of performance improvement has recently been identified by the health care sector as the model that best addresses quality, the authors chose to focus a majority of this chapter on the application of performance improvement principles in home care. Home health agencies vary greatly in the systems and methods they use to measure quality. The information in this chapter provides basic concepts that will enable the nurse to evaluate quality in her own agency.

DEFINITION OF TERMS

Quality Management

Modern quality management is a way of looking at the process of production. First used in industry, it includes such concepts as production processes, insights into the nature of quality with both successes and failures, and methods used to plan, improve, and control quality. Although the term *quality improvement* is often used synonymously with quality management, quality management is a larger concept, dealing with the varied activities of an integrated program that includes but is not limited to quality assessment and improvement, infection control, utilization management, and risk management/safety.

What is often missing in an organization's quality management program is the integration of *all* quality management components. These areas are so dependent on each other that the whole is enhanced by integration of the component parts. In other words, if an agency's quality management program does not address all of these areas, it may be seriously lacking a view of its total quality.

Quality Assessment and Improvement (QA/I)

QA/I is the systematic monitoring process that identifies opportunities for improvement in client care delivery, designs ways to improve the service, and continues to evaluate and follow up actions taken on those opportunities for improvement. In the QA/I component of the quality management process, a home care organization improves client care by increasing the probability of positive client outcomes by assessing governance, managerial, support, and clinical processes. The approach to improving processes is coordinated and integrated with all agency functions, which requires the attention of all managers and clinical leaders of the home care organization. Most governing, managerial, clinical, and support staff are motivated and able to carry out the assessment process using this framework.

Using QA/I techniques allows the organization the opportunity to identify more frequently the factors that improve client outcomes rather than only looking at mistakes and errors that are found in the quality assurance activities. As a result of these QA/I activities, without neglecting serious deficits in knowledge or clinical skills, the home care organization's principal goal is to improve the processes in which everyone is involved.

Infection Control

A four-component infection control program is the most successful in controlling infection and is important to a comprehensive quality management program. The four critical elements of an effective program are (1) surveillance, (2) intensive control, (3) an adequately trained employee who knows infection control, and (4) a well-trained staff knowledgeable about infection control. Surveillance by objective (SBO) is recognized by the Centers for Disease Control and Prevention (CDC) as an effective means of surveillance where different surveillance systems are designed to monitor and control various types of infections.

Quality Control

Quality control is the process through which actual performance is measured, actual performance is compared with goals, and the difference between the actual measurement and the goals is acted on. Operational techniques and statistical methods are used to predict quality. Home care organizations generally perform quality control activities on clinical laboratory services, equipment provided to clients and used in providing care, and pharmacy equipment and preparations. Examples of quality control activities include performing high and low control checks on a blood glucose monitoring device or performing routine and preventive maintenance on pumps provided to clients for infusion.

Utilization Management

Basic utilization management activities include the review and assessment of the use of professional care, services, and procedures for need and appropriateness. The evaluation of need and appropriateness includes looking for patterns of underutilization as well as overutilization. Utilization management programs should employ a plan with stated program objectives and screening criteria.

Risk Management/Safety

Risk management/safety programs occupy an important place in the broad definition of management and are devoted to minimizing the adverse effects of accidental loss on an organization. These programs involve a process of planning, organizing, leading, and controlling activities of an organization to minimize the adverse effects of accidental losses on an organization at a reasonable cost.

Total Quality Management/Continuous Quality Improvement

Some organizations call their quality improvement programs *total quality management* (TQM) or *continuous quality improvement* (CQI). The choice of these terms is often based on the basic philosophy or originator of the organization's quality program. Whatever terms are used, the goal is the same: to expand traditional quality processes to include all clinical, administrative, and support functions to improve the quality of health services.

Performance Improvement

The concept of performance improvement is based on a framework for improving organizational performance. Performance improvement offers a broad look at how performance can be improved while recognizing that a home health organization does not operate in a vacuum. The external and internal issues that affect a home care organization's performance are varied. External issues that affect a home care organization's function include political, social, economic, and other societal forces that must be addressed in order for an organization to fulfill its mission. Internal issues affecting a home care organization include those important governance, management, clinical, and support activities that affect client care and outcomes. Within the performance improvement framework is a cycle for improving organizational performance.

To improve organizational performance over time, the home care staff must systematically and scientifically design, measure, evaluate, and redesign the processes that affect organizational performance. The end result is an improvement in the overall organization by improving the processes. The cycle can be carried out as part of everyday activities that involve a variety of people and roles or can be delegated to a specific improvement team that is composed of individuals who are responsible for a process, carry it out, and are affected by the outcome of that process. A home care organization's performance of important functions significantly affects client outcomes, the cost to produce those outcomes, and perceptions and judgments by its customers as to the quality and value of its services. Simply stated, performance improvement is a well-executed, systematic process of continuous improvement that includes cycles of planning, execution, and evaluation.

Measurement

Measurement is used for a multitude of purposes in home care. One purpose is to provide baseline data about a process. Measurement may use specific indicators for ongoing data collection. Once assessed, the data can identify when a process requires further investigation and analysis. A second purpose of measurement is to decide when a process requires further improvement, and a final purpose is to demonstrate the effect of an improvement action. The results of measurement are an organizationwide and organization-specific internal reference database. Measurement can occur at one point in time or be repeated over time. The data and frequency of all data collection will be determined to be appropriate to the activity or process being measured.

COMPONENTS OF QA/I

In order to measure the quality of care a client receives, three areas have traditionally been assessed: (1) structure, (2) process, and (3) outcome (Barlow, 1989). The interrelationship of these three components forms the essence of any QA/I program. Any of these elements studied individually cannot provide the evaluator and the agency with the necessary data on which to base decisions regarding the quality of care that clients receive. The three elements work together to provide a thorough measurement of the quality of services provided. This section examines the three elements of a QA/I program—structure, process, and outcome—and follow with a discussion of their interrelationships.

Structure

Structure is the setting or framework in which the nurse-client relationship exists. It is the employing agency, not the home where the actual nurse-client interaction takes place. Structure includes:

1. the philosophy or mission statement of an agency
2. agency objectives
3. the organizational structure of an agency
4. agency staffing patterns
5. employment criteria for the agency
6. available resources, such as equipment and supplies
7. agency communication patterns
8. any other organizational characteristic of the agency (Wisnom, 1989)

Mission Statement

When evaluating the structure of an agency, one must begin by evaluating the mission statement or philosophy of the agency. What are the beliefs about the clients to be served and the type of nursing care to be delivered? For example, does the philosophy suggest that ill people cared for in the home are the primary clientele served by the agency? If so, is this consistent with the types of clients actually served by the agency? If the philosophy suggests that nursing care in the home is provided from a collaborative framework, does the agency employ other professionals and paraprofessionals to facilitate this collaboration? If nurses are expected to collaborate regularly with professionals outside the agency, are there adequate time and resources (telephone, secretarial support) to accomplish this objective? Examination of structure often involves looking for a match between what is written and what actually occurs within the agency.

The Agency's Objectives

Following an examination of the mission statement or philosophy of an organization, evaluation of the agency objectives takes place. Agency objectives are statements of the goals of the agency. Often, agency philosophies are abstract in nature, including words and phrases that may not have much meaning to the clinical practitioner. Objectives are used to translate into practice the intent of the mission statement or philosophy, from which they are derived. In evaluating the agency's stated objectives, the nurse tries to determine if the objectives of the organization are reflective of the stated beliefs identified in the philosophy. For example, if the philosophy suggests that the client is an active member of the heath care team, do the objectives reflect an active role for the client in the planning and implementation of care?

Organizational Structure and Staffing Patterns

The third and fourth areas of structural evaluation are examination of the organizational structure and staffing patterns of the agency. Both of these variables have a significant impact on the type and quality of nursing care provided. As discussed in Chapter 1, the organizational structure of the agency can be identified by examining the agency's organizational chart. Line and staff relationships, as well as reporting mechanisms and supervisory relationships, can be identified. The staffing patterns and the methods used to recruit skilled employees and to assign specific responsibilities within the agency may not be readily identifiable from reading the organizational chart. It may be necessary to interview the individual responsible for hiring within the agency to determine the desired staffing pattern for the agency. In times of severe nursing shortages, the desired staffing pattern for the agency may be very different from the actual staffing pattern.

Employment Criteria

Another structural aspect that must be evaluated is the agency's employment criteria. The employment criteria of the agency should be consistent with the role requirements of the nurses in the home care setting. For example, if the philosophy suggests that one of the roles of the nurses within the agency is to develop new nursing knowledge through research, the nurses hired by that agency should have the skills, either through experience or education, to conduct or participate in clinical nursing research. Similarly, if the agency uses a case management approach, the nurses hired as case managers should possess the skills to function in that role.

Available Resources

Any resource, such as equipment or supplies, that the agency uses may be assessed as part of the structural evaluation because adequacy of resources often affects client care directly. A resource can be defined as something as simple as a policy manual. Does the agency have a policy manual and is there easy access to it by staff members? An agency that does not have enough stethoscopes for the nurses to use cannot expect nurses to take blood pressure measurements for their clients. In this situation, the quality of care the nurses can provide is directly affected by a structural aspect of an agency. Office supplies and resources are included in the evaluation of the structural aspects of an agency.

Communication Patterns

The communication patterns used throughout the agency form another structural aspect that must be assessed in a QA/I program. In large health care agencies, many organizational problems can be attributed to inadequately developed communication systems. Home care agencies often face problems with communication, not because of their size, but because their staff members are independent in their practice and infrequently see each other to communicate on issues of concern. In these situations, written communications, such as memos, policy statements, and procedure instructions, are used to ensure that all staff members concerned receive the same message. When evaluating the communication patterns within an agency, all forms of communication (e.g., memos, newsletters, announcements, and verbal communication) must be considered. Assessment of the structural aspects of an agency provides the necessary foundation for the evaluation of the next two elements involved in QA/I.

Process

Evaluation of the process aspect or dimension of the QA/I program focuses exclusively on the activities of the nurse. Process is the sequence of events and activities of nursing care. It involves the clinical performance of the nurse, including the degree of skill, the interactions between the nurse and the client, and the degree of client involvement in the care provided.

Assessment of the process dimension of QA/I involves examination of the use of the nursing process to determine if it is used appropriately in working with clients and families. Process evaluation includes review of the activities carried out by the nurse or her designee in order to help clients meet their specific health care goals. It must be remembered that the process dimension not only examines the activities of the primary care nurse, but it also examines the activities of all other professionals and paraprofessionals involved in the implementation of the interventions described in the client care plan. For example, evaluation of the process dimension in QA/I involves reviewing the activities of the home health aide to determine if the services provided were appropriate, timely, and supervised by a professional.

Record Audit

There are many ways in which the information regarding the activities and events of nursing care can be measured. The most common type of process evaluation, the nursing audit, is defined as "a method of evaluating the quality of care through the appraisal of the nursing process as it is reflected in the client care record" (Phaneuf, 1976). Audits can be retrospective or concurrent. A retrospective audit is done with records for clients who have been discharged from the agency. An evaluation of the total implementation of the nursing process can be made because the client has already received all care and has been discharged from the agency. Concurrent audits are done using charts of clients who are currently receiving care from the agency. These clients may be newly admitted to the agency or may be approaching discharge from home care services.

The chart is the central index of information of all aspects of client care and is, therefore, used for the audit. As such, charting is the most effective method of documenting and communicating all vital information. The chart becomes a reflection of the quality of care the client receives and the measure of the level of professional practice of the home care nurse. Because the chart is used to evaluate the quality of care a client receives, the importance of accurate and comprehensive documentation on the chart cannot be overemphasized.

A nursing audit is accomplished with the use of a nursing audit tool. This tool or instrument is developed by the agency and is based on the expected standards of care. When a chart is selected for review, usually at random, the nursing audit tool is used to provide the format for evaluation of all services provided. The reviewer examines what is documented in the record against the criteria detailed in the nursing audit instrument. An example of a specific criterion on a nursing audit instrument is "All nursing entries are signed." Using the nursing audit instrument, the chart is reviewed to determine if all nursing entries are signed by all the nurses who provided care to this client.

Audits may be internal or external. The internal audits are completed by other practicing nurses or supervisors employed by the agency who have not cared for the client directly. External audits are conducted by professionals with (it is hoped) home care experience, who review the records of their disciplines using the same formalized audit tool. The external audit is felt to be an objective measure of process quality.

Because the nursing audit instrument provides the format used to appraise the implementation of the nursing process with specific clients, it will be helpful for the nurse to examine the nursing audit instrument used in her agency. This will give the home care nurse an idea of the criteria used to evaluate a client record. A judgment regarding the quality of client care provided will be based only on what is written in the client care record; therefore, nursing audits reinforce the importance of accurate and complete documentation. If the record does not reflect that specific assessments, interventions, or evaluations were performed by the nurse, it will be assumed by the reviewer that they were not done. The record may indicate there were deficiencies in the care provided when, in fact, the deficiencies were in the documentation of care.

Following the review of the record using the audit instrument, the reviewer will identify the next step in the auditing process. For example, if no major deficiencies and appropriate care were found, there may be no further action taken on this record except to give positive feedback to the nurses involved. If there were minor deficiencies found in the record, the supervisor may discuss these with the specific nurse so that the nurse can improve the quality of her practice. If major deficiencies have been identified, the chart may have to be referred to a secondary review committee, which could make suggestions for policy decisions to avoid similar problems in the future. The process for determining to whom the chart will be referred following review is made by the agency and can be described by the nursing supervisor.

Supervisory Evaluation

If an agency is Medicare-certified, a quarterly review of the clinical records is required by the Medicare Conditions of Participation. The individuals performing the clinical record review should be appropriate health care professionals representing the scope of services provided by the organization within the last quarter. This review need not be performed at a joint, sit-down meeting, but rather may be completed at separate times. The clinical record review includes:

- A random selection of active and inactive cases within the last quarter that encompass the scope of services provided to determine whether established policies are followed in furnishing services directly and/or under contract. If a specific service, such as occupational therapy, was not provided in the previous quarter, that discipline need not conduct a clinical record review.
- A review to determine the extent to which the organization and its staff comply with accepted professional standards and principles that apply to professionals furnishing home care services. These include, but are not limited to, the federal Medicare Conditions of Participation; state practice acts; and commonly accepted health standards established by national organizations, boards, councils, and the organization's own policies and procedures. The professionals review the case based on a set of standards identified by the agency. Using a record review tool, the reviewer compares the standard with what is written in the record.

Nurses should not review a home care case in which they were professionally involved. The clinical record review process will be documented with the client's identification number used for recording purposes. The consolidated quarterly clinical record review results should be presented at the subsequent professional advisory board meeting and shared with all staff.

Another method of process evaluation is supervisory evaluation of staff performance. Most likely, in addition to reading the nurse's clinical records and having case conferences, the supervisor will want to make joint visits with the home care nurse to evaluate directly the nursing care being provided to clients in the home. This is a useful learning experience for the new staff nurse because the supervisor will be able to give feedback on the care provided and evaluate the nurse's charting based on that home visit. It is important that the nurse view this joint visit as an opportunity to improve her clinical practice skills. The nurse should be open to the suggestions and constructive criticism made by the supervisor. The nursing supervisor's role is to discuss different perspectives and approaches to the delivery of care to clients and not to be punitive in judgments.

The process dimension of the QA/I program, focuses on the activities of the nurse, often there is a great deal of anxiety on the part of both the evaluator of care and the nurse whose record is being evaluated. The evaluator, either from within the agency or outside, often feels anxious about identifying deficiencies on the record of a colleague or even a friend. Although it may be difficult to review a colleague's records, it must be remembered that peer evaluation is part of the role of a professional. Also, it must be remembered that a nursing audit is done for the purpose of improving the quality of care that clients receive, not for the purpose of identifying individual staff weaknesses. The process evaluation often identifies staff strengths, not just individual nurses' weaknesses.

Outcome

The third phase of a QA/I program centers on the assessment of outcomes. The outcome dimension of the QA/I model program focuses on assessing the measured change in the client's behavior as it relates to the care provided. Outcome measures examine the end results of nursing care and measure behavioral changes in the client rather than examine the process used by the nurse to effect that client change. For example, an outcome criterion might be "the client will be able to change his own dressing using appropriate technique."

In order to evaluate this criterion, the nurse would determine if the client can perform this procedure, which is the outcome of care. The evaluator would not be concerned about how the client learned the appropriate technique for the dressing change but rather would evaluate the client's ability to perform the designated procedure. In order to measure outcomes, basic criteria must be defined. These criteria are developed from the standards of care and identify behaviors that the client should achieve as a result of nursing intervention.

Outcome criteria are measurable statements that reflect the intent of a standard and relate to specific diseases that will be encountered in home care practice. For example, a standard for a client with chronic obstructive pulmonary disease (COPD) might be, "The client will remain free from exacerbation of illness." This general statement needs some measurable criteria to make it meaningful to the practitioner. Criteria for a client with COPD might include the following:

- The client's temperature will remain within normal limits.
- The client will be able to identify a low-sodium diet and plan nutritious meals within those parameters.
- The client will be able to plan his or her activities of daily living, integrating rest periods with necessary activity.
- The client's significant other will be knowledgeable regarding the prescribed care regime for the client.

The behaviors of the client with COPD at discharge would be evaluated against these identified criteria as one way to evaluate the care provided.

Some home care agencies choose not to base their outcome measures on criteria related to specific diseases but rather to identify an overall goal of client care and evaluate client outcomes based on that goal. Client classification systems have been developed to measure changes in client behaviors based on level of dependence or ability for self-management. For example, a home care agency might identify independence as the goal of client care for the agency. This would first be reflected in the philosophy or mission statement for that particular agency (structure). Nursing care would focus on those activities that foster independence in clients (process). The agency would then identify the criteria that relate to independence. Client behaviors at discharge would be evaluated against those identified criteria (outcome). Because these criteria would not relate to a specific disease, they could be used to evaluate all client outcomes, regardless of the diagnosis. Examples of "independence" criteria could include the following:

- The client will be able to perform his or her activities of daily living without assistance.
- The client will have the necessary skills and possess sufficient knowledge to manage his or her medical care regime.
- The client will identify those areas in which support is needed from others and secure that assistance.

Soliciting information from the client can also supply data for the assessment of care provided. A face-to-face interview with the client can be conducted to ask such questions as "What did you like about the nursing care you received?" or "Were there specific problems with the care you received?" This technique is not used often because, many times, the client is not the best judge of how effectively the nursing process was utilized to meet the identified health needs. As a

nonprofessional, the client is unable to evaluate the subtle aspects of professional practice that are essential parts of quality care.

In addition to face-to-face interviews, anonymous surveys and questionnaires can be sent out by the agency. Although the information obtained through surveys and questionnaires can be useful, often this method of collecting QA/I data suffers some problems with thoroughness. The clients who respond tend to be either very happy with the care provided or extremely dissatisfied. Therefore, the agency obtains only data reflective of very positive or very negative perceptions. A second problem with surveys is that clients may not be totally honest in their responses if they feel that they could be identified by their responses in some way. Even if there is little identifying information requested on the questionnaire, people may respond in a socially acceptable manner. As a result, the data obtained from clients need to be evaluated and utilized with a recognition of the problems inherent in this data collection strategy.

Interrelationship of Structure, Process, and Outcome

Once data have been collected on the structure, process, and outcome aspects of care, interpretations must be made about the quality of care provided. This is the most important element of QA/I, because it is through this evaluative process that suggestions for change and improvement are made in various areas of the agency. The strengths of the nursing staff can also be identified through this evaluative process.

It is important to remember that quality of care cannot be evaluated through the examination of only one phase of the QA/I model program. For example, by examining only the process aspect, which focuses on the activities of the nurse, the evaluator will learn valuable information regarding the implementation of the nursing process but will not be able to determine the effectiveness of those interventions on the client's behaviors. Similarly, by examining only the outcome aspect of the QA/I model, one would be able to evaluate the changes in the client's behaviors but would lack information about the nursing activities that assisted in that change (Carron, 1988).

Every nurse has experienced a situation in which a client would not modify his or her behaviors to reflect the teaching that was done. Regardless of the interventions performed with this client, the behaviors did not reflect the amount of time, energy, and expertise put into the client's care. By evaluating the outcomes only, the evaluator may suggest that the care provided was deficient. After evaluation of the process and outcome elements, the evaluator would see that the nursing process was implemented appropriately and that the client outcomes were not a result of inadequate nursing care.

In summary, QA/I has always been a concern of nurses and the nursing profession. Factors within the nursing profession, such as standards of care, and pressures from outside the profession, such as third-party payers, have combined to focus increased attention on QA/I in home care nursing. A typical method of assessing quality of care is through the examination of the structure, process, and outcomes elements of nursing practice. The interrelationship of structure, process, and outcome in the evaluation of the quality of nursing care provided cannot be overemphasized. Examination of all three aspects is essential to provide the evaluator and the agency with an accurate picture of the quality of care provided.

Process and Outcome Measurement

For each process and outcome of care and service identified, a well-defined, specific, objective problem statement that has measurable criteria should be developed. These measures will reflect processes of care (e.g., procedures or techniques or outcome of care, such as infection rates) that are reasonably expected to be related directly or indirectly to client outcomes. The measures will be related to the process of care and may include clinical criteria (e.g., clinical standards, practice guidelines, or critical pathways).

Process measures describe the behavior of the staff or client/caregiver at the desired level of performance or the actual processes used in the delivery of care.

Outcome measures describe the results of the care or services in terms of changes in the staff's or client's activities or behavior, either short term or long term. Outcome measures that relate to sentinel events may be monitored through the organization's incident reporting system.

QUALITY AND NURSING IMPLICATIONS

Quality involves the accountability of the provider delivering care to clients and measuring the quality of that care. One of two questions that must be answered when addressing QA/I is "What is being assessed?" QA/I involves the examination of nursing practice so that all clients will receive care that is equal to or better than the standard of care for clients who have like characteristics. Standards of care are comprehensive guidelines that define the ideal nursing interventions or be-

haviors to be performed in specific situations. This means simply that if the home care nurse is caring for a client with a specific illness, there are certain required interventions to be performed. For example, if the nurse is caring for a client with a myocardial infarction (MI) and the standards of care for clients with an MI include assessment of the peripheral vascular status, the client's peripheral vascular status must be assessed on each visit. Sources for the standards of care include nursing textbooks, journal articles, the American Nurses Association (ANA), and precedent established through judgments in court cases.

The second question is "To whom is the nurse accountable?" The nurse is primarily accountable to the client for the quality of care that is provided. The client has the right to expect the highest quality of care available within the constraints of applicable rules and regulations. The delivery of home care is client specific, and, as such, the client should play as active a role as possible in the delivery of that care. As the recipient of care, the client pays the greatest price for inadequate or inferior care, not only in dollars but also in risk to health.

The nurse is also accountable to the employing agency, which expects a certain degree of excellence in professional practice, and to the third-party payers, who pay for the services that are performed and who expect a professional level of treatment in exchange for the expense of a registered nurse. Since the advent of Medicare, home health agencies have been required to monitor the quality of care to clients in various ways in order to attain and maintain status as Medicare-certified agencies. Other third-party payers, such as private insurers, have also required the implementation of QA/I programs for home health agencies.

Another category of accountability is the nurse's professional peer group, which demands that high-quality care be provided. Although the home care nurse is independent in practice, peer relationships are an important element in professional growth and job satisfaction. Peers can be helpful in discussing a difficult or challenging client situation and in providing emotional support. As a member of a professional group, the nurse must also be willing to provide emotional support and professional consultation to her colleagues.

PERFORMANCE IMPROVEMENT AS THE BASIS FOR HOME CARE QUALITY ACTIVITIES

As the health care environment becomes more complicated and customers, providers, and payers demand more cost-effective and accountable services, it is important to establish a balance among cost, quality, and access. The environment in which nurses practice exerts a large amount of pressure both externally and internally on a home health agency and its employees to constantly look for new ways to provide efficient and effective home care services. When a home health agency puts emphasis on improving quality throughout the entire organization, the outcome can be an elimination of waste, a reduction in costs, and an overall improvement in productivity, employee morale, clinical outcomes, and client satisfaction. Although this sounds almost too good to be true, other businesses and industries have instituted performance improvement methods with phenomenal results.

Although instituting performance improvement principles on a daily basis is relatively new to the home care industry, home care organizations can achieve positive results, similar to those in other businesses. Home care nurses in all levels of the organization can make a positive impact by actively participating in performance improvement activities.

Because performance improvement principles are becoming prevalent in home care and the Joint Commission has identified performance improvement as a foundation in its home care standards, this section educates the new nurse on the principles and practices of performance improvement.

PRINCIPLES OF PERFORMANCE IMPROVEMENT

Home care organizations that have been successful in improving the quality of care and service, while reducing variation in processes, operate on the following basic concepts and characteristics:

1. *Client-focused quality and value.* Quality and value are key strategic components that demand constant sensitivity to emerging client desires and health care marketplace requirements. The client is the preeminent definer and judge of the quality and value of the organization's products and services. Client-focused quality and value also demand ongoing awareness of new technology and new modalities for the delivery of home care services.
2. *Leadership.* Organizational leaders work together to set the direction and provide a clear mission, expectations, and values. Leaders take part in the creation of strategies, systems, and methods for achieving excellence in client care services. Leaders serve as role models in participating and im-

proving the home care organization and its services.
3. *Management by fact.* Facts and data needed for organizational improvement can be of many types, including client, staff, administrative and business, and payer and customer satisfaction. The data collected from measurement activities are used to make operational and clinical decisions.
4. *Staff participation and development.* Improvement activities are conducted by all staff and may include participation on a performance improvement team or contributing to the development of new home care services.
5. *Continuous improvement.* A well-executed, continuous improvement process that has clear goals about what to improve is fact based and incorporates measures and/or indicators; includes cycles of planning, execution, and evaluation; and is nonjudgmental, focusing on key processes. The approach to improvement becomes part of the daily work life for the entire staff and not just something to do to meet external requirements, such as accreditation or licensure.

TRANSITION TO PERFORMANCE IMPROVEMENT

The staff nurse will in some way be involved in measuring the quality of care provided by the home care organization. The quality of services may be reviewed by measuring the processes and/or outcomes of care. The home care organization should collect data on process and outcome performance improvement activities that address all home care services provided either directly by the agency or services contracted with another organization through written agreement.

For services provided through a written agreement, the organization may obtain process measurement results by using one of two methods. The agency may collect its own data on care or service provided to its clients by the contracted organization and initiate action when opportunities for improvement are identified. The second way of collecting information is to obtain process measurement results that contractors have compiled from their own quality process. This is valid only if the contracting agency's clients are included in the sample evaluated by the contracted provider.

When the home health agency is going to provide a new home care service, change locations, or significantly modify existing functions or processes (such as installing a new computer system), effective, extensive processes should be designed. The design of process activities should be based within the context of the organization's mission, vision, and plans, as well as the needs and expectations of clients, staff, purchasers, payers, accreditors, regulators, and others. The design also should consider current knowledge about organizational and clinical activities, relevant historical data, and up-to-date resources that provide valid comparative information. A comprehensive improvement in organizational performance uses the phases of (1) design, (2) measure, (3) assess, and (4) improve.

Design

When a new process is designed within a home care organization, consideration must be given to how this new process affects the organization's mission, vision, goals, and strategic plans, as well as its effect on the needs and expectations of clients, staff, and others. Other factors to consider when designing a process are the performance of the same process by other organizations and the appropriate and applicable practice guidelines and standards.

Measure

In a performance improvement framework, measuring requires that a systematic process of collecting data that addresses both process and outcomes be used. Additionally, important issues identified by the home care organization, client and staff expectations, and quality control activities that are currently being implemented by the agency must be considered when determining what is to be measured and by what methods. Although the Joint Commission standards from the *Accreditation Manual for Home Care (AMHC)* no longer require that a specific number of indicators per category of service be measured, they do state that all of the important client-focused and organizational functions listed previously, with the exception of the improvement of the organizational performance standard, should be measured by the agency's performance improvement system (Joint Commission, 1995).

Assess

The assessment phase of the agency's performance improvement process analyzes the data collected in the measurement phase. This analysis should be conducted by using statistical control techniques to identify opportunities for improvement. Intensive assessment should also be conducted when certain undesirable events occur (such as a client who experiences an ad-

verse drug reaction), when care is given that is not covered by a physician order, or when an incident occurs that affects a client or staff member. From the analysis of this data, specific processes and/or outcomes can be identified that need improvement.

Improve

The improvement phase of the performance improvement process identifies how the process or outcome will be improved by developing a specific plan for improvement. Usually, a trial action plan is instituted with ways to measure the effectiveness of the change over time. If it is found that the trial action plan is not effective, a new trial action plan is begun until the process is improved and there is a reduction in the variation of the process.

MEASUREMENT OF ORGANIZATION PROCESSES

The home care organization should measure the performance of processes in all its functions on a continuing, systematic, and organizationwide basis. Within the functions, processes of importance should be identified and prioritized as follows:

- *High Risk.* This category includes clients who are placed at risk of serious consequences or deprived of benefit if care or service is not provided correctly, is not provided when indicated, or is provided when not indicated. These processes may include administration of infusion therapy and surveillance of infections.
- *High Volume.* These are processes that occur frequently or affect large numbers of clients. These processes may include client assessment, identification of problems and planning of care, performing invasive treatment and procedures, and education of clients and caregivers.
- *Problem Prone.* These are processes that tend to produce problems for clients or staff. These processes may include billing accuracy and timeliness and completeness of documentation by staff.

THE BOARD OF DIRECTORS' ROLE IN PERFORMANCE IMPROVEMENT

The home care organization's governing body, usually known as the board of directors, is ultimately responsible for the quality of the client care service provided by the organization; therefore, it must see that all performance improvement activities are implemented in a systematic way throughout the organization. Performance improvement activities the board of directors are responsible for include but are not limited to:

- Ensuring that adequate resources are allocated for the assessment and improvement activities of the organization's key functions by establishing process improvement initiatives that focus on monitoring and evaluation activities.
- Ensuring that someone is administratively responsible for the entire performance improvement system and allowing that person to assign certain performance improvement activities to other staff members, such as a performance improvement coordinator.
- Ensuring that all key organization management staff undertake education concerning the approaches and methods of process improvement.
- Ensuring that all staff are provided training in the approaches and methods of performance assessment and improvement. This training must be consistent with the general principles of quality management.
- Ensuring that additional training is provided on a just-in-time basis for individuals who will participate in performance improvement teams and who need additional knowledge on process measurement and the principles of statistical process control. This training may be provided by the team leader or outside resources to ensure that all team members have the same knowledge base.
- Ensuring that, as part of the annual organization evaluation, the effectiveness of the performance improvement system is assessed to determine if it has made an impact on the quality of client care.

THE LEADERS' ROLE IN PERFORMANCE IMPROVEMENT

Leaders have a crucial role in ensuring that performance improvement activities are carried out organizationwide. Leaders:

- are ultimately responsible for the quality of client care/service provided by the organization and for implementation of the performance improvement activities
- ensure that all staff undertake education concerning the approaches and methods of process improvement

- assess the effectiveness of the performance improvement system to determine if it has made an impact on the quality of client care
- ensure that adequate resources are allocated for the assessment and improvement of the organization's key functions by establishing process improvement initiatives
- assign certain performance improvement activities to other staff members, such as a performance improvement coordinator

THE STAFF NURSE'S ROLE IN PERFORMANCE IMPROVEMENT

As part of a new nurse's orientation, an overview of the home care organization's approach to performance improvement should be shared. All staff should be involved in performance improvement activities at some level, either by providing input and feedback on how the organization's current performance could be improved or by participating as a member of a performance improvement team. The staff nurse should be aware of the organization's mission, vision, and long-term strategic plans. It is through these plans that priorities are set for performance improvement. It is here that the role of home care staff nurse becomes critically important.

No one knows the client care process and outcomes better than those providing direct client care. Performance improvement teams should be initiated that include individuals from throughout the organization. It is important that the performance improvement teams be interdisciplinary, including staff from all service specialties, as well as including, if appropriate, nonclinicians, such as billing staff members. The teams should use scientific problem-solving methods throughout the organization to examine the issues and identify areas for improvement. The teams should facilitate the performance improvement process and report results to the governing body.

All staff nurses participating in performance improvement activities will be responsible for adhering to the organization's confidentiality policies. Results of performance improvement activities and reports should not contain any identifiable client or staff information and, if necessary, information should be coded or reported in aggregate numbers.

JOINT COMMISSION HOME CARE STANDARDS RELATIVE TO PERFORMANCE IMPROVEMENT

The Joint Commission will provide accreditation to home health organizations that meet or exceed the guidelines found in the *AMHC* (Joint Commission, 1995). Although the Joint Commission standards do not require that an organization adopt a specific CQI or TQM program, the standards have selectively incorporated several core concepts of these methods and philosophies. The standards also do not require that an organization adopt any particular management style or any specific type of quality management method. Additionally, although the Joint Commission requires that an organization implement a process improvement system, there is not a mandate to adhere to any specific process improvement model (such as the Joint Commission's ten-step model).

This freedom of choice in a quality management approach for home care organizations means that Joint Commission performance improvement standards are written in language that allows home care organizations flexibility and creativity in meeting the intent of the standards in a cost-effective manner. To assist in the transition to performance improvement, the aggregation rules for the improving organizational performance (IOP) standards have been made lenient so that the weighting of the IOP standards is not as stringent as it was previously, and it will be more difficult for an organization to receive a Type 1 recommendation, which is a recommendation that must be acted upon. Full compliance with the IOP standards will be phased into the survey and scoring process at a pace consistent with the home care industry's readiness.

The *AMHC* is structured into two sections, client-focused functions and organizational functions. This structure represents a shift from previous department-based standards toward functional-based standards. The *AMHC* outlines important functions that all home care providers must implement to be accredited. These 11 functions are as follows (Joint Commission, 1995):

Client-Focused Functions:

1. rights, responsibilities, and ethics
2. assessment
3. care, treatment, and services
4. education
5. continuum of care

Organizational Functions:

6. improved organizational performance
7. leadership
8. management of the environment of care
9. management of human resources
10. management of information
11. surveillance, prevention, and control of infection

These standards stress that home care agencies should use performance improvement as a framework for managing quality of the entire organization. The standards require that a planned, systematic organizationwide approach to performance improvement be collaborative among all disciplines and services.

The leadership section of the *AMHC* also has standards that relate to the role of leaders in performance improvement activities (Joint Commission, 1995). These standards require that all staff assigned managerial responsibilities participate in performance improvement activities. Leaders must also understand the approaches and methods of performance improvement and ensure that processes and activities throughout the organization are continuously and systematically assessed and improved. The responsibility for taking action on recommendations generated through performance improvement activities needs to be assigned and defined in writing. On an ongoing basis, leaders will analyze and assess the effectiveness of their contributions to improving the organization's performance. Although customer satisfaction does not need to be addressed as an indicator, it will continue to be measured and results incorporated into the planning process. In all performance improvement activities, customer needs and expectations should be an essential consideration.

PROGRAM EVALUATION

The Medicare Conditions of Participation require that a home health agency produce an annual program evaluation that provides information regarding the organization's total operations. This annual evaluation is conducted to ensure the appropriateness and quality of the services provided by the organization. Findings from an agency's annual evaluation are used to verify policy implementation, to identify problems, and to establish mechanisms to resolve identified problems or revise policies. The annual evaluation is usually completed by designated staff in conjunction with the agency's professional advisory committee. To adequately evaluate the agency's client care services, both staff and consumers may have input into the evaluation.

The annual evaluation process may be completed at different times of the year, depending on each agency's schedule, and will include but not be limited to:

- A review of the organization's overall performance improvement system, which includes:
  - objectives of the performance improvement system
  - scope of the performance improvement system

−organization of the performance improvement system
  a. appropriateness of designated authority and responsibility
  b. effectiveness of the flow of information and reporting
−adequacy of all monitoring activities
−evidence of the resolution of identified problems
- A review of various aspects of agency operations, which includes:
−organization and administration
−policies
−clinical records
−statistical and financial information
−program development and projection
−exposure control plan and infection control policies
−safety management and the emergency preparedness plan
- The minimal data to be considered in reviewing the above operational aspects, which includes:

−number of clients receiving each service offered by the agency
−number of client visits and/or hours of service
−reasons for client discharges
−statistical breakdown of client diagnoses
−sources of referrals
−number of clients not admitted and for what reason
−total staffing requirements for each service offered

CONCLUSION

The days of improving quality of client care only through clinical record review exist no longer. As home care organizations move toward improving client care and improving process and outcomes through the principles of performance improvement, the staff nurse will be able to be a participant in the process and make a significant contribution to quality client care.

TEST YOURSELF

1. Review the mission statement or philosophy of your agency to determine the types of clients served and the roles and responsibilities of the home care nurse.

2. Review the objectives of your agency to see if there is congruence between what is written in the philosophy and the stated objectives.

3. Examine the organizational chart for your agency. See if you can identify the relationships between members of the organization. For example, who is your immediate supervisor? To whom does your supervisor report? To whom does the executive director (CEO) report?

4. Review the employment criteria for your agency. Are employment criteria for specific agency positions identified?

5. Try to identify all the methods used by your agency to obtain information about the process aspects of the QA/I process.

6. Review the outcome measure instrument used by your agency. Do you feel comfortable writing outcomes based on your agency's system? How are client outcomes evaluated? And by whom?

7. What is the staff nurse's role in improving organizational performance?

8. What is the difference between quality assurance, quality assessment and improvement, quality control, and performance improvement?

9. List and describe at least four principles of performance improvement.

10. What is the board of directors' role in performance improvement?

11. Briefly describe the Joint Commission's home care standards that pertain to performance improvement.

REFERENCES

Barlow, A. (1989). Comprehensive quality assurance. *Caring, 7,* 17–19.

Carron, M.K. (1988). Comprehensive quality assurance: Inception through evaluation. *Caring, 7*(1), 17.

Deming, W.E. (1982). *Quality, productivity and competitive position.* Cambridge, MA: Massachusetts Institute of Technology Center for Advanced Engineering Study.

Donabedian, A. (1966). Evaluating the quality of medical care. *Milbank Fund Quarterly, 44,* 78–93.

Joint Commission on Accreditation of Healthcare Organizations. (1995). *Accreditation manual for home care: Volume I.* Oakbrook Terrace, IL: Author.

Juran, J.M. (1988). *Juran on planning for quality.* New York: Free Press.

Phaneuf, M. (1976). Documentation of the side effects of medications. *Home Healthcare Nurse, 5*(4), 36–38.

Wisnom, B. (1989). Quality assurance: Is your practice effective? In S. Dittman (Ed.), *Rehabilitation nursing.* St. Louis, MO: Mosby.

Client Teaching in the Home

OBJECTIVES

Upon completion of this chapter, the reader will be able to identify:

1. Types of learning that clients experience
2. Steps of the teaching-learning process
3. Sources from which data about a client can be collected
4. Characteristics of a well-written objective
5. Various teaching methods that can be used to implement the teaching plan
6. Application of teaching and learning principles to selected client populations
7. Potential problems in client teaching
8. Items necessary to document client teaching

AGENCY-SPECIFIC MATERIAL NEEDED

- Teaching aids available for use with client
- Blank client care record
- Descriptions of the demographic characteristics of the client population served by the agency
- List of literacy support programs in area

KEY CONCEPTS

- **Writing goals**
- **Approaches to client teaching**
- **Teaching the client with low literacy skills**
- **Teaching the client in poverty**
- **Documenting client teaching**

INTRODUCTION

It is widely recognized that one of the many professional roles of the nurse involves client education. In home care nursing, this responsibility is even more pressing because of the limited number of visits with the client and family and because the major responsibility for the health care of the client rests with someone other than the nurse. As a managed health care delivery system evolves in which the number of home visits is limited not by the provider of care but by the payer, the need to teach clients, assess their ability for self-care, and discharge them from service in a timely manner becomes more pressing. The primary role of the nurse case manager will be the self-care education of clients and their families. Client education is one of the components that Medicare considers a skilled service and is, therefore, reimbursable. The other covered skilled services are direct care services and observation and assessment of the client's condition. Home care nurses have identified client education as being frequently underutilized and underdocumented in practice (Jackson & Johnson, 1988). It is imperative that home care nurses gain a working knowledge of the teaching-learning process and be able to implement it with clients and families in the home setting.

The teaching-learning process, like the nursing process, can be examined in terms of the activities that occur at each step of the process. This chapter explores the teaching-learning process, in general, followed by an assessment of learner readiness. The chapter also examines teaching intervention strategies and the process for evaluating teaching strategies used, including specific examples and illustrations.

BLOOM'S THREE FORMS OF LEARNING

Many learners have sat through an inservice program or a class in nursing school and listened to a presenter for a period of time and realized when the presentation was finished that they had no idea what the instructor had been trying to teach. That experience is an important lesson about the teaching-learning process. Although the goal of all teaching is learning, very often the instructor and the student fall short of this goal. The process of giving information does not ensure that learning has taken place. Learning occurs when a person is able to do something he or she was not able to do before.

The home care nurse is involved in client education that has the potential to change some aspect of the client's behavior. The nurse can never assume that teaching alone will result in a behavior change. When making choices about their health, clients may choose to continue unhealthy behaviors, even if they have the knowledge of why they should change and have the means to do so. The three forms of learning, as described by Bloom (1969), include the cognitive, affective, and psychomotor domains. In order to understand the teaching-learning process, the three forms of learning are reviewed briefly.

Cognitive Domain

The cognitive domain deals with "recall or recognition of knowledge and the development of individual abilities and skills" (Bloom, 1969). There are six major categories in the cognitive domain, as follows:

1. Knowledge: recalling facts, methods, and procedures
2. Comprehension: combining recall and understanding to grasp the meaning of information
3. Application: using information in new, specific, or concrete situations
4. Analysis: distinguishing between parts of information and understanding the relationship between them
5. Synthesis: putting the parts of information together in a unified whole
6. Evaluation: judging the value of ideas, procedures, and methods by using the appropriate criteria (Stanhope & Lancaster, 1992)

These six categories form a hierarchy based on the degree of difficulty of the tasks at the various levels of learning. For example, a learner must know the four basic food groups (knowledge) before he or she can develop a balanced meal plan for the day (application). Similarly, a client must be able to follow a prescribed meal plan, including the four food groups (application), before he or she is able to substitute different foods on a basic exchange list (analysis).

Affective Domain

The second domain, as described by Bloom, is the affective domain. This kind of learning involves "changes in interests, attitudes, values and the development of appreciations and adequate adjustment" (Bloom, 1969). Although it is not as obvious as learning in the cognitive domain, nurses are frequently involved in the teaching-learning process in the affective domain. For example, the nurse who spends time during each visit discussing with the diabetic client the value of wearing slippers instead of going barefoot is teaching in the affective domain. The purpose of this teaching is to change the client's attitude toward going barefoot with a resultant change in behavior toward wearing slippers. Affective learning occurs at four levels, depending on the learner's knowledge and commitment. The levels are:

- *Level 1.* The learner is willing to listen and be attentive. For example, a home care nurse was working with a client, teaching the importance of diet in the client's recovery from coronary bypass surgery. On the first visit, the client was very interested in hearing what the nurse had to say and asked questions.
- *Level 2.* The learner becomes an active participant in the process. Based on the previous example, on the second visit, the nurse found that the client had completed a diet history and had a friend purchase a copy of the *American Heart Association Cookbook.* Evaluating this behavior, the nurse determined that the client had become an active participant in the learning and was not just listening passively.
- *Level 3.* The learner attaches value to the information and demonstrates a commitment by practicing the newly learned skills. On the third visit to this client, the nurse could see that the diet history showed that the client was following the diet creatively by using the new recipes and complying with the diet's restrictions.
- *Level 4.* The learner internalizes the ideas or values. This may be evidenced by extended practice of the new behavior. The client in the example would have, at this point, integrated the new behavior into his lifestyle and be found to have learned this information completely. The client not only understood the special diet but was able to suggest healthy eating strategies for others. The diet teaching goal of the nurse's care plan in this example had been reached because there was a clear change in the behavior of the client based on a change in values or attitude toward this special diet.

Psychomotor Domain

The third and final domain, as described by Bloom (1969), is the psychomotor domain. The psychomotor domain includes visible, demonstrable performance of skills that require some kind of neuromuscular function. Home care nurses are almost always involved in

this domain as they teach clients and their families. The home care nurse's sole responsibility could be to teach a family how to administer insulin to a newly diagnosed diabetic client, a goal specific to the psychomotor domain.

Three conditions must be met before psychomotor learning can take place:

1. the learner must have the necessary ability
2. the learner must have a sensory image of how to carry out the skill
3. there must be opportunity for practice (Spradley, 1990)

To illustrate these conditions, consider a situation in which a new amputee needs to learn the process of crutch walking. In order for the amputee to be able to crutch walk, he or she must have the necessary ability. This means that there must be one intact leg and a fair amount of upper body strength. This client must also have a mental picture of what crutch walking looks like and how the skill is performed. Once the client knows how to perform the skill, there must be the opportunity to practice crutch walking with the home care nurse or therapist in order for psychomotor learning to take place.

Clearly, cognitive, affective, and psychomotor forms of learning are not mutually exclusive. It is almost impossible to teach a client and family about wound care (psychomotor domain) without discussing the concepts of asepsis (cognitive domain) and influencing their values and attitudes about cleanliness (affective domain).

So, how does the home care nurse determine which domain(s) pertain to each client situation and develop the teaching plan? This can be done only by applying the concepts of assessment, planning, implementation, and evaluation to the client and family situation. For effective client teaching to occur, the home care nurse must assess the needs of the client and family in each domain and structure teaching to meet identified needs.

ASSESSMENT

Just as in the nursing process, the first step in the teaching process involves assessment. Assessment of both the learner's readiness to learn and the nurse's ability to teach is a critical component of this step of the process. The assessment phase of the teaching-learning process provides the foundation for all the steps that follow. Without adequate and accurate data from the assessment, the decisions made and the steps to follow in the remainder of the process will, most likely, be confusing and unproductive for both the nurse and the client.

Assessment of the Learner

The most significant portion of the assessment phase of the teaching-learning process involves assessment of the client's and family's readiness to learn. Many factors affect the client's readiness to learn. These factors include the client's:

- perceived needs
- interests and concerns
- educational background
- maturational level and age
- degree of motivation
- cultural, social, religious, and economic factors

For example, a client living below the poverty level might be unwilling to learn a new procedure for the care of peripheral vascular ulcers because he or she cannot afford to purchase the supplies needed to perform the procedure. The client resists the teaching of the nurse, recognizing that his or her economic situation precludes the client from implementing the teaching done by the nurse.

Assessing Motivation

Motivation is a factor that affects significantly a client's readiness to learn. The motivation of the learner is the actual desire to learn. There are two types of motivation that affect the learning process in clients. The first type, *intrinsic motivation*, is derived from values, attitudes, and the perception that there is an unmet need. A client who wants to learn about exercise in order to integrate an exercise program into his or her daily life may be operating from internal motivation. Perhaps this client has recently become aware of the value of exercise to a healthy lifestyle. Perhaps this attitude toward the client's own health has recently changed. The motivation for learning comes from within the client, not from an external source.

The second type of motivation is *extrinsic motivation*, which stems from such outside forces as family pressure, a change in health status, or environmental factors. Following the above example, if this client's desire to learn about an exercise program is the result of an employer's dictum that he or she should get in shape or be fired, this client's motivation to learn would be external. External motivation is very common in health care situations. Often, some health crisis is the impetus for a client's desire to learn. The client who suffers a myocardial infarction is often highly motivated to learn a low-fat diet in the first few weeks after the attack.

Once the impact of the crisis becomes less acute, however, the motivation also becomes less significant and the client's interest can diminish.

Motivation to learn varies with each client, and any motivation to learn is a valid one. If a client has identified a learning need, it will be helpful if the home care nurse can first identify the client's motivation for learning, because reinforcement of that motivation should be integrated into the teaching plan.

Using Data Sources

There are many sources of information that can be used to determine the client's readiness to learn. In addition to identifying the client's readiness to learn, assessment of the learner will involve the determination of the learning needs of the client. The nurse can determine what the client's learning needs are by using the same data sources used to assess the client's readiness to learn. If a client has recently been discharged from the hospital, valuable information regarding the learning needs of the client and the teaching already accomplished can be obtained from the discharge planner or the primary nurse involved with the client in the hospital.

The best source for collecting data about the client will be the client. As a result of the initial and subsequent home visits, the nurse will gather information about factors that have the potential to influence learner readiness both by talking to the client and by observing his or her behavior. Additional data can be obtained from the client's family and significant others involved.

Although the client will often identify his or her learning needs, the nurse must be able to identify existing as well as potential needs not identified by the client. Through the use of an organized approach (whether it is based on the physiological systems or on the work of a specific nursing theorist), the home care nurse is often able to identify knowledge deficits that may indicate the need for the development of a teaching plan.

Existing learning needs of clients are often evident through the assessments made on the initial home visit. For example, during the initial health assessment as part of the admission process, the home care nurse might observe that the client is obese. This would be an indication that diet teaching might need to be included in the care plan even though the client has not identified nutrition as a problem.

Potential learning needs are not always evident to the home care nurse. In order to identify potential learning needs in clients, the home care nurse must know the developmental tasks appropriate for the age of the client being seen in the home. If a home care nurse is seeing an elderly man for wound care following surgery and discovers that the client was recently widowed, potential learning needs might be identified as a result of examining the client's ability to deal with this developmental crisis. Although this would not be the primary purpose of the home visit, a teaching plan addressing this potential learning need could be integrated into the plan dealing with wound care.

Another source of data that can be useful in determining the client's readiness to learn is the client care record, including the nursing care plan and information from the other health care professionals involved in the client's care. If the client received teaching in the hospital, the professionals involved in that teaching may be instrumental in identifying the client's response to previous teaching, as well as the learning resources used.

Assessment of the Teacher

All too often in the teaching-learning process the focus is on the learner and the information to be conveyed. The characteristics of the teacher also play a crucial role in the teaching-learning process. It is important that the home care nurse assess her own teaching abilities carefully before developing a teaching plan for a client. There are four areas that the nurse should assess about herself when developing the teaching plan. These are:

1. the knowledge of the material to be taught
2. the ability to assess the cultural, economic, social, and religious factors
3. the nurse's skill in teaching
4. the potential impact of the nurse's value system on the effectiveness of the teaching

Assessing how much the home care nurse knows about the material to be taught is integral to the teaching-learning process. Clearly, if a nurse knows very little about a specific medication, the amount she can teach the client about the side effects and methods of administration of the medication will be minimal. Once the home care nurse has identified a gap in her own knowledge, she can examine the literature, consult with other professionals, or use teaching aids provided by the agency to fill in that knowledge deficit.

As previously discussed, there are many factors that influence the client's ability, readiness, and motivation to learn. Some of those factors include the client's cultural, economic, social, and religious backgrounds. Home care nurses must examine carefully their own ability to assess these factors in clients as they relate to the teaching-learning process. Considering the example of medication teaching, home care nurses must have

the skills to assess a client's ability to purchase the prescribed medications before implementing a teaching plan to foster compliance in taking the medication. A client who is financially unable to purchase the medication will be noncompliant regardless of the amount of knowledge that he or she has about the medication.

The home care nurse's skill in teaching must also be considered in the assessment phase. Some nurses come to home care with a great deal of teaching experience, whereas others are novices at using this type of intervention. The nurse's skill in teaching may influence the teaching strategies used and affect how comfortable the nurse is in implementing the teaching plan. In the preceding example, a home care nurse who is a novice at teaching might feel more comfortable with a highly structured presentation to the client on the medication, its administration, and the side effects, while an experienced teacher might informally discuss the material with the client, using a handout on the medication as a guide.

The last area of assessment of the teacher involves examining how the nurse's value system might affect the teaching to be done. As in all areas of nursing practice, the values of the nurse must be recognized as an important variable in the implementation of a teaching plan with clients. In the preceding example, the nurse might be teaching a client about a medication that is part of the client's treatment for drug abuse. If the home care nurse does not recognize her own negative feelings for drug abusers, the implementation of the teaching plan could be seriously compromised. Perhaps the client will sense the negative attitude and feel that it reflects a dislike for him or her personally. Perhaps the nurse's negativism will be evident in a lack of enthusiasm for the material being taught. The nurse's inability to assess her own values related to the teaching to be accomplished will certainly affect the teaching-learning process of the client and the nurse.

Following this self-assessment and the assessment of the learner, the home care nurse is ready to move into the second phase of the teaching-learning process, the planning phase.

PLANNING

Setting Objectives

Once the home care nurse has completed the self-assessment and the assessment of the client and family, an effective plan for teaching the client can be developed and implemented. Working with the client and family, the home care nurse needs to identify those behaviors to be acquired by the client as a result of the teaching process. These behaviors are called objectives or goals.

In addition to guiding the development of the teaching plan, learning objectives serve four other important purposes:

1. They clearly describe to the client what is expected.
2. They provide a means for evaluation.
3. They allow for coordination of various disciplines in the implementation of the teaching plan.
4. They provide a means of organizing client teaching that will facilitate efficient use of time (Jackson & Johnson, 1988).

There are two characteristics that must be considered in the development of the objectives. An objective must be *client centered* and *measurable*. Because an objective is a statement of intended outcome rather than a summary of material to be presented, objectives are always written in terms of the behaviors the client will accomplish as a result of the teaching, *never* in terms of what the teacher will do to facilitate the learning. Objectives describe the results of teaching rather than the means of achieving those results. For example, a client-centered and measurable objective would be:

> After completion of the teaching plan and the client's verbalization of content about digoxin administration, the client will record his pulse on a flow sheet every morning before taking his digoxin.

An example of a nurse-centered objective, which is of little use in evaluating the teaching, would be:

> The nurse will teach the client how to take his pulse and why the pulse should be recorded before taking digoxin.

The latter statement does not reflect the desired change in the *client's* behavior; therefore, the nurse does not have a means to measure whether the teaching was effective.

The most useful objectives are clear and succinct, leaving little room for interpretation and misunderstanding on the part of the reader. Unfortunately, there are many words used that are open to a wide range of interpretation on the part of the reader. For example, what does it mean when the nurse wants a client to know the four basic food groups? Does the nurse want the client just to be able to say that he or she knows the four food groups or does the nurse want the client to be able to identify a sample 24-hour intake, with selections from each group? Exhibit 7–1 presents a list of action words that are open to few interpretations and

Exhibit 7–1
ACTION WORDS USED TO WRITE OBJECTIVES

• To write	• To compare
• To count	• To identify
• To list	• To record
• To define	• To recite
• To administer	• To state

that can be used to write objectives. The following are some examples of objectives that are client centered and measurable:

- After completion of the teaching plan about the four food groups, the client will be able to:
  1. Identify the four food groups.
  2. List five foods that are part of each group.
  3. Plan a day's meals integrating the concept of the four food groups.
- After completion of the teaching plan on care of the abdominal wound, the client will:
  1. Wash hands before beginning the dressing procedure.
  2. Assemble all necessary equipment before beginning the procedure.
  3. Remove the old dressing using unsterile gloves.
  4. Apply the new dressing using the principles of aseptic technique.
  5. Wash hands following the dressing procedure.
  6. Accurately record the amount and type of drainage on a flowsheet.

The first set of objectives is clearly related to the cognitive domain, whereas the second set of objectives relates more closely to the psychomotor domain of learning.

Developing a Teaching Plan

Following the development of the learning objectives, the home care nurse can develop the teaching plan. The planning phase involves creating a plan for the learning experience that meets the objectives that were developed. Designing the plan includes:

1. identifying the material to be covered
2. determining the sequence of the material
3. selecting the teaching methods that will be used to deliver the specified material

This part of the plan should include a list of the tools (e.g., media, pamphlets, tapes) that can be used to enhance the presentation. A written teaching plan will allow for coordination of the teaching with the various disciplines that may be involved. Relevance of the subject matter to the client is an important factor in the learning process. Learning takes place more readily and is retained longer if the learner feels that the material is immediately useful. If the client has identified a particular learning need, the nurse is challenged with showing how the learning plan will meet that identified need. When there is little or no recognition that a learning need exists, the greater challenge of helping the client see the lack of skill or knowledge as a problem confronts the home care nurse. With this in mind, *clarifying the learning need* becomes the first step of a teaching plan. Once the learning need is clarified, the home care nurse is faced with making the subject matter relevant to the client's needs.

The home care nurse need only examine the objectives developed in the previous phase of the teaching-learning process to identify the material covered in the teaching plan. Material that helps the client achieve the identified objectives is the material that needs to be included in the teaching plan. For example, if the nurse, in consultation with the client, identified an objective involving the client's ability to identify the side effects of a particular medication, the nurse would then need to teach the client about the side effects as part of the teaching plan. Following the example about the client's ability to change an abdominal wound dressing, if the nurse wants the client to be able to remove the old dressing using an unsterile glove, the nurse needs to include information concerning:

- why it is necessary to use an unsterile glove to remove the dressing
- how to put on an unsterile glove
- how to remove the dressing
- how to discard safely the old dressing material

All this information is derived from the one objective related to the client's ability to remove the old abdominal dressing.

Teaching Methods

Making a teaching plan relevant to the client also involves planning the method(s) used to deliver the material. Among the many different teaching methods that can be used by the home care nurse, the most traditional methods used in the home are *lecture* and *discussion* between the nurse and the client and family. Most commonly, the home care nurse combines the two approaches to teaching, allowing for some time when material is presented to the client followed by a two-way exchange between the nurse and the client and family. Although it can be an excellent method of imparting information efficiently, as a single strategy the lecture is limited because it creates a passive learning environment. A discussion teaching strategy gives the learner the opportunity to ask questions, make comments, and receive feedback in order to enhance understanding. This active participation moves the learner further into the learning process.

Demonstration, another teaching method often used for teaching psychomotor skills, is most effective when accompanied by explanations of why the procedure is done in a certain way and by discussions to allow the learner to be more active. Demonstration can give the learner a clear sensory image of how a skill should be performed. When using demonstration as a teaching strategy, it is most helpful to demonstrate with the same kind of equipment the client will be using. The client should have ample opportunity to practice the skill being learned with the nurse present to correct the technique whenever necessary and provide constructive criticism and positive feedback.

Using audiovisual aids is another method of teaching. Audiovisual materials can be used in the teaching plan to enhance the material presented by the teacher. Audiovisual material includes pamphlets, booklets, films, flip charts, audio and videotapes, and demonstration models. These materials are often available through books and through local chapters of health-related agencies in the community, such as the American Red Cross, the American Heart Association, or the American Cancer Society.

Before using any audiovisual aid with a client, the home care nurse must review the material to determine its usefulness in the teaching plan and develop a working knowledge of the material in the presentation. Often, home health agencies have a library of audiovisual materials that are quickly accessible to the nurse; the home care nurse should check with her supervisor.

All written material should be reviewed with the client to determine if the client understands the information being presented in the pamphlet or brochure. It is not enough just to hand the client a brochure or booklet and expect him or her to go over it unassisted. The nurse should take a few minutes and read important areas with the client, highlighting some points by circling or underlining to be sure that the client reads at least some of the material.

Examples of educational material that can be used with a client are found in Figures 7–1 and 7–2. When using this client education material, the home care nurse will use the information as a guide for teaching. The nurse will review the entire document pointing out

Anticoagulation Information Sheet

GENERAL INFORMATION

- Take Coumadin at the same time each day.
- Report for your blood test on the scheduled date.
- Observe for any signs of bleeding.
- Avoid aspirin products and multivitamins containing vitamin K.
- Inform health care provider of any dietary changes.
- Avoid or limit alcoholic intake.
- Be safety conscious to avoid accidents and injury.

REMEMBER

Report any of the following to your physician or nurse:

- nosebleeds
- bleeding from mouth or gums
- coughing up blood
- blood in urine and/or bowel movements
- abnormal vaginal bleeding
- easy bruising
- cuts that will not stop bleeding

ABOUT ANTICOAGULATION MEDICATIONS AND ASPIRIN

You should avoid the use of aspirin and aspirin-containing products. We have listed for your convenience several common products containing aspirin.

Common Aspirin-Containing Products

Alka-Seltzer	Empirin
Anacin	Excedrin
Ascriptin	Fiorinal
Aspergum	Fizrin
Bromo-Seltzer	Midol
Bufferin	Nytol
Congespirin	Pepto-Bismol
Coricidin	Percodan
Darvon Compound	Sominex
Dristan	Vanquish

However, you should **always** read the label of **all** medications before you take them. If you see these ingredients listed—aspirin, salicylate, acetylsalicylic acid, and ASA—do not take that medicine.

Aspirin-free products, such as acetaminophen, Tylenol, and Datril, can be safely used.

If you have any questions about what is in a medication, check with your physician, nurse, or pharmacist.

Figure 7–1 Patient Education Sheet on Anticoagulation. Source: *Ambulatory Care Nursing Policies & Procedures*, Supplement 4, Leigh Emery, Suzanne P. Noone, and Lynn O'Neal, eds., Aspen Publishers, Inc., © 1992.

Giving Yourself a Subcutaneous Insulin Injection

INSULIN ADMINISTRATION*

In order to offset the effect of food on your blood glucose level, insulin should be taken about 30 minutes before a meal.

To inject insulin subcutaneously, wash your hands thoroughly and remove your prescribed insulin from the refrigerator if it's stored there.

1. Warm and mix the insulin by rolling the vial between your palms.
   CAUTION: Never shake the vial. Check the expiration date; then read the label to make sure the medication is the correct strength and type. Use an alcohol swab to cleanse the rubber stopper on top of the vial.
2. Before drawing up the insulin, inject an equal amount of air into the vial. With the bottle right-side up, push the needle into the center of the rubber cap of the insulin bottle.
3. Push the plunger down so that all the air in the syringe is transferred into the bottle.
4. Turn the bottle upside-down with the needle still in it; slowly pull the plunger back to two or three units more than your dose and allow the insulin to flow into the syringe.
5. Flick your finger against the syringe lightly to remove any air bubbles.
6. Push the plunger to your exact dose; this will force any air bubbles out through the needle.
7. Remove the needle from the bottle carefully.
8. Put the syringe down, making sure the needle does not touch anything.
9. Select an injection site. Use the fatty tissue of your upper arms, abdomen, thighs, or buttocks. It is necessary to rotate your injection sites, leaving at least an inch between injections. Repeated use of one injection site can cause the tissue to become fibrous. Fibrous tissues absorb insulin poorly. Raised, toughened areas or deep skin indentations indicate overuse of an injection site.
10. Wipe the site with an alcohol swab.
11. Pinch the skin with one hand, or stretch the skin taut. Either is acceptable.
12. With your other hand, grasp the syringe on the barrel (like holding a pencil). Plunge the needle into the skin, straight down (90-degree angle), up to its hub.
13. Release the injection site and grasp the plunger, slowing pulling back to see if any blood appears. (If this does happen, discard everything and start again. The newer needles are so short that there is little likelihood of reaching a blood vessel.)
14. Inject the insulin by pushing on the plunger.
15. Pull the needle out of the skin, then apply pressure over the injection site with an alcohol swab.

*Courtesy of Hospital Home Health Care Agency of California, Torrance, California.

continues

Figure 7–2 Patient Education Sheet on Subcutaneous Insulin Injection

Figure 7–2 continued

Many people reuse their disposable syringes and needles without any problem. If you do reuse a disposable, recap the needle immediately after use. The needle will become dull after about two injections.

Dispose of used needles and syringes carefully to prevent accidents to others. The following tips are also important:

- Destroy your used needles and syringes in a manner which makes each unit unfit for reuse in any way.
- Be cautious: Conceal the discarded needles and syringes in a well-sealed, impervious, opaque container.

INJECTION SITES**

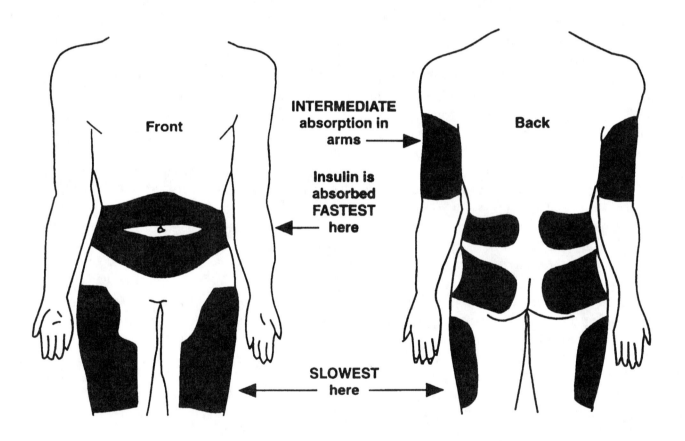

**Courtesy of Medical Center Hospital of Vermont, Burlington, Vermont.

specific points that are particularly relevant to that client. For example, on Figure 7–1, the nurse may highlight specific aspirin-containing products that the client took prior to beginning anticoagulant therapy. After this document is used as a teaching guide, it can be left in the client's home. The client and significant other can review the material as needed or consult it if they have a particular question.

Printed educational materials are particularly helpful when they include pictures or diagrams that enhance the verbal instructions of the home care nurse. Figure 7–2 shows exactly where the client can administer insulin. The client can consult this diagram if there is a question about insulin administration sites.

It is important to remember that the use of audiovisual aids is also dependent upon the client's ability to see, read, or hear. The inability to read may not be readily apparent to the home care nurse but must be assessed before using any written material as part of the teaching plan. In the course of reviewing written materials with clients, the nurse often can determine that the client is having difficulty reading. If the nurse thinks that the client would not be offended by the question, she may ask the client candidly if he or she is having difficulty reading the specified information. If the nurse decides that the client might be offended by the question, the nurse may ask him or her to relate in the client's own words, what the document says. If the client cannot perform this task, the nurse can, in a nonjudgmental way, substitute another teaching strategy for the one that involves reading. If may be that the client is unable to read or understand the contents of the document or perhaps the print in the document is too small for the client to see clearly. Any or all of these factors can affect the client's use of a teaching aid in the learning process. Whatever the cause of the difficulty, the nurse should substitute another teaching strategy for this client and document the assessment in the progress notes and on the client care plan.

In summary, when developing the teaching plan, it is important to remember that learning experiences should provide for the maximum involvement of the client and family. Learning will be enhanced with the active participation of the client in the teaching-learning process. Research has shown that an individual remembers 10 percent of what is read, 20 percent of what is heard, 30 percent of what is seen, 50 percent of what is heard and seen, 80 percent of what one says, and 90 percent of what one says and does (Patterson, 1962). As this research shows, the more of the client's senses that are involved in the learning process, the more likely it is that learning will occur.

IMPLEMENTATION

Implementation of the teaching plan is carried out just like other nursing interventions. Following the first step, assessment of the learner and the teacher, and the second, development of objectives and a teaching plan, the home care nurse should be prepared to implement the teaching plan with the client and the family. The home care nurse must consider certain factors in the implementation phase of the teaching plan. One of the first considerations is to find an environment conducive to learning in which to carry out the teaching plan. In collaboration with the client and family, the home care nurse must select a noise-free setting that contains the equipment necessary to perform the teaching. Unrelated sound or movement from television or other family members in the home will inhibit the learning process by distracting the teacher or learner or both. If learners say the television does not bother them, the nurse can say that it bothers her and that she would prefer it if it were turned off. In this way, the nurse has made the most positive environment possible without making the client feel uncomfortable.

It may be helpful for the home care nurse to ask the client where they could go in the home to do the teaching so that they would not be distracted by household noise. If access to a sink is important to the nurse's teaching plan, she should let the client know that the teaching needs to take place either in the kitchen or near the bathroom. Because the setting influences all the teaching that takes place, it must be chosen very carefully and be consistent from visit to visit.

In implementing the teaching plan, certain strategies make the teaching process smoother and facilitate learning on the part of the client. These strategies include:

- Approaching the teaching situation with confidence and enthusiasm. This gives the client the message that the nurse has the knowledge to teach something and that what the nurse has to teach is important.
- Taking time in the presentation and allowing for questions, repetition, and reinforcement as needed.
- Providing lots of positive feedback (praise) to the learner throughout the presentation. Rewards are sometimes helpful, although they should be used in limited situations. An example of a reward sometimes used by home care nurses is spending extra time with a client, either taking him or her for a

walk or engaging in some other activity that is out of the ordinary for this client.

- Allowing the client to practice the new skill or use the new information without delay. Learning is reinforced through application.
- Avoiding the use of medical jargon in the teaching process. The use of technical terms can be overwhelming to the client. Try to talk in plain language, repeating if necessary.
- Being sensitive to the client's cues during the teaching process. The nurse might have planned to teach about the diabetic diet and foot care during one home visit, but the client seemed exhausted after just learning about the diet. In this situation, the nurse would modify the timetable for teaching based on the client's ability to learn. Little learning will take place when the client is tired.
- Requesting client input throughout the teaching program, asking the client to share what he or she knows about the subject and how it relates to his or her lifestyle and current family situation.
- Summarizing teaching frequently, especially just before ending the teaching session.
- Letting the learner know the progress that was made based on the identified objectives.
- Planning for any subsequent teaching sessions that will be needed.

Remember, a good teacher uses this outline:

- Tell them what you are going to tell them (introduction).
- Tell them (implementation of the plan).
- Tell them what you told them (summary of points covered).

The preceding list covers some suggestions that will help the home care nurse develop the art of client teaching. Because teaching is an art, creativity in one's approach to the teaching process enhances teaching effectiveness. For example, a home care nurse may need to motivate a cardiac client to reduce his or her intake of sodium. One approach would be to tell the client that he or she has too much sodium in the diet and suggest that he or she implement a low-sodium diet. A second, more creative approach would be to take a diet history and show the client, using table salt, how much sodium he or she consumes in a day from all the foods he or she eats. The second approach is bound to have a greater impact on the client and result in a more motivated learner. Teaching and learning are facilitated through the use of creative approaches.

CLIENTS WITH SPECIAL LEARNING NEEDS

In working with clients in the community, the home care nurse often sees those clients with special learning needs, such as low literacy skills, fatigue that affects the ability to learn, or low motivation. In addition, physiological, psychosocial, economic, and educational factors may provide unique challenges to the development of a meaningful and realistic teaching plan. Adult learners, clients with low literacy skills, and clients who live in poverty are three populations whose specific characteristics influence the teaching-learning process. Specific approaches to these groups are discussed in this section.

The Adult Learner

Home care nurses see clients of all ages in the home, but most of their clients and the agency's caseload will be over 65 years of age. This population has unique characteristics and needs relating to the teaching-learning process. With an understanding of the adult learner, the home care nurse can design and implement a teaching plan that will meet the learning needs of the client.

The teaching of adults is a field of its own called *andragogy*. The theory of teaching adults is based on four assumptions that differ from the process of teaching children. These assumptions suggest that as people grow older:

1. Their concept of self shifts from one of dependency to one of self-direction.
2. They possess a wealth of experience that can be drawn upon in situations.
3. Developmental milestones become an impetus for learning.
4. Orientation to learning shifts from future to present and from subject to problem (Knowles, 1980).

These four assumptions form the basis for the examination of life. The teachable moment for an adult is when the material and skills to be taught are consistent with the developmental tasks of the adult at that point in his or her life (Stanhope & Lancaster, 1992). The final characteristic of the adult learner, and the one that affects the teaching plan most directly, is that adults pursue learning for mostly pragmatic reasons. They want to learn in order to be able to do something better or do something they could not do before this time. They may also want to gain information in order to make a decision. The major emphasis of the adult learner is definitely on practical, applied knowledge and skills. The teaching plan must be designed to meet those practical needs of the client. For example, in teaching clients about a diabetic diet, adult learners will be more interested in and retain more information about the food that should be included in their diets and how that relates to their lifestyle than about the chemical composition of the carbohydrates and fats. Taking into account their unique characteristics, adult learners are just as capable of learning new skills and acquiring knowledge as any other learner. The home care nurse must remember that the degree of illness will play a role in the learning ability of all clients, not only adult learners. Such factors as degree of pain or fear influence a client's ability and willingness to learn. A client preoccupied with pain is not likely to be able to focus his or her attention on what the nurse is trying to teach. Similarly, a client with a new colostomy must get over the fear of looking at his or her stoma before the nurse can teach him or her to change the colostomy bag.

Considering the physiological needs of the client, the home care nurse can design a meaningful and rewarding learning experience for the adult learner. In developing the learning experience, the nurse must assess the previous learning experiences of the adult client. The nurse can use the same methods to assess the previous knowledge and skills of the adult learner that she would use to assess any other client. These assessment strategies are discussed in the previous section, Assessment.

The Client with Low Literacy Skills

Twenty-three million American adults may not be able to comprehend what a health professional is trying to tell them. These are adults who are either illiterate (cannot read or write) or functionally illiterate (they do not have the literacy skills needed to function effectively in today's society). One out of every five American adults is considered functionally illiterate and generally has a reading skill below the fifth-grade level. Given the huge numbers of people with low literacy skills, the home care nurse can expect to be providing care to many of these clients in her practice (Doak, Doak, & Root, 1985). It is important to make the distinction that a lack of comprehension skills or an inability to read does not reflect the client's intelligence or the ability to learn (Peragallo-Dittko, 1994). Clients with low literacy skills have often mastered unique ways of learning without having to read the written word.

Because one of the primary roles of the home care nurse is client education, the client with low literacy skills provides some unique challenges. For clients whose reading, writing, listening, and speaking skills are not well developed, traditional methods of client education may not be appropriate. Research has shown that much of the material published for use by health professionals in client education requires at least an eighth-grade reading level. Poor readers and people who do not read at all usually do not ask questions to obtain information. They may not have the skills necessary to develop the question, or they may feel embarrassed by a poor vocabulary. Most people with low literacy skills will cope with new situations by agreeing to whatever is asked of them. For example, when asked, "do you understand?" they may reply "yes" even if they do not understand. This will prevent them from having to explain what they didn't understand. These clients also may not have well-developed problem-solving skills and may have difficulty in classifying information into categories. For example, the client with low literacy skills might have difficulty developing a system for taking several different medications during the day (Hussey & Gilliland, 1989).

Home care nurses need to be aware of three factors that contribute to reading difficulty. These factors are:

1. frequent use of polysyllabic words
2. the use of technical terminology
3. the use of complex sentence structures (Peragallo-Dittko, 1994)

As nursing professionals, it is easy to get caught up in teaching clients by using language that is complicated and difficult for a nonprofessional to understand. For the client with low literacy skills, the language needs to be simple and clear and the sentences need to include only one subject. An example of a complex sentence with polysyllabic words might be, "The sodium in your diet has an effect on your heart and your ability to breathe effectively." Instead, you might want to say, "The salt that you eat makes your heart have to work too hard. The salt also makes water get into your lungs so you have trouble breathing."

When teaching clients with low literacy skills, the nurse may need to make changes in the material and the process of the teaching plan in order to help the client achieve the identified objectives. Assessment of the client's literacy skills is the first step in determining the teaching plan to follow. Imagine the frustration on the part of the home care nurse following a teaching plan that was based solely on written pamphlets and instructions when she finds out that the client was unable to read what was left as a teaching aid. The home care nurse's frustration is rivaled only by the frustration and embarrassment felt by the client.

Determination of the client's literacy skills can be done very informally be reviewing written material with the client. Through subtle questioning about the content of written material, the nurse can determine the client's ability to comprehend the written word. Clients become expert at creating defense mechanisms or manipulating the situation to avoid reading or writing. Some responses from the client that reading or writing is problematic for the client may be "I forgot my glasses at home," "I want my husband/wife/significant other to read this first," or "Would you read it for me? My eyes are tired."

Asking the client to describe the written material, in the client's own words, is helpful in determining if the client is having difficulty reading or understanding the material in the document used as a teaching aid. If the home care nurse has a question regarding the client's skill in reading, a direct question may be indicated. Most clients respond positively to an honest, caring approach and may even be relieved to share this information so that they can feel more comfortable throughout the learning process. If the client is unable to read, part of the intervention might be a referral to a program that could remedy this problem.

The three strategies identified as central to teaching clients with low literacy skills emphasize client participation and assisting clients in the problem-solving process. They are:

1. Teach the smallest amount necessary to reach the objective.
2. Make your point as vividly as possible.
3. Provide for repeated reviews.

The first strategy involves *teaching the smallest amount necessary to reach the stated objectives*. Most clients want to learn just enough to allow them to perform the necessary skills. Knowledge for the sake of knowledge is not important to clients with low literacy skills and should be omitted from the teaching plan. Once the nurse has identified the material to be included in the teaching program, it should be reexamined for order and amount of information contained. It may be helpful to teach the skill first, when the client is fully attentive and then go back to provide some information about the skill later in the visit. For example, when teaching wound care, it would be helpful to teach the skill at the beginning of the visit when the client's attention is at its peak and then teach aseptic principles after that.

The second strategy of teaching clients with low literacy skills is *making the points as vividly as possible*. The home care nurse can improve vividness by:

- making the sentences short and precise
- illustrating the spoken word with drawings and examples
- organizing the material with headings and groupings
- organizing the material as a list rather than in narrative form
- summarizing important points

For example, it is much clearer to say, "Change your foot dressing every day," than "The foot dressing needs to be changed every day." It is often helpful to link new information with old to facilitate recall of material. If a new skill can be shown to be similar to a skill the client already can perform satisfactorily, learning is enhanced. For example, in demonstrating a wound dressing, the use of a bulb syringe could be likened to the use of an eyedropper or even a turkey baster.

The third strategy used in teaching clients with low literacy skills involves *providing for repeated reviews*. As for all clients, periodic reviews allow for the determination of whether information has been retained or whether misunderstandings have developed throughout the teaching process. Pictures that the client can review independently can be helpful in reinforcing material between visits. There may be a family member or significant other willing to reinforce the teaching if he or she is included in the initial teaching with the client. In addition to reinforcing the material learned, continued reinforcement provides opportunities for continued rewards. Encouraging words are essential in facilitating the learning process.

Teaching strategies may need to be altered with this population of clients. Demonstration and psychomotor practice should replace written information. Diaries and records, which are often used to evaluate adherence to the recommended care regime, may be too difficult for the client with low literacy skills to maintain. If a client has difficulty processing sequence information, a calendar may have little meaning and, therefore, will not be useful as an evaluation strategy. The client with low literacy skills will benefit from restating or demonstrating the learned material frequently to either the nurse or a family member. The client should be asked to describe what has just been learned, in his or her own words, or demonstrate the skill just acquired. Comprehension occurs when a client can restate what has been learned in his or her own words. Frequent repetition of the learned material or demonstration by both the home care nurse and the client improves the client's ability to recall the new material. The more that clients can rehearse and see themselves in real-life situations, the greater the chances for long-term memory.

Because of the magnitude of the literacy problem in the United States, the home care nurse can expect to see many clients with low literacy skills in practice. Although this population presents some challenges to client education, the modification of traditional teaching strategies will result in a more positive teaching-learning episode. These modifications will yield tremendous benefits in the area of client comprehension and, therefore, will increase the possibility of adherence to a recommended care regime on the part of the client.

The Client in Poverty

Low-income families are seen frequently by the home care nurse in practice. Many factors combine to put the low-income client at risk for numerous health problems. These factors, such as overcrowded living conditions, limited education, and difficulty in using available resources, make problems seem overwhelming for the family and the home care nurse alike. Poverty, a relative term, reflects a judgment made on the basis of standards prevailing in the community. For the purpose of this discussion, the client to be addressed is one who lives in a chronic state of poverty that spans many generations and is an accepted way of life. Because of limited education, this client is often unable to find meaningful or regular work. Feelings of low self-esteem are reinforced by the inability to maintain regular employment.

Clients who live in a chronic state of poverty often have four distinctive life themes that tend to characterize their behaviors. These life themes are (1) fatalism, (2) orientation to the present, (3) authoritarianism, and (4) concreteness (Aleman, 1982). These four life themes combine to make teaching clients in poverty a challenge for the home care nurse. All these life themes affect the material and method of teaching to be used by the home care nurse. Consideration of these life themes is essential to making the teaching process meaningful for the client living in a chronic state of poverty. However, with some extra planning and an innovative approach to interventions, teaching can be effective and rewarding.

Fatalism

This results from a strong feeling of powerlessness. Often, clients have many external forces, such as their caseworker, the food stamp program, or the welfare office, controlling their lives. Because they often feel at the mercy of these external forces, they lose all motivation to learn. Recognizing that motivation is a critical element in the teaching-learning process, the home care nurse must help the client find either an internal or external motivation for learning.

Orientation to Present

The second life theme, orientation to the present, is seen as a result of the client having to spend a great deal of time obtaining such basic needs as food, housing, and fuel. After these tasks are accomplished, little time or energy remains for planning for the future. Because the availability of resources to meet basic needs is not assured, the client becomes preoccupied with the present, unable to plan ahead or delay gratification. For the home care nurse trying to teach this client, the existence of this characteristic provides unique challenges. The benefits of a behavior change that will improve long-term health status are not likely to be valued by the client with an orientation to the present. Furthermore, the client occupied with meeting basic needs may not be interested in the teachings of the home care nurse. Recognition of this life theme is essential in planning the teaching-learning process with low-income clients.

Authoritarianism

This is the third life theme often seen in clients in poverty. Decision making in these families is often situational and based on authority. The person in charge makes the decisions for others. The home care nurse must identify the person in charge and, once identified, enlist that individual's support and assistance. The home care nurse can increase her credibility and effectiveness with these clients by establishing a liaison with the influential people in the client's community, therefore being seen as an authority to the client.

Concreteness

This is the final life theme often seen in clients in poverty. In these clients, life is seen to be very concrete and activity oriented. Action is valued; emotions are expressed in visible, tangible ways. Listening tends not to be a reinforced skill. Everyone may talk at once, trying to be the loudest to get the desired attention. This life theme has direct implications for the teaching-learning process. The home care nurse can best meet the learning needs of clients through an action-oriented teaching plan, with little emphasis on learning through listening. Perhaps demonstration could replace oral instructions for these clients to meet most effectively the specified learning need. These clients should be actively, tangibly involved in each step of the teaching-learning process.

EVALUATION

Just as it is in the nursing process, evaluation is the final step in the teaching-learning process. Although this step is critical to determining the success of the teaching, it is often forgotten or ignored. There are two areas that can be addressed in evaluation of the teaching-learning process: (1) evaluation of the teaching effectiveness and (2) evaluation of the teacher performance.

Evaluation of Teaching Effectiveness—Evaluating the Learner

Evaluation of the teaching effectiveness can be done by examination of the objectives that were developed at the beginning of the process. The objectives are statements of the anticipated client behaviors that should be present at the conclusion of the teaching. As the home care nurse examines the identified objectives, a determination of whether the client met the objectives can be made. Determination of what the client learned can be made by return demonstrations, written tests, documentation of the client's behaviors in progress notes, and examination of self-reported information, such as diaries and logs. Although all these methods are useful, the most frequent evaluative measure used by the home care nurse is oral questioning of the client. The home care nurse will often say "Tell me what you had for breakfast this morning and lunch and supper yesterday" to determine the effectiveness of the diet teaching that was performed. If the client has met the objective, the teaching plan can be considered successful.

If the objectives were not accomplished, there are four areas to examine to determine why the stated objectives were not met.

1. Perhaps the objectives were unrealistic or too complex for the client to meet in the time available.
2. If it is impossible to determine if the learner has met the objectives, the learning objectives may not be client centered or measurable.
3. The teaching strategy may not have been appropriate for the learning objectives. For example, if an objective called for the client to learn a new skill and the teaching method was exclusively the lecture, the teaching strategy was not appropriate for the learning objective.

4. Perhaps the learner was not motivated to learn what was included in the teaching plan. This points to the need for inclusion of the learner at each step of the process, including the development of the objectives. The home care nurse should also determine if the instructional aids were useful and suitable. If it was determined that the teaching was unsuccessful or incomplete for any reason, the entire process begins again, starting with assessment.

Evaluation of Teacher Performance

Evaluation of the performance of the teacher is important for both the client and the professional development of the home care nurse. The home care nurse may simply want to ask the client for feedback on her effectiveness as a teacher. Peers and supervisors may be asked to review the teaching plan on the client record to provide insight on the home care nurse's strengths and weaknesses as a teacher. If an in-depth evaluation is needed, a supervisor or peer can make a joint visit with the home care nurse to assess the teaching more thoroughly. Most likely, most information about the effectiveness of the teacher will be obtained through self-evaluation on the part of the home care nurse. Following implementation of the teaching plan, the home care nurse may reflect on her familiarity with the subject taught and the degrees of confidence, openness, and mutual respect that were displayed to the client. All these factors will have an impact on the degree of success of the teaching-learning process for both the client and the home care nurse. The evaluation phase may end the nurse-client relationship, or it may lead to the identification of further problems to be addressed. It can never be assumed that because teaching was done, learning has taken place. Evaluation must be done as the final phase of the teaching-learning process.

Potential Problems in Teaching

Client teaching, like other areas of nursing practice, does not always go as smoothly as the home care nurse would hope. There are often unforeseen circumstances that affect the client's receptivity to the teaching plan or affect the nurse's ability to effectively deliver the anticipated intervention. The nurse can learn from mistakes. Difficulty in teaching may be encountered at any point in the teaching-learning process; common potential problem areas are identified and strategies to deal with these problems are discussed in this section. The common problems in the teaching-learning process are:

- failure to negotiate goals
- client overload
- poor timing of client teaching
- poor use of audiovisual aids
- failure to validate all areas of client information

Failure to negotiate goals can lead to the nurse and client working toward different and often conflicting ends. Goals are established by mutual agreement between the client and the nurse and are a dynamic part of the teaching-learning process; that is, they need to change as the client situation changes. Periodic renegotiation of goals between the client and the home care nurse is essential.

The specific characteristics of the client are important in the teaching-learning process. It must be remembered that the nurse is sometimes teaching a client with a reduced attention span and endurance resulting from some past or present illness. Sometimes the client will be in pain or distracted by fatigue or anxiety. *Client overload* will result from presenting too much material in too short a time. If possible, shorter sessions occurring more frequently will help to avoid this problem.

Sequencing of the activities in the visit must also be considered. Often difficulties that relate to the *poor timing of client teaching* arise in the teaching process. For example, if a home visit involved a complicated wound dressing and a teaching session, it might be better to perform the teaching first, before the client becomes distracted with the wound care.

Audiovisual aids can be an asset to the home care nurse in the planning and delivery of client education. *Poor use of audiovisual aids* does little to facilitate learning and may even impede the learning process. The home care nurse must always review the material before using it with a client. Important points in the media should be stressed or highlighted for the client. Never rely solely on an audiovisual aid to perform the teaching. Aids should be used to supplement or enhance the presentation, not as a substitute for teaching.

Failure to validate all areas of client information is the final potential problem area to be discussed. When the nurse makes assumptions about a client's motivation, previous knowledge, or level of understanding about the client's illness, the nurse will be basing important decisions on information that may be false. This can lead to an inefficient use of the nurse's time and a frustrating learning experience for the client. The best way to find out what the client knows about his or her illness is to ask. In every step of the teaching-learning process—assessment, planning, intervention, and evaluation—the nurse must validate all information

about the client with the client. In this way, the nurse can be sure that her decision is based on accurate information.

Although not an exhaustive list, these few potential problem areas are seen frequently in the home care setting. The home care nurse should consider these areas when devising and implementing a teaching plan for a client.

Client Compliance

Webster's New Collegiate Dictionary defines compliance as "the act or process of complying to a desire, demand or proposal or to coercion." As professionals, home care nurses hardly want to think of their role as involving coercion. Although nurses want their clients to adhere to their recommended care regimes, that adherence, ideally, should come as a result of an understanding by the client that certain behaviors are more beneficial to his or her health status than others. As a result of a therapeutic relationship in which health teaching is conducted, the client should gain the necessary knowledge and skills to make wise choices about his or her health based on the developed care regime.

Variables That Affect Compliance

Client compliance is a complex behavior that is affected by many variables. A key factor in achieving client compliance is the *nurse's relationship with the client*, including a respect for the client's values, individuality, and autonomy. The client must be viewed as a partner in the teaching process rather than as a passive recipient of information (Leff, 1986). Compliance increases if the client and nurse share their concerns and goals for care.

A second factor that influences compliance is a *clear understanding by the client of the relationship between the prescribed care regime and the prevention or treatment of illness*. Once that relationship has been established, the nurse is often charged with helping the client to see the importance of the desired change in relation to the client's short- or long-term health status. This is a necessary and often difficult step on the road to compliance, especially when the changes involve behaviors that have been long standing.

Strategies To Increase Compliance

Contracts between the nurse and the client may be helpful in this process because the client can clearly identify the desired behaviors. There is not a clear relationship between knowledge and compliance. In other words, there is no assurance that a client will comply with a prescribed diet just because he or she has the necessary information to plan a healthy meal appropriately. Recognizing this limitation, certain techniques or strategies can be used to increase compliance. These strategies include:

- *Simplify the care regime.* The home care nurse should always begin with the simplest activities and build to more complex actions. Also, any activities included to reduce the overall complexity of the client situation will enhance compliance.
- *Allow change to occur slowly.* Compliance will be improved if the client is allowed to make changes in his or her life slowly. This allows the client to adapt his or her lifestyle to the prescribed change without major disruption.
- *Enlist family support.* A client's likelihood of compliance is increased if the family is supportive of the change. Family support is often necessary because a behavior change in the client may affect the family members.
- *Increase client supervision.* Increased supervision of clients can be accomplished by scheduling more frequent home visits for follow up and practice of the skills or by enlisting the caregivers' help in working more closely with the clients. Increasing the frequency of home visits must always be done with consideration for the reimbursement potential for the visit.

Recognizing that client compliance is not always associated with increased education, the home care nurse must consider the preceding strategies in order to enhance the potential for compliance. It must be stressed that the first and most significant variable in promoting compliance is a *therapeutic relationship between a nurse and client* in which the client plays an active role in the decision making and the goal setting with regard to the plan of care.

DOCUMENTATION

Following the implementation and evaluation of the teaching plan, the home care nurse must carefully and thoroughly document each stage of the teaching plan. The need for documentation of client teaching for the purpose of continuity of care and as part of the nurse's responsibility as a health care professional is readily apparent. Assessment of the client's knowledge deficit and documentation of client teaching are both crucial elements in determining the reimbursement of the

home visit through third-party payers, such as Medicare. Documentation of a carefully outlined teaching plan, description of the teaching to be done, and the client's and family's responses to that teaching is necessary to demonstrate that the teaching that was done was indeed reimbursable. In attempting to help clients reach the goal of independence, client education is one of the most frequent interventions used by home care nurses. Although used often as part of the care plan, client education is frequently undocumented or underdocumented by the practitioner.

It is suggested that teaching is probably one of the most underdocumented skilled services because most nurses in home care do not recognize the scope and depth of the teaching they do. The teaching is often done in an informal, conversational, and sometimes reactive manner. Nurses tend to view much of their teaching as commonsense suggestions. Yet, such suggestions are based on the nurse's professional education and experience (Omdahl, 1987).

In order to document effectively the process of client teaching, the home care nurse must first know what constitutes a skilled teaching visit. Under the Medicare program, specific criteria have been established that determine whether a teaching visit is reimbursable. In general, home health benefits under Medicare are reimbursable for intermittent skilled services for a client in the acute or subacute phases of an illness. Chronic care, even when it is skilled, is not considered reimbursable by Medicare. Given this general criterion, three factors can be used to determine if teaching visits are reimbursable under the Medicare program:

1. examination of the person who conducted the teaching
2. the teaching is reasonable and necessary
3. the teaching is new and related to the client's condition

The first criterion used by Medicare to determine if the teaching visit is reimbursable is an *examination of the person who conducted the teaching.* Skilled care, which requires professional health training, is performed by registered nurses (RNs) or licensed nurses (LPNs or LVNs) and physical or speech therapists (PTs, STs). Teaching that requires the expertise of one of these health care professionals is considered reimbursable under the Medicare program. When the nature of the service is such that it can be performed adequately by a person without professional training, that service is not reimbursable regardless of who performs it. For example, if the home care nurse taught a client about a diabetic diet, that teaching would be reimbursable because it required the professional training of the nurse to accomplish. On the other hand, if the professional nurse told a client with edema to elevate his or her feet, that would not be considered skilled care because most nonmedical people have enough knowledge to do this in the event of swelling (Jackson & Johnson, 1988). It also must be remembered that the teaching of a skill to a client or family member, as well as the performance of that skill, may be considered reimbursable. When a home care nurse teaches a family member a skill, after the skill is mastered, the family member functions as the skilled provider. In a situation in which the family member becomes unable to perform that skill for the client, performance of the procedure will be considered a skilled service if performed by the nurse (Jackson & Johnson, 1988).

The second criterion used to determine if the teaching visits are reimbursable by Medicare is the *reasonableness and necessity of the teaching.* To be considered reasonable and necessary for the treatment of an illness or injury, the services must be consistent with the nature and severity of the individual's illness or injury, his or her particular medical needs, and the accepted standard of practice for clients with like conditions (Health Care Financing Administration, 1989).

Examination of the nature and severity of the illness is the first stage in determining the amount of teaching needed. For example, a client who has been a diabetic, administering insulin for 20 years, would not require an extensive teaching plan about insulin administration unless it could be determined and documented by the nurse that severe knowledge deficits and misunderstandings were present.

The home care nurse must be especially careful that the teaching that is done is *related to the client's condition* and is not reinforcement of previous teaching. As mentioned, reinforcement is a necessary part of the teaching-learning process but repeated teaching (often called reinforcement) is generally not reimbursable unless client changes that justify the intervention are noted by the nurse. For example, if the client's blood pressure had increased and the physician changed the medication, this change would indicate that new teaching should be provided. Another example would be if a 2-g sodium diet was taught to a cardiac client and the physician changed the diet order to a low-sodium diet, reinforcement of a low-sodium diet would be indicated. When documenting client teaching, the nurse should try to avoid using such words as *reinforced, reviewed,* or *reminded.* Whenever possible, link reinforcement of previous teaching with documentation about new teaching that was performed. Remember, Medi-

care *may* reimburse for one visit to reinforce teaching, but reimbursement would not extend further.

Client compliance with the new information learned is another factor in determining whether teaching visits are reimbursable. The purpose of the teaching-learning process is to help the client improve function and manage disease. If the home care nurse determines that the client continues to be unable to manage his or her disease following implementation of the teaching plan, a determination must be made for the reason for the lack of compliance. Evaluation of the teaching plan will help determine if the teaching strategies used were inappropriate and thereby blocked learning. In some cases, the client will achieve the desired objectives if more time than originally allotted is provided. If the client will not comply with instructions even though learning has been determined to have taken place, further teaching visits would not be reimbursable. Periodic reevaluation of the client's progress toward a specified learning objective is essential to the reimbursement process.

Considering all the factors that are evaluated to determine if a service is reimbursable under the Medicare program, the home care nurse must document all assessment and teaching clearly and as specifically as possible. One of the major flaws in documenting teaching is that the home care nurse writes about teaching in general terms. In order to facilitate clarity of documentation, the home care nurse must ask, "Why am I telling the client this?" and "What impact should this teaching have on this client?" (Omdahl, 1987). In order to make the documentation clear and specific, therefore increasing the likelihood of reimbursement for the teaching visit, the following ten items can be included in the client record:

1. date and time of the teaching session
2. to whom the teaching is directed (if not the client, why?)
3. client's health status
4. specific instructions given
5. teaching method used
6. client's level of comprehension
7. barriers to the teaching process
8. goals that were met during the teaching session
9. evaluation of the teaching session
10. plans for the next teaching session (Jackson & Johnson, 1988)

Inclusion of all this material in the written narrative notes may result in a rather lengthy submission, but it is all material that needs to be included to justify Medicare services. Some agencies use flowsheets or check-

Problem/knowledge deficit	Objectives/goals
1.	Upon completion of the teaching, the client will
2.	a.
3.	b.
4.	c.
5.	d.
	e.

Date						
Time						
Who was taught						
Response to teaching / Goals met						
Teaching intervention						
a.						
b.						
c.						
d.						
e.						
f.						
CODE P: Instructions provided, learning progressing, continues to need teaching C: Instructions provided, teaching completed N: Instructions provided, noncompliant	Signature/Title					

Figure 7–3 Teaching Flowsheet

lists to facilitate quick, yet complete charting. A flowsheet may be adequate for recording basic information regarding the teaching episode, but the nurse must realize that a flowsheet can and should be supplemented with narrative charting as the need arises. If all the preceding items can be included on the flowsheet, no narrative charting is needed. If not, a narrative note to supplement those areas not addressed on the flowsheet is indicated. Figure 7–3 is an example of a teaching flowsheet. The home care nurse should discuss the use of flowsheets with the nursing supervisor.

CONCLUSION

Client teaching is one of the most frequently used interventions by the home care nurse. As one of the skilled services reimbursed by Medicare, it is essential that the home care nurse develop expertise in teaching clients. The teaching-learning process is analogous to the steps of the nursing process. Documentation is an essential, yet often overlooked step of the teaching-learning process and is essential for reimbursement of teaching by Medicare.

TEST YOURSELF

1. Mrs. Brown is a frail 76-year-old woman who lives with her 68-year-old, unmarried sister. Both are retired schoolteachers and are able to live comfortably on their pensions and Social Security. Mrs. Brown was discharged from the hospital following a two-week stay for treatment of a peripheral vascular ulcer. Before her hospitalization, Mrs. Brown bumped her leg on her bedpost. At first, the bump resulted in a one-inch abrasion. The wound opened and started weeping, and Mrs. Brown treated herself with baking soda compresses and Tylenol. By the time she saw her doctor, the wound was three inches around and one-half inch deep with purulent yellow drainage. She also had a fever of 101.6°F. Mrs. Brown is diabetic and is treated with oral hypoglycemic agents.

   Mrs. Brown was referred for home care services for wound care to the partially healed ulcer. Because the client is diabetic, the doctor feels that the healing time will be prolonged, with total time of approximately three months. Orders for home care include teaching the client and caregiver the wound care procedure.

   a. What are the main issues that need to be addressed as part of the initial assessment for Mrs. Brown?
   b. Identify three objectives or goals for this teaching plan.
   c. Develop a teaching plan in order to accomplish the wound care instruction.
   d. What unique characteristics of this client situation must be taken into consideration in implementing the teaching plan?
   e. Think about a teaching session that could take place with this client and then document all the significant elements of clients who are labeled "noncompliant."

2. What are the strategies you can use to make the teaching-learning experiences positive for both the client and yourself?

3. What techniques have you found successful in teaching clients who are labeled "noncompliant"?

4. Mrs. Jones is a 27-year-old woman who lives with her three children under the age of five. Her husband and father of the children is absent and does not give them financial support. Mrs. Jones has barely been able to make ends meet on welfare. She completed eight years of school and is unemployed with no family financial support because her mother, sister, and aunt are also on welfare. Mrs. Jones just found out that her middle son, John, is diabetic.

   a. What areas of assessment would be most important for this family?
   b. What are some potential problems in teaching this family about John's care?
   c. Write two goals for this family that relate to learning a diabetic diet.
   d. Develop a teaching plan to bring into account the unique needs of this family.
   e. What teaching strategies might be most effective in teaching this mother about the care of her newly diagnosed diabetic son.

REFERENCES

Aleman, A. (1982). Nursing care of the multiproblem poor family. *Home Health Care Nurse, 1,* 34–38.

Bloom, B. (1969). *Taxonomy of educational objectives.* New York: McKay.

Doak, C., Doak, L., & Root, J. (1985). *Teaching patients with low literacy skills.* Philadelphia: Lippincott.

Health Care Financing Administration. (April 1989). *Medicare home health agency manual pub. 11.* Washington, DC: Author.

Hussey, L., & Gilliland, K. (1989). Compliance, low literacy and locus of control. *Nursing Clinics of North America, 25,* 605–611.

Jackson, J., & Johnson, E. (1988). *Patient education in home care.* Gaithersburg, MD: Aspen Publishers.

Knowles, M. (1980). *The modern practice of adult education.* Chicago: Follett.

Leff, E. (1986). Ethics and patient teaching. *The American Journal of Maternal-Child Nursing, 11,* 375–378.

Omdahl, D. (1987). Preventing home care denials. *American Journal of Nursing, 8,* 1031–1033.

Patterson, O. (1962). *Special tools for communication.* Chicago: Industrial Audio-Visual Association.

Peragallo-Dittko, V. (1994). *A core curriculum for diabetes education.* Chicago: American Association of Diabetes Educators.

Spradley, B.W. (1990). *Community health nursing.* Boston: Little, Brown.

Stanhope, M., & Lancaster, J. (1992). *Community health nursing.* St. Louis: Mosby.

Strategies for Effective Clinical Management

OBJECTIVES

Upon completion of the chapter, the reader will be able to identify:

1. Phases of contracting in home care
2. Components of a home care critical path system
3. Roles a case manager assumes in a managed care system
4. Ways nurses can have effective relationships with case managers
5. How home care management information systems affect clinical operations

KEY CONCEPTS

- **Setting up realistic expectations with clients**
- **Nursing's role in a home care critical path system**
- **How case managers work in a managed care system**
- **Developing the home care nurse's relationship with a case manager**
- **Home care management information systems**

AGENCY-SPECIFIC MATERIAL NEEDED

- Tools used by the agency to monitor client outcomes
- Critical paths used in the agency, if applicable
- Information for staff relative to agency managed care contracts
- Agency policy on working with and reporting to case managers
- Management information systems manual

INTRODUCTION

Effective home care practice is dependent upon understanding specific elements of the system in which the home care nurse practices, clinical management strategies, and variables that affect the ever-changing delivery of home care. In this chapter, the home care nurse is introduced to the concepts of contracting and critical paths, both very useful in the nurse's everyday clinical practice. Because home care nurses will increasingly provide care to clients who have case managers through their insurance provider, health maintenance organization (HMO), or other managed care entity, this chapter goes on to discuss the role of the case manager and how to develop a positive relationship between the case manager and the home care nurse and agency. Finally, recognizing the important relationship between home care nursing practice and home care information, as well as the increased use of computer systems in home care agencies, a description of management information systems (MIS) in home care and the nurse's role in working with them is given.

CONTRACTING IN HOME CARE

The most significant function of a home care nurse is the promotion of healthy behaviors through the identification of client needs and the development of plans to meet those needs. The client's and family's active participation in the assessment and planning phase of the therapeutic relationship has been shown to be effective in helping the client learn and practice healthy behaviors. Contracting can be used by the home care nurse to promote the active role of the client in all phases of the nursing process. This section includes a description of the concept of contracting, followed by a description of the phases of the contracting process. A discussion of the advantages of contracting, in the home care setting concludes this section.

The Concept of Contracting

Contracting is defined as any working agreement between the nurse and the client that is continually being renegotiated (Sloan & Schommer, 1982). It is an agreement between the client and the nurse that provides the framework for planning and evaluating the interactions that are occurring. It accomplishes this by identifying what each person in the relationship can expect from the other person in the relationship. It covers what behaviors the nurse can expect from the cli-

ent and what behaviors the client can expect from the nurse.

The concept of legal contracts is familiar to everyone. Nursing contracts differ in that they are not legally binding and are much more flexible than legal contracts. Contracts are used primarily to increase the role played by the client in the health care process. Through the identification and formalization of the client's role in the individual health care plan, the cooperative relationship between the nurse and the client strengthens.

Phases of the Contracting Process

Contracting is a learned process between the nurse and the client. All parties must have an understanding of the process of contracting for this strategy to be effective. Both nurse and client have significant responsibilities in each step of the process, mandating active involvement of both parties through the entire process. Sloan and Schommer (1982) describe eight phases that make up the contracting process, as follows:

1. *Exploration of need.* This phase involves the assessment by both the client and the nurse of the client's health needs and problems. Identification of the client's perspective regarding his or her health status and treatment plan is an essential component of this first phase.
2. *Establishment of goals.* Through discussion, the nurse and the client establish mutually agreeable goals for the purpose of alleviating the identified health problem or need. Goals should be realistic and attainable; the tendency to set overly ambitious goals should be avoided. Goals should be recognized as dynamic, which means that they can be renegotiated if they are unrealistic or are no longer relevant.
3. *Exploration of resources.* In this phase, the nurse and the client define how each can contribute to achieving the identified health goal. The nurse and the client should work together to identify appropriate resources, such as significant others, community services, and other professionals, that can play a role in alleviating the identified health need.
4. *Development of a plan.* Activities designed to meet the specified goals are developed in this phase of the process. If there is more than one goal, the nurse and the client collaborate to develop a priority list of identified goals. Identifying activities

to meet one goal at a time, beginning with the one with the highest priority, prevents the client from feeling overwhelmed by the contracting process and the implementation of the plan.

5. *Division of responsibilities.* In this phase, the nurse and the client decide who will be responsible for which activities. At first, the client may feel fearful in assuming activities identified as the professional responsibility of the nurse. As a client experiences success in managing his or her situation, the client will feel more at ease in assuming greater responsibility for his or her own health care.

6. *Agreement on a time frame.* As in all areas of goal setting and intervention, a time frame for accomplishment of goals must be determined. At the initial visit, the home care nurse should work with the client to develop a plan that outlines the anticipated frequency of home visits based on doctor's orders and the nursing assessment. This planning is conducted in all agencies, and nurses are required to complete this for various forms and for their own case management plans; often, however, nurses do not share this important information with the client. For example, the home care nurse, in collaboration with the client, might plan to make home visits three times per week for two weeks, two times per week for two weeks, and then one time per week for four weeks. Both client and nurse should agree on the established time frame and the specific goals to be accomplished at each step of the eight-week period. By doing this, both the client and the nurse know what is expected and how they are progressing on the goals developed.

7. *Evaluation.* Assessment of progress toward the goals or accomplishment of the goals is done in this phase. The nurse and the client evaluate the progress to date, both in terms of the client outcome and the interventions used to facilitate that outcome.

8. *Renegotiation or termination.* Based on the evaluation, the nurse and the client determine if the contract needs to be renegotiated or terminated. If the goals have been met, the contract can be terminated. If the goals have not been met, the contract can be modified and renegotiated. Any part of the contract may require modification. Perhaps the goals were too ambitious or the interventions inappropriate to meet the designated goals. In some cases, the nurse may have to assume tasks previously assigned to the client with the client assuming responsibility for other activities. Different strategies can be tried before contracting is abandoned.

Nursing contracts can be formal or informal, depending on how comfortable the nurse is with this intervention strategy, the client's readiness to assume responsibility for self-care, and the agency's policy. Formal contracts between the nurse and the client involve written identification of goals, including each person's responsibility in achievement of the goals, and signature of the written document by both parties. Less formal contracts, often used in home care situations, involve verbal identification of goals, including identifying each person's responsibility toward achieving those goals. In an informal contract, the nurse and the client develop a plan and come to an oral understanding regarding each party's responsibility in the contract. Client goals and the methods selected for achieving them, then documented in the nursing care plan, form the written evidence for implementation and evaluation of how the contract was achieved. Contracting takes time and effort on the part of the nurse and the client, but it is more than worth the time and work required at the beginning of the home care nursing relationship.

Some clients are afraid to assume an active role in their health care. If a client does not feel ready to take an active role, contracting may not be an appropriate strategy to use at the onset of care. Some clients prefer to relinquish all power to the professional involved in their care. These clients tend to be passive recipients rather than active participants in their health care. Clients with minimal cognitive abilities often find difficulty with the concept of contracting. There must be an appreciation of the concept of commitment in order for contracting to constitute an effective intervention strategy.

In some cases, the home care nurse can persuade a hesitant client to accept the process of contracting. Through an explanation of the process, the client may see that contracting is not as difficult as it may sound. Clients may also be persuaded to try contracting if they know that they can get out of the contract at any step in the process. Unlike legal contracts, there is no binding effect to the nursing contract. Clients may also be persuaded to try contracting when it is described as a means to attaining their health care goals quickly and efficiently. In today's climate of cost containment and reimbursement limits, contracting is a useful tool in moving both the client and the nurse to the identified goal in an efficient manner.

The role of the nurse in the nurse-client relationship will be altered when employing the concept of contracting. The nurse must be willing to relinquish her control as the powerful expert. In a hospital, the nurse is usually in control of care, and the patient is a passive recipient. In home care, the nurse and the client share equal authority in the relationship. The concept of contracting involves empowerment of the client, a concept that may frighten some professionals.

Contracting is most effective when there exists the potential for a long-term nursing relationship (more than two visits) between the client and the care provider. It is difficult to work through all the steps of the contracting process in one or two visits. As the nurse becomes adept at the contracting process and the client becomes accustomed to playing an active role in his or her health care, the contracting process can be accomplished in a shorter period of time.

Contracting involves the active participation of the client and the nurse in the planning, implementation, and evaluation of the nursing care provided. This care centers on a common goal, with interventions geared toward the achievement of that goal. Contracts can be formal or, as seen most commonly in home care, informal. Benefits of contracting for the client and the nurse include the following:

- Time is saved in the long run by setting up a contract with the client at the onset of care.
- Contracting allows everyone, especially the client, to know what is going to happen and the timetable on which it is going to happen. This gives clients a sense of security. Clients will know how long they will be receiving services and have an estimate of what the current goals are.
- Contracting keeps the nursing process goal directed and focused, thereby increasing the likelihood of reimbursement by third-party payers, such as Medicare, Medicaid, and private insurance.

Advantages of Contracting in Home Care

There are several reasons why contracting is an important intervention strategy in the practice of home care nursing. First, by the development of a plan through contracting, the roles and expectations of the nurse and the client become clarified. Increased clarity often enhances the nurse-client relationship. When each person is aware of his or her role and responsibility in the therapeutic relationship, the chance of meeting designated goals effectively increases.

Second, in home care nursing, the relationship between the client and family and the nurse is unlike that seen in an inpatient facility, such as a hospital. In the

hospital, the nurse assumes the responsibility for providing for the majority of care given to clients. In the home, the home care nurse's role is to teach the client or family member how to provide the necessary care to improve or maintain the client's level of health. The nature of the care delivery system dictates that clients and families play an active role in the health care provided. Contracting is a process in which that active role is given due recognition. Other advantages to using contracting in the home care setting include:

- The client plays an active role in his or her health care, rather than remaining a passive recipient of the care provided.
- Client empowerment and self-esteem are increased as success is experienced in self-care.
- New sets of coping strategies and decision-making skills are developed for the client.
- The possibility of achieving health goals identified by the client and the nurse increases because all parties are clear about the goals to be reached.
- Clearly defined goals, made achievable in measurable terms, can be used to motivate a client toward achievement of those goals.
- Increased focus on the interventions and evaluation of the intervention is possible, thereby increasing the likelihood of reimbursement by third-party payers.

In summary, contracting is an intervention strategy in which the nurse and the client (1) identify goals, (2) determine activities to achieve those goals, (3) identify who will assume responsibility for accomplishing those activities, and (4) evaluate the achievement of the goals. Contracts between clients and home care nurses can be very formal, with all steps to the process written with signatures of each party on the written document. More commonly, contracts are informal, oral agreements in which each step of the process is negotiated between the nurse and the client, and an oral evaluation is used to measure attainment of the goal.

CRITICAL PATHS IN HOME CARE

Home care agencies are increasingly using critical paths as a way to outline the various components of the client's care plan; measure the visits and personnel necessary to work with the client in reaching goals; and provide the nurse, client, and family a document, in writing, of the ways the outcomes can be reached. These critical paths are closely related to the process of contracting. With a written document that outlines all the nurse and client are to do to reach the mutually desired outcomes, the nurse can perform the components of contracting in a more efficient way based on the standards of care. This section outlines the components of the critical path system that can be used in an agency.

The Development of Critical Paths in Home Care

Zander (1988) states that a critical path identifies the timing of key interventions so that desired outcomes can be achieved. A critical path can also be seen as the optimal sequencing and timing of interventions (number of visits) by health care professionals (nurses, therapists) for a particular diagnosis or procedure. The critical path identifies key tasks or events as they relate to client problems rather than to a nursing or medical diagnosis. Critical paths use agency resources and personnel more efficiently, provide high-quality care, ensure timely progression of the care, and provide a way to measure the client's outcome.

Critical paths were initially used in industry in the 1950s to look at the cost, time, and resources needed to produce a product. Recently, hospitals began to apply the same critical path process to diagnoses and procedures that were costly in order to save money in response to the implementation of diagnosis-related groups (Corbett & Androwich, 1994). The use of critical paths with selected acute care diagnoses and procedures has resulted in reduced inpatient lengths of stay, a reduction in costs, better coordination of services, and improved client and family participation in care. Critical paths have also been useful in increasing the quality of documentation so that the exact care the client was receiving is as clear as the outcomes achieved.

Like hospitals, home care agencies are pressured to decrease costs, continue to document quality outcomes, and also increasingly to compete with agencies who have implemented a critical path system. There are two main motivations for home care agencies to implement a critical path system. First, the increased involvement of home care in managed care and case management contracts has meant that the home health agency must have progressive documentation not only of the care that was provided but also of the indication that client outcomes were achieved within a predetermined period of time for a certain amount of money.

Although this is certainly an issue when an agency is dealing directly with the payment source, it is also important because most managed care providers compare home health agencies when determining who will receive contracts to provide service for their clients. For example, critical path information for clients with con-

gestive heart failure (CHF) from your agency may be compared with the same information from other home care agencies that also have contracts with the managed care company. This review entails not only evaluating the kind of care provided but the amount of resources (type of personnel and number of visits) needed by each agency to achieve the same outcome. The information provided on the critical path, used with financial data of the cost per visit or episode of care from each agency, can then be used by the payer to compare the cost-effectiveness of each home care agency.

The second reason home care agencies have been increasing their use of critical paths is the need to look at the management of a client's care across settings, for example, in some cases, from hospital to rehabilitation facility to home care. The number of hospital-based home health agencies has increased significantly in the 1990s. Many of these agencies are linking their home care client's time on service and care provided with that of the hospital. For example, if a client comes into the hospital for a hip replacement and a critical path is used during the hospitalization, when the hospital discharges that client to its home health agency (or any home health agency) it wants to monitor how that client's care and cost progress during his or her time on home care. If the client had gone from the hospital to a rehabilitation facility and then was admitted to the home health agency, there might be three critical paths that allow monitoring the client from initial surgery until the final outcome of functioning back in society.

With the potential for payment for health care services to be in a "lump sum" for each diagnosis or procedure, and because many payers require providers to obtain prior authorization for covered services, the services expended and the dollars charged for all the client's health services (in this case, hospital, rehabilitation center, and home care) must be closely monitored. This is being done in many areas by the implementation of a critical path system (Gooldy & Duncan, 1994).

Components of a Home Care Critical Path System

Using critical paths in home care is much more than just completing an additional piece of paper on the client or revising the care plan used in the agency. Additionally, because of the complexity of home care and the numerous variables present, the implementation of critical paths in a home health agency is more complex than in an acute care facility. A home care agency must implement a critical path *system* that is organized and documents that the care provided by the agency is delivered in the most cost-effective manner. The system identifies client and family educational needs, and the interdisciplinary interventions to meet those needs, and plans them on a timeline to achieve the most cost-effective, desirable outcome. The critical path system is implemented throughout the home health agency with an interdisciplinary focus, not just in the nursing department. It is important to note that some agencies implement critical paths as their nursing and clinical documentation systems for visits whereas others use these forms as pieces of information in addition to their care plan documents. The agency has the choice of how to use the system and the many pieces of information. The various components typical in a critical path system are discussed in this section (American Health Consultants, 1994).

The Critical Path

A critical path system has, as a centerpiece, a document known as a critical path. The format for a critical path is usually the same throughout the agency, and the content is developed by examining the specific clinical activities needed for a client with a specific diagnosis or procedure. A critical path is similar to a standardized care plan; however, it has an added timeline that in home care is usually visits or weeks of care.

An example of the three components of one company's critical path product is found in the critical path agency forms in Appendix F. In this example the HomeCare-Path Assessment Visit and the HomeCare-Path Visit represent the standard format used in all the agency's critical paths. The third form in Appendix F, CHF—HomeCare-Path—Visit #1, has taken the format and made it specific to a client with CHF. The sections on Nursing Intervention/Education and Patient Outcome are specific to the nursing care expected to be given to this client on the first home visit. The sections marked Other are included so the nurse can personalize this path to the needs of the specific client.

A "detour" from the critical path is called a *variance*, which you will see on the lower right corners of the forms in Appendix F. Variances can be positive or negative and are essentially something that has transpired (either planned or unplanned) that affects the care being provided on that visit, which will, in turn, affect the client's outcome. Variances can be caused by:

- Client and family: For example, a family member may be unavailable to learn how to perform a key care management activity
- Clinician: For example, the physician revises the plan of care

- System: There may be an equipment failure. For example, the accucheck breaks down, which interferes with the timely progress of the plan of care
- Community: There may be a lack of community resources to support the family and client at home

Co-Path

Because most home care clients do not present with only one diagnosis, it is often necessary for the nurse to address the client's care needs taking into consideration multiple diagnoses and procedures. The co-path was developed and is used in most critical path systems to allow the nurse and other providers to address those interventions and outcomes that affect the client with more than one diagnosis. For example, the client may have CHF as a primary diagnosis, but because of a secondary diagnosis of diabetes mellitus also needs teaching and monitoring of this condition. In this case, the client would have a path for CHF and a co-path for diabetes.

Outcomes

In the reforming health care delivery system of the 1990s, the focus on client outcomes will continue to be at the center of care. Home care agencies, and especially home care nurses because of their role as coordinators of care, are challenged to find ways not only to measure outcomes but also to identify what specific interventions were most important in reaching those outcomes. Nurses historically have had difficulty in understanding outcomes as opposed to processes of care. Chapter 6 discusses structure, process, and outcome in the context of the overall provision of care to the agency's clients. When examining outcomes in an agency's critical path system, it is important that the nurse be comfortable with the definition of an outcome and understand how to measure it.

Variance Tracking Reports

The variances that occur while caring for clients are tracked for the total group of clients seen for a specific diagnosis or procedure by use of a report, often called a *variance tracking report*. On this sheet, the types of variances mentioned earlier—client and family, clinician, system, and community—are categorized to identify agency trends. For example, it may be noted that in a group of agency clients whose main diagnosis is CHF, nurses reported variances because they routinely had to make additional visits because the client's oxygen was not set up properly or was not there at all. These variances would be seen on the variance tracking report under the category of system and then tracked further to see who was the primary vendor responsible for these problems. Because the agency was expending more resources (personnel and visits) simply because the equipment was not there, the agency may then take steps to address the problem with the vendor. If the problem was solved, the variances, and therefore costs, should decrease. If the number of variances specific to this problem did not decrease, the agency might stop doing business with this vendor. The tracking of variances is not only an important aspect of the critical path system but is also used in the home care agency's quality management program and can be used to direct quality improvement activities.

The Nurse's Role in Critical Paths

Critical Path Team Member

When an agency is developing critical paths for certain clients, it is important that clinical nurses who care for these types of clients be a part of the initial creation of the system. Because critical paths are focused on the clinical care the client is given, nurses must have input into the content of the critical path as well as the number of visits it will take to accomplish the client outcomes. Just as important as development, the ongoing evaluation of the system, once implemented, must have input from direct service nurses, not just management. Nurses who sit on these committees can be the facilitators and educators of the other staff during initial and ongoing implementation of the system in the agency.

Case Manager

Many home care agencies are giving the primary nurse who sees the client the responsibility of being a case manager to the clients in her caseload. When a critical path system is used in an agency, it is the case manager or primary nurse who is responsible for completing the critical path, identifying the variances, and monitoring the frequency and duration of care the client receives. Additionally, the agency nurse who is coordinating the client's care is the main contact person to communicate with everyone connected with the case, especially the payer. This is especially true when working with clients whose care is covered by HMOs, managed care companies, and any payer that requires prior authorization or is working under a capitation agreement where care is provided for a set amount of money.

The home care nurse, therefore, completes the majority of the paperwork associated with a critical path system. It is very important that the nurse understand how the system is to be implemented and the specific definitions of the types of variances recorded. Additionally, the accuracy of the documentation by the nurse is crucial to the effective use of a critical path system. The computer expression "garbage in, garbage out" can be applied to the nurse's role in documenting on the critical path system. If the nurse does not write the correct information consistently similar to others who are working with the system, the validity of the data will be compromised and the agency will not be able to accurately track the effect of its services.

In summary, the use of critical paths is increasing in home care. Nurses are essential components of the system and are responsible for seeing that the data used in the system are accurate and timely. A critical path system can be an important aspect of evaluating the agency's clinical and financial performance as well as a tool integral to the agency's performance improvement and quality management programs.

THE CASE MANAGER IN HOME CARE

Changes in the health care delivery system are the hallmark of the 1990s. Because motivation for change has been brought about by the need to control costs, payers have been focusing on preventing illness, providing community-based care, and controlling the type and amount of care a client receives. These actions fall under the broad term of *managed care,* and, although initially used by insurance companies, they are being used increasingly by all payers, including state and federal governments.

In a managed care system, beneficiaries (clients who are covered by an insurance plan or other payment source, such as an HMO) are required to get prior approval for needed care from the payment source. When approval is received, the payer often dictates to the provider (for example, the home health agency) the type, frequency, and duration of services that can be provided based on client information and consultation with the physician. As you have learned, home health agencies already have to provide services in the complicated environment of local, state, and federal rules and regulations as well as certification standards and regulations. With managed care payers, there is yet another layer of rules, regulations, and personnel an agency must work with to obtain services for clients. The person who interacts with the agency to approve and monitor the services and acts as a gatekeeper for the client to receive services is called a case manager. This section gives an overview of case management, the case manager's role, and how the home care nurse can effectively interact with this gatekeeper.

Definition of Case Management

The definition of case management from the Certification of Insurance Rehabilitation Specialists Commission (1993) is: "Case management is a collaborative process which assesses, plans, implements, coordinates, monitors, and evaluates the options and services required to meet an individual's health needs, using communication and available resources to promote quality, cost-effective outcomes."

The philosophy of case management from the same source is as follows:

> Case management is not a profession in itself, but an area of practice within one's profession. Its underlying premise is that when an individual reaches the optimum level of wellness and functional capability, everyone benefits—the individuals being served, their support systems, the health care delivery systems, and the various reimbursement sources. Case management serves as a means for achieving client wellness and autonomy through advocacy, communication, education, identification of service resources, and service facilitation. The case manager helps identify appropriate providers and facilities throughout the continuum of services, while ensuring that available resources are being used in a timely and cost-effective manner in order to obtain optimum value for both the client and the reimbursement source. Case management services are best offered in a climate that allows direct communication between the case manager, the client, and appropriate service personnel in order to optimize the outcome for all concerned. Certification determines that the case manager possesses the education, skills, and experience required to render appropriate services based on sound principles of practice.

Although very familiar and similar to what home care nurses do, the scope of practice for a certified case manager (CCM) covers a much broader spectrum of care and services for a client. The CCM coordinates care through the entire continuum of care: prehospital, hospital, subacute, nursing home, home health, outpatient, clinic or office visits, and life care. The CCM must concentrate on the big picture and stretch the benefits and resources to cover all services and settings, for both immediate and future needs of the client. This is an important point to remember when negotiating services for a client, as home care nurses can become too narrow-minded and only consider the client's home care needs. Unlike the Medicare program, managed care policies have limits in coverage.

Where traditionally case managers perform utilization review (U/R) or audit functions, they do not want to be viewed just as a person who controls the money spent on the client. Many insurance companies have separated the U/R department from case management. As CCMs grow in numbers and employment settings, they are very focused on *care* management. This means they are looking not only for cost-control mechanisms but for quality services with positive client outcomes. They are creative in using resources and combining a variety of care settings and services to obtain the best care as efficiently as possible.

Who Is a Case Manager?

The roots of case management are in community and public health nursing. Public health nurses have traditionally coordinated care for clients with catastrophic and communicable disease conditions. Over the years, this case management role evolved from public health to workers' compensation plans where nurses focused on high-risk and high-dollar cases, such as head and spinal cord injuries. The uncontrolled rising costs of health care and the subsequent emergence of managed care have extended the case manager role to other health care settings. Case managers are now found in every insurance company where they may manage the care of all clients or just those representing the high-risk or high-dollar cases (Knollmueller, 1989).

Case managers are primarily registered nurses (RNs) who come from a variety of clinical backgrounds. Many are certified rehabilitation registered nurses (CRRNs) or certified insurance rehabilitation specialists (CIRSs). RN case managers also have specialty backgrounds in pediatrics, infusion therapy, oncology, and maternal-child health, depending on the company they work for and the client population with whom they deal. Case managers who are not RNs may be physicians; physical, speech, or occupational therapists; or medical social workers. Presently, few case managers have home care backgrounds and therefore need the guidance of experienced home care professionals to plan and evaluate home care services.

The CCM process was started in 1991 and has had a positive effect on standardizing the profession. Prior to this certification, there was much confusion about case management practice. The lack of standards or established boundaries for case managers led to wide variations in practice resulting in a friction between physicians, providers, and clients. The CCM certification process has set standards of practice, defined minimum qualifications, and clearly defined the case management process and philosophy.

To apply for the CCM examination, one must:

- Hold a current RN license or other health care professional license or hold a national certification in a health and human services profession
- Have six months to two years of qualifying case management experience
- Have two to four years of qualifying clinical experience

The application process is lengthy and requires specific documentation from previous supervisors or employers to ensure that case manager candidates have minimal accepted background and experience. The exams are given presently two times a year in test sites across the country. If the exam is passed, the certification is good for five years. Certification can be renewed automatically with proof of eight hours of CCM-approved continuing education units, or the CCM may retake the exam for certification renewal.

Where CCMs Are Employed

Case managers work in the following settings, and new areas are being identified constantly:

- workers' compensation carriers, where case management was started and where many rehabilitation nurses and therapists are employed
- HMOs
- preferred provider organizations (PPOs)
- managed care organizations (MCOs)
- traditional health insurance companies providing fee-for-service contracts
- hospitals
- physician offices and clinics
- community-based programs, such as Community Care for the Elderly or special Medicaid programs (differs by state)
- self-insured employers
- case management companies, which are in the business of case management and may contract their services out to any of those listed above
- independent case managers, who are self-employed and may contract their services with any of those listed above (most often found in rural, outlying areas)

What CCMs Expect from a Home Health Agency

Honesty and Integrity

CCMs expect the home care nurse to be honest about the services the agency can offer and those it cannot. You should say what you can do and then do what you say. For example, CCMs expect that the agency will have the clinical expertise on staff if it accepts a high-tech IV referral.

Flexibility

CCMs expect you to be flexible in staffing patterns and hours of care delivery. If the client (the customer) requests early morning or late evening services or visits at the workplace, you should be able to accommodate that request. CCMs may ask the home care nurse to do an evaluation visit only and then discuss why the services can or cannot be done in an outpatient setting versus home care. They may often authorize services only for very short periods of time, such as week by week or visit by visit. This will require ongoing collaboration with the CCM on the continued need for services. If the family is involved in the care, the home care schedule may depend on the family's availability day by day or week by week.

Negotiation

CCMs expect you to be open to negotiations on the level of care, frequency and duration of care, and the charges for care. Negotiation is defined as "to carry on business, to confer or bargain, to discuss with a view towards reaching agreement, to bring discussion." It implies that each side has something the other side wants. In this situation, the CCM has the client referrals you want and you have the services the CCM wants for clients. All negotiations must include what the physician, client, and family want as well. Decisions must be based on desired outcomes agreed to by all.

Verifying insurance policy coverage is not the same as negotiating the care with the CCM. Verification of the policy is usually done by an administrative person to determine whether the policy is current and how to submit claims. Negotiation of services with the CCM determines the policy coverage, authorizes the services, and may result in further out-of-policy services if that proves to be the most efficient means to achieve the desired outcomes.

Communication

CCMs expect to be able to speak to a nurse when they call a home care agency and preferably to the nurse who is knowledgeable in the care of the client. They want to speak to the nurse who can make decisions about the care and services to be provided. They want to be kept informed of the client's progress or decline on a frequent basis. Some will require written reports; others will require telephone reports.

Most of your communication with CCMs will be by telephone. Much misinterpretation can occur without the benefit of eye-to-eye contact and the observance of body language. Special care should be taken to ensure that good communication is always happening. Try to call the CCM when you are in a quiet place and can devote attention to the subject of the conversation. Frequent telephone conferences should occur, and you will want to set up the schedule and time for these from the beginning. It is very beneficial to have the key home care staff present for these conferences so the CCM can communicate directly with the primary home care nurse.

It is important to document all verbal communication and to ensure no misunderstandings have occurred. Summaries of case conferences and any negotiations for services should be put in writing for the client record and for the CCM's file.

On-call or after-hours communication may also need to occur. Determine with CCMs from the beginning how they can be reached or how they want to handle situations that need their input or approval and may arise outside of business hours. Tips for communicating with CCMs are:

- *Do* communicate with CCMs at the agreed-upon time and in the agreed-upon manner.
- *Do* communicate when you've made a mistake, missed a visit, or if a problem arises.
- *Do* communicate immediately if the client has been hospitalized or expires.
- *Don't* expect that the CCM will remember to call you to authorize further care.
- *Don't* leave your office without a designated person to take the CCM's call if you are expecting a call.

Teamwork

CCMs expect teamwork to occur in your agency and with all other providers who are involved in the client's care.

Support

CCMs expect your support for the care management plan and that you recognize their broad scope of coverage. They expect that you will not take sides if problems arise with the physician or client and family.

Positive Outcomes

CCMs expect that you will reach the outcomes or goals agreed upon to the satisfaction of all: client, family, physician, CCM, and payer.

What CCMs Are Concerned About

Successful work with CCMs requires an understanding of the things they are accountable for and therefore are most concerned about.

Customer Satisfaction

The people who are insured by the insurance company must be pleased with the health services they receive. The insurance industry is very competitive, and employers will switch companies for reasons other than cost if the insured are unhappy. If there is a loss of participants, the CCM could be held accountable and lose his or her job; therefore, CCMs want the clients to be happy with the care and services received.

Physicians are customers as well and must order all care for the client. A CCM must be sure that the physician is consulted, agrees to the care plan, and is happy with the services provided to the client. Additionally, home care services should be easy for the physician and his or her office staff to use. The providers of care, such as hospitals, home health agencies, and clinics, are also the CCM's customers and must be happy with the plan or they may not want to service the clients.

Confidentiality

Laws regarding patient information differ by state, but all are very sensitive in the areas of mental health, substance abuse, human immunodeficiency virus (HIV), and acquired immune deficiency syndrome (AIDS), and regarding any information that could be damaging to an individual's reputation or employment. The CCM may not give you specific information about a client until the agency has accepted the client for service and a release of information consent form has been signed by the client.

Managed Care Liability

CCMs cannot restrict access to necessary or appropriate care because of cost, or in any manner consider, or appear to consider, cost over outcomes. CCMs do not work in a vacuum. They must confer directly with the insurance company and/or client's physician regarding case management determinations and suggestions both at the onset of care and throughout the care continuum. The physician maintains control of the care ordered at all times. Additionally, CCMs cannot require the client or physician to accept the case management recommendation in lieu of any other treatment or by threatening nonpayment or noncoverage.

Negligent Referral

Negligence in referrals can arise from the referral itself and also from the failure to refer when the care is needed. CCMs can be held accountable for negligence in the following areas:

- referral to a practitioner who is known to be incompetent
- inappropriate substitution of inadequate therapy for an adequate but more expensive one
- decision to stop treatment inappropriately where the decision was a "substantial factor" in bringing about injury or harm to the client
- referral to a practitioner or facility clearly inappropriate for the needs of the client

Recommendations given to CCMs to prevent negligent referrals are:

- Investigate the providers or practitioners to whom you refer clients. Check licenses, certifications, and accreditations. Verify evidence for the skills and services that are advertised.
- Seek references from other CCMs, clients, and physicians.
- Perform thorough evaluations of the client's history and health needs.
- Communicate regularly with the client, family, and providers of care.
- Hold regular case conferences. Carefully evaluate satisfaction and outcomes to head off problems early.
- Know the limits of your expertise. Seek experts in areas outside your experience and training.

Fraud and Abuse

With the changes in health care reform, fraud and abuse laws are increasing in number and scope. The CCM literature advises CCMs to adhere to the same guidelines as Medicare and Medicaid regarding conduct, regardless of payer source. These laws are discussed in Chapter 10 and center around prohibiting filing of false claims, excessive charges, kickbacks, bribes, or rebates in exchange for referrals.

Experimental Treatment

CCMs cannot automatically deny coverage for services when a treatment is determined to be experimental. Company policies must specify the sources of information the CCM must review before making the determination that a treatment is experimental. For example, CCMs must usually consult Food and Drug Administration determinations, other insurance company determinations, and published medical literature.

Rehospitalizations

Perhaps the most frustrating thing for a CCM is a client's rehospitalization or frequent hospitalizations. The hospital is the most costly setting for care, and rehospitalization raises questions about whether the care provided prior to the hospitalization was appropriate. All parties involved in the client's care must recognize the importance of understanding realistic outcomes for care and communicating appropriately if the care is not allowing progression toward those outcomes.

How To Develop a Relationship with a CCM

The discussion of the role and function of CCMs is provided to help the home care nurse understand the various responsibilities of CCMs in order for the nurse to work more effectively with them. For every home care nurse, especially experienced ones, working in a managed care environment is a challenge because it calls for a different approach to providing home care than the traditional Medicare model. Increasingly, Medicare clients are enrolling in managed care plans and HMOs so that the home care delivery model for these clients is changing to one of working with CCMs. Often home care nurses feel threatened by CCMs. The nurses feel they are best prepared to determine the needs, frequency, and duration of services because they see the client and family directly and the CCM deals with everyone only on the phone.

For a home health agency to be successful in obtaining and keeping managed care contracts, the staff nurse (direct care provider) who delivers care to the client (customer) must work closely with the CCM. Whether you are a nurse who currently works with managed care clients or not, you need to understand the principles of this delivery system and the impact it has on your agency and clients. The following suggestions are presented to assist the home care nurse and managers in thinking of ways to be successful in this new environment:

- Educate yourself and your staff. Read everything you can find on managed care and share it with those with whom you work. Attend managed care conferences and educational seminars and subscribe to periodicals written for CCMs and the managed care industry. The more you understand and keep up with the trends and changes, the less fear you'll have.
- Decrease and control costs in your workplace. Make sure all your systems and processes are as efficient as possible. Make sure all staff members are as productive as possible.
- Increase your client referral base or census. Managed care will require a larger volume of clients to make up for the reduction in revenues.
- Identify trade associations in your area and attend meetings and networks.
- Network with CCMs in your area. Share current home care information with them and ask them to provide educational programs to your staff.
- Identify the top ten employers in your area and find out who provides their insurance coverage. Explore the plan and opportunities for home care services.
- Provide community education programs to groups other than the Medicare population to educate them on the advantages of home care.
- Be alert for the growth and spread of Medicare managed care plans. The Health Care Financing Administration (HCFA) has set up an Office of Managed Care. The purpose of this office is quality assurance and regulation of HMOs and other plans dealing with Medicare and Medicaid.

All areas of health care in the United States are undergoing major change. Reductions in costs, greater efficiency, and improved, measurable client outcomes are going to continue to be the focus of this change. Home health care is an integral component of achieving the changes necessary, but not without a great deal of change in the way services are currently provided. As home health organizations reorganize, restructure, and rethink how things are done, the home care nurse increasingly will need to be flexible in creating and living with the changes. As CCMs play an increasing role in managing home health care for clients, the home care nurse will need to continue to find new and creative ways to work with them as the gatekeepers for client services.

MIS IN HOME CARE

Home care practice in the 1990s has become increasingly reliant on computers. The home care nurse is often expected to collect information from the client, enter that information into some type of computer (laptop, hand-held), and send the data to the home care agency so that bills are developed, payroll is generated, and information about client care and outcomes can be collected. An understanding of the way information is collected and how it is used by the home care agency is essential to successful clinical practice and overall effectiveness of the nurse's job performance (Muellin, 1986). This section will present an overview of integrated home care MIS with an emphasis on clinical applications and the role of the home care nurse in working with these systems.

The Home Care Nurse's Role with Computers

For the home care agency and the professional staff nurse to meet the challenges of reducing costs while improving client outcomes, using a home care computer system that reduces the burden of documentation and streamlines the work of the agency's business department is essential. Many home care nurses are fearful about using computers or are concerned about their ability to use them effectively. Home care nurses with basic keyboard skills will find accessing and entering data to be an easily learned routine. For those with limited computer experience, the home care agency will provide on-the-job training so that everyone with computer responsibilities feels comfortable with this method of documentation. Most computer systems used in home care are designed for nurses with little or no computer background.

Learning any new skill can be frustrating, especially if the nurse feels the pressure of productivity expectations. The agency should account for a decrease in productivity for a limited time while the nurse is learning to use the computer or system. Like the addition of any new technology in nursing practice, there will be less efficient functioning during the learning period.

Some nurses are fearful of using a computer because they are concerned about destroying the computer database, losing data, or unintentionally changing data. This database holds all the client information, including clinical, billing, and demographics. Most computer systems have password security features that permit the nurse access to just those portions of the computer system relevant to her clinical practice. Other parts of the database will be restricted, such as billing and finance files. Additionally, there are usually other data integrity safeguards, such as field edits, that require you to enter correct information in one section before letting you move on to the next field. To protect against losing data, agencies back up data entry on separate files on a daily basis to secure client documentation. In this way, if a file is damaged or lost, only that day's entries are affected. These protections allow the nurse to feel more comfortable in using the system and less fearful that a mistake on her part can affect the client's entire information record.

Most laptops and hand-held computers are very durable and withstand most of the usual daily wear and tear. Computers are sensitive to heat, bumping, and power failures, experiences common to the home care setting. It also must be remembered that computers are costly items; the home care nurse should keep the computer locked in the trunk of her car when it is not in use.

When information is collected by the nurse and input at the client's home, it is called a point-of-care documentation system. Technological developments in home care have resulted in the emergence of new methods of documenting all components of client information. In addition to using the standard keyboard way of entering data, wands or pens can be used in some systems to input data on a screen; these systems are called pen-based documentation. Using this type of system alleviates the intimidation of using a keyboard.

Visit data can also be recorded using touch-tone phone lines or client swipe cards, similar to credit cards. These cards can be programmed to hold insurance and clinical data. Swipe cards pose a problem in home care when the nurse does not have the device necessary to read the card. In addition to agency MIS, electronic data initiatives are being developed to electronically link home care agencies with other providers in the community (such as hospitals, clinics, and physician offices) to improve client outcomes and reduce costs. Regardless of what type of system your agency uses, it is important to have an understanding of the system so you can feel comfortable and understand your responsibilities.

Integrated Home Health MIS

Most home health agencies that have a computer system have at least billing and some clinical capacities. It is essential for staff nurses to appreciate integrated MIS from the standpoint of both clinical practice and overall agency demands. For current and future health care delivery, a system that balances cost and quality, as well as produces greater efficiencies throughout the organization, is crucial to an organization's survival.

All too often professional staff perceive the administrative pressure to reduce cost as a priority over clinical practice, setting up tension between professional and administrative staff. Given the realities of spiraling health care costs, competition to provide cost-effective home care services, and the likelihood that health care reform will shift financial risk to the provider, administrative and clinical staff need to share the challenge to reduce costs while they improve clinical outcomes. Part of the solution to meeting this challenge is the implementation of computer systems that integrate and merge departments and information within an agency.

Fully integrated MIS should tie together basic operations in an agency by minimizing the need to reenter shared data, maximizing the accuracy of data, and improving turnaround of forms and output time for each department. From the initial referral to discharge, client data are routinely gathered in integrated MIS for care planning, service requests and scheduling, billing, statistics, finance, quality improvement, management reports, payroll, inventory, and purchasing. The nurse can see the importance of the accuracy and timeliness of the data collected on visits. All agency departments depend on the accuracy, completeness, and thoroughness of the data collected by the nurse.

How Information Flows through Home Care MIS

After a client referral is received by the agency, it is registered in the computer database. After this activity, client assignments and scheduling occur, which build the client's multilevel database. When a client is admitted by the nurse on the initial visit, physical and psychosocial assessments are completed, and these form the foundation for care plans; service orders; HCFA Forms 485, 486, and 487; and other information that makes up the client's home care record. Additional service data and financial data are simultaneously gathered on other forms, such as travel route sheets, visit notes, and billing and consent forms. These data elements are then keyed into the client's database using a unique client identifier, such as a medical record number or Social Security number. Nonclinical data are stored for billing, payroll, financial reports, accounts payable, and the general ledger that records all agency transactions.

Service requests that are entered into the system can be tied or integrated to inventory, purchasing, and actual scheduling of staff. Scheduling on the system will in turn, after verification, generate the bill at the appropriate time. Bills from the system are electronically sent to the fiscal intermediary for payment in a paperless system. The flowchart in Figure 8–1 illustrates the inter-relatedness of departments and their functions. Notice how the arrows integrating activities and departments go in several directions and require data from more than one source.

The Nurse's Role in MIS

The role of a staff nurse is pivotal in ensuring accurate, timely, and appropriate data collection using either direct entry point-of-care devices or worksheet forms entered later in the office by clerical support staff. Fully integrated home health MIS will not only capture, sort, and distribute data to the appropriate departments, but will also streamline data collection throughout the agency.

A database registers baseline client data and adds to or modifies that baseline over time. Some data remain constant and should be entered only once during the entire length of time the client is on service. These data elements would be start of care (SOC) date and client date of birth, Social Security number, sex, and provider address. Other data elements are relatively stable and require infrequent modification; address and living arrangement are examples. Some data elements are constantly changing; examples of these elements are medication and service orders, goals, and clinical findings. The computer software system that eliminates rewriting stable data and allows for easy modification of changing data will increase efficiencies and decrease costs both by decreasing entry time and avoiding data entry errors. For example, many of the fields on HCFA Form 485 remain constant, whereas others need only slight revision on recertification. Most MIS packages generate HCFA Form 485 from registration or intake data that are modified by the admitting staff after the first home visit. Similarly, when a home care nurse needs to complete recertification, she should not be

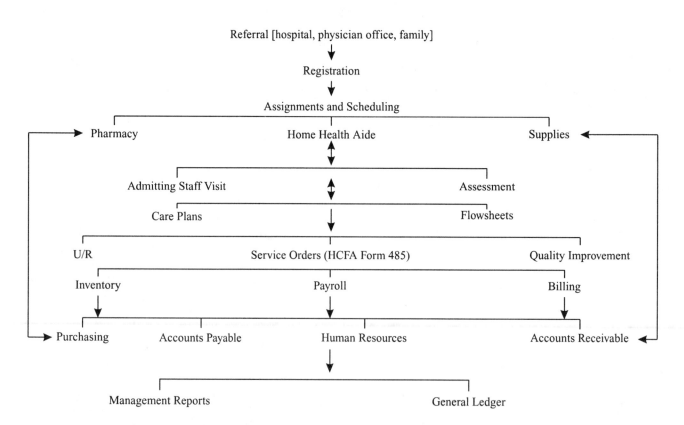

Figure 8–1 Generic Integrated Home Health Management Information System

required to reenter stable data but only revise those fields with changes. Software systems generally print a worksheet of the most current information in the database and a copy of the most recent certification or recertification for reference. This allows the nurse to update the worksheet and enter the information into the computer to produce a new HCFA Form 485. With some software packages, the same streamlining efficiencies can be accomplished for revision of care plans, medication, and visit flowsheets using either the worksheet method or a copy of the previous computer output or form. Other forms, such as physician verbal orders and summary reports, can also be generated by MIS. At a time when reduction of the paperwork burden has been a primary goal, these kinds of streamlining in MIS packages have saved tremendous amounts of pre- and postvisit recording time, thereby saving money and increasing the nurse's job satisfaction and productivity.

Clinical Modules

Software systems today are generally developed with a core package of applications for regulatory compliance that include HCFA Forms 485, 486, and 487 and the Universal Billing-92 form (UB-92). Separate modules are then added to enhance the core package to capture more sophisticated internal data that affect other agency operations and to anticipate regulatory changes or requirements that may happen in the future. Clinical modules may be installed as part of the core package when an agency first purchases its system or they may be purchased separately at a later date.

The better MIS clinical modules will systematically follow the nursing process rather than make the nurse conform to the computer's data entry pathway. Clinical modules are now available that standardize assessments with "hard coded" or predetermined phrases from which the nurse can choose rather than free text fields that require the nurse to type in the basic wording, much of which is repetitive in all client situations.

For example, under lung sound assessment you might see a list of possible assessments with additional descriptors. You simply check the appropriate box and then move on to the next phrase until lung sounds are fully described. The assessment programming will require you to fill out the past medical history, a review of systems, and environmental and psychosocial assessments leading to problem identification in either nursing or medical problem terminology. The system may even include decision trees prompting you to identify the client problems. Again, the information collected can be directly entered by the home care nurse or docu-

mented on assessment worksheets for entry by clerical staff. Hand-held point-of-care devices do eliminate the need for entry later, but some argue that well-designed worksheets are just as efficient for the staff. Exhibits 8–1 and 8–2 are examples of standardized skilled nursing assessment forms that are entered later into the agency database. These forms have both hard-coded parameters and free text options for the nurse. The parameter "DME/Supplies (485-14)" indicates integration of this data element with HCFA Form 485, Field 14. Once these assessment data are entered into the computer database, a hard-copy health history and problem list with goals and interventions are printed for the clinical record. This is illustrated in Exhibit 8–3.

Some clinical modules can now identify problems from assessments and develop a standardized care plan with specific interventions, goals, and outcomes to track improvement. These software packages offer critical path care plans that specify recommended care plan interventions and visit frequencies, and track variance from the expected outcomes. The degree of sophistication of the care planning and evaluation programming will vary significantly in clinical software programs. Regardless of the type of clinical module you are currently using, all agencies will need to plan how to standardize care and client outcomes using either an automated or manual system.

MIS and Quality Improvement

MIS also help the agency evaluate the quality of care it is providing to its customers. In the past, agencies regularly conducted client evaluation summaries in traditional quality assurance record reviews, objectively measuring outcomes in terms of home care utilization, hospital recidivism, or the ability to self-manage. Other outcome parameters or health status indices, such as functional, cognitive, and behavioral changes over the course of care, were difficult, if not impossible, to gather. These outcome parameters are now being included in MIS software packages.

The agency that can summarize client health indices over time will be in a good position to respond to reimbursement and other health reform changes. The computer software system standardizes these measurements by requiring all nurses to describe their clients using the same terminology and the same system. The agency can then retrieve the data and analyze them for quality improvement information.

As the client database expands over the length of stay, standard management reports can be generated that provide information about the agency's performance. These reports can be broken out by specific client

Exhibit 8–1
SKILLED NURSING ASSESSMENT FORM: HEALTH HISTORY

Allergies: "Tetracycline, silk tape"

[X]   Angina:
[ ]   Arrhythmias: "pt. states he had arrhythmias for about 30 years with exacerbation three years ago, was started on Lanoxin at that time"
[ ]   Arteriosclerosis:
[X]   Heart Disease:
[ ]   Hypertension: "was hypertensive 10 years ago and has taken Lopressor last 5 years, D/Ced last hospitalization"
[ ]   Murmur:
[ ]   Myocardial Infarction:
[ ]   Palpitations:
[ ]   Phlebitis:
[ ]   Postural Hypertension:
[ ]   Stroke/CVA:
[ ]   Asthma:
[ ]   Bronchitis:
[ ]   Emphysema:
[ ]   Frequent URI:
[ ]   Lung Disease:
[ ]   Pneumonia:
[ ]   Tuberculosis:
[ ]   Gastric Abnormalities:
[ ]   Intestinal Abnormalities:
[ ]   Peptic Ulcer Disease:
[ ]   Kidney Disease:
[ ]   Prostate:
[ ]   Diabetes:
[ ]   Hyperthyroidism:
[ ]   Hypothyroidism:
[X]   Blood Transfusion:
[ ]   Cancer: "prostate"

Equipment Needs:

[ ]	Hospital Bed	[ ]	Eggcrate Mattress	[ ]	AP Mattress
[ ]	Bedpan	[ ]	Urinal	[ ]	Bedside Commode
[ ]	Suction Machine	[ ]	Bedrails	[ ]	Braces
[ ]	Walker	[ ]	Cane	[ ]	Crutches
[ ]	Wheelchair	[ ]	Chair Lift	[ ]	Dressings

Action Taken To Obtain Equipment:
DME/Supplies (485-14):
Equipment Needs Comments:

Courtesy of Management Software, Inc., Springfield, Missouri.

Exhibit 8–2
SKILLED NURSING ASSESSMENT FORM: VITAL SIGNS

Color/Temperature:

Body Size:

Skin Color:
Skin Temp:
Oral Temp:
Rectal Temp:

[ ] Average   [ ] Obese
[ ] Thin   [ ] Malnourished

Pulse:
A: R:

Blood Pressure:
Left: Right:

[ ] Irregular
[ ] Weak
Characteristics:

Lying
Sitting
Standing

Respiration:
Characteristics:

Weight/Height
[ ] Gain   [ ] Loss
Amount of gain/loss:
When gain/loss:
Normal Weight: Height:

Courtesy of Management Software, Inc., Springfield, Missouri.

Exhibit 8–3
PROBLEM LIST OUTPUT FORM

Condition: Oncology

Problem: ONC: Anxiety: Cancer Diagnosis, Treatment—Set: (date)

Status: Anxiety related to diagnosis of cancer, prescribed treatment regimen

Goals: Verbalize feelings, ways to deal—Set: (date)

Status: Will verbalize awareness of feelings and identify ways to deal with them

Interventions: Teach measures to relieve anxiety—Set: (date) Disc:

Type: Teach measures to promote relief of anxiety

Date: _____ Signed: _____

Courtesy of Management Software, Inc., Springfield, Missouri.

groups, ICD-9-CM diagnostic categories, client acuity, a specific nursing group, or even an individual nurse to analyze the relationship between client problems, delivery of care, and client outcomes. Some clinical software modules provide this kind of customized management report, whereas other systems require an interface or connection with a report writer to retrieve the specific client and staff variables from the database. Use of quality report, with a specific client diagnostic group is briefly described in the next section.

In addition to assessments, problem lists, care plans, flowsheets, and evaluation forms, some clinical modules offer other supports for caregiving and documentation. Computer "libraries" are either built into the software or connected as stand-alone packages to agency MIS. If the nurse is using a point-of-care documentation device, she can often access these libraries on her computer at the client's bedside. These libraries can provide drug information, client instruction materials, anatomy and physiology refreshers, or normal lab values to help you perform care, conduct teaching, and evaluate a client's clinical condition.

Data and Information Needs

The data that are collected by the home care nurse provide the essential information needed for the operation of the agency. A new era of quality management has become a fact of life for the health care industry, home care included. Existing software vendors or companies that write MIS software are just now beginning to integrate cost and outcome data at the client level for aggregate analysis. When clients with similar characteristics are grouped, the agency can determine the care needs of that group of clients. Managed care organizations no longer want to reimburse home care agencies on a fee-for-service basis but rather in a fixed capitated amount (usually a per client per month fee) regardless of the amount of service the client requires. Agencies must be able to analyze their historical utilization by client groups to determine what is a reasonable fixed reimbursement that does not jeopardize the quality of care. Here is where integrated MIS provide the necessary data to project client costs.

For a home care agency to meet the challenges of health care reform, integrated home care MIS must be able to correlate cost and outcome data at the client level with an adjustment for case mix or severity of illness. Unfortunately, the home care industry lacks good predictors of utilization based upon client characteristics, and the variation in practice patterns across the country is wide. The use of standardized care plans, generally set up by medical diagnosis, are appearing in newer software packages, but not all clients "fit" the

standard care plan. The home care nurse must clearly document the reason why a client does not fit into the standardized care plan or critical path. Good MIS will track the clients who do not fit and their variances for quick summary statistics.

How do managed care and capitation affect the home care nurse? If a new reimbursement structure dictates the plan of care, the most important question is what resources and tools are available to the home care nurse to achieve the desired outcome in the allotted time. It is important to ask the following questions:

- Are there MIS assessment and care planning guidelines that map out the course of care?
- How can you use these guidelines most effectively to efficiently provide care?
- How much flexibility is there in tailoring the plan of care should the client fall behind in the prescribed plan of care, and how do you document the reasons for the variance from the prescribed plan of care?

Take, for example, the new diabetic. Does the average standard care plan account for your client who has retinopathy, lives alone, and cannot draw up his insulin, prepare a diabetic diet, or inspect his feet for recurring ulcers because of poor vision? How many more visits do you need to accomplish the clinical, knowledge, functional, and behavioral outcomes for your client?

In some cases, the client may never be able to achieve independence with diabetic care and may require long-term home care, which poses yet another challenge for reimbursement and quality improvement documentation. Many kinds of information management challenges are facing every home care agency. The successful agencies will respond with highly integrated MIS and nursing staff that are receptive to adapting to the changing home care practice.

The home care nurse of today must understand various strategies that will allow her to practice more efficiently and effectively in the challenging and ever-changing world of home care. The art of contracting and the use of critical paths can assure the nurse and the agency that care is being delivered consistently and with the client and family's full participation. Working with case managers in a managed care system means that nurses must constantly be working on their communication skills as well as their clinical knowledge of how the client is reaching important outcomes of care. As home care agencies rely more on computer systems and nurses get more involved with point-of-care documentation, the nurse must attain and maintain computer skills that will allow her to be as productive and efficient as possible.

TEST YOURSELF

1. Case example: Mr. Jones is a 60-year old man who was discharged yesterday from the hospital following an aortic valve replacement. Surgery and the postoperative course were uneventful except for two periods of arrhythmia that occurred one day before discharge. Mr. Jones was referred to home care for diet teaching and assessment of his cardiac status. Before surgery, Mr. Jones was a long-distance truck driver for a major moving company. He plans to return to this job as soon as his doctor permits, because he is only three years from retirement. Because Mr. Jones spends weeks away from home, he eats many of his meals at fast-food restaurants and diners. He feels that this way of life is inevitable, given his job and its requirements.

    Mr. Jones has been married for 35 years and has two grown children who live out of the house. His wife would like to see him change his eating habits but is unwilling to confront him on this subject because she sees him as "the boss."

    a. What things would you need to consider before setting up a contract with Mr. Jones?
    b. Describe the main points about contracting you would discuss with Mr. Jones.
    c. Outline the contract you would develop with Mr. Jones.

2. What problems do you think you will find in contracts with clients and their families?

3. If your agency uses critical paths, review the specific diagnoses and procedures they are written on and determine why your agency chose these specific categories.

4. Using a chart from your agency of a client who was recently admitted with a diagnosis of CHF, complete the example of a critical path for the first visit in Appendix F using the information on your client's record. How are the two documentations similar? How are they different?

5. Identify five companies in your community that employ case managers. Do any of them have contracts with your agency?

6. Using the suggestions listed in this chapter for developing a relationship with a case manager, what are the areas you feel you need the most assistance with as you learn to communicate with case managers?

7. What does customer satisfaction mean to you? How do you measure it? How does your agency measure it?

8. If your agency has a management information system, follow the steps involved from when the nurse completes the initial computer data client information sheet in the home until HCFA Form 485 is sent to the physician for signature.

9. Identify the ways computer information gets from the clinical side of your agency (nursing, therapy) to the business side that creates a bill. Who are the people responsible for these functions, and where do you as the nurse "fit" into the flow of information and paper?

REFERENCES

American Health Consultants. (1994). *Hospital home health.* Atlanta, GA: Author.

Certification of Insurance Rehabilitation Specialists Commission. (1993). *CCM certification guide—certification for case managers.* Orlando, FL: Author.

Corbett, C., & Androwich, I. (1994). Critical paths: Implications for improving practice. *Home Healthcare Nurse, 12*(6), 27–34.

Gooldy, J., & Duncan, B. (1994). Home care's role in clinical pathways. *Journal of Home Health Care Practice, 6*(2), 63–69.

Knollmueller, R. (1989). Case management. What's in a name? *Nursing Management, 20,* 38–40.

Muellin, J. (1986). Strategic importance of MIS for home healthcare. *Computers in Healthcare, 7*(6).

Sloan, M., & Schommer, B. (1982). The process of contracting in community health nursing. In B. Spradley (Ed.), *Readings in community health nursing* (pp. 241–248). Boston, MA: Little, Brown.

Zander, K. (1988). Nursing case management: Strategic management of cost and quality outcomes. *Journal of Nursing Administration, 18,* 23–30.

Home Care Nursing Strategies for Success

OBJECTIVES

Upon completion of this chapter, the reader will be able to identify:

1. Ways a home care department can be organized
2. Definition of caseload management
3. Ways to be more efficient in home care nursing practice
4. Three leading causes of stress for home care nurses
5. Ways in which the home care nurse can manage stress
6. Definition and purposes of supervision
7. Expectations of supervision from the perspectives of both the staff nurse and the supervisor
8. Roles and functions of the supervisor
9. Strategies for professional development of the home care nurse

KEY CONCEPTS

- **Home care delivery strategies**
- **Productivity**
- **Stress management**
- **Definition of supervision**
- **Key supervisory roles**
- **Supervisor as orientation coordinator**
- **Professional role development**

AGENCY-SPECIFIC MATERIAL NEEDED

- Productivity standards and ways of evaluating productivity
- Professional reference material available (e.g., books, journals)
- Nurse personnel evaluation schedule, policies, and forms
- Schedule and policies on inservice and continuing education

INTRODUCTION

The field of home care nursing can be professionally challenging for the nurse, especially working with clients and families in the home and community. The home care nurse must understand that the relationship with clients is important, but that there are also interpersonal aspects of the job that require equal attention. Additionally, if the nurse is not aware of the work stressors unique to home care nursing, she is likely to experience burnout and frustration that can have an impact on her personal as well as professional life.

This chapter explores organizational models of home care nursing units as well as caseload and workload management, productivity, and time and stress management–all crucial aspects to becoming an effective home care nurse. How to work effectively with your supervisor and issues related to professional goal development are also discussed. Guidelines and exercises included in this chapter can help the nurse to succeed in these important areas.

HOME CARE NURSING DELIVERY STRATEGIES

The importance of the staff nurse's understanding of the organizational structure and function of the total agency early in her orientation is discussed in Chapter 1. Once that understanding takes place, it is then essential that discussion focus on the organization of the nursing department or unit within the agency. Because nursing plays the pivotal role in a home health agency, the nursing department should be organized so that work is carried out effectively and efficiently and so that the nurse is supported in the tasks she performs in caring for clients.

Organizational Models for Nursing Units

All nurses are familiar with the standard models of nursing care delivery—primary, functional, team, and case method—based on their student or work experiences. These models are generally used in home care agencies but often with different objectives, because home care is provided outside an institution and is a more independent practice. The various delivery models are presented, outlining the ways they are used in a home health agency. It is important to remember that these models focus solely on the responsibilities of nursing personnel in an agency—registered professional nurses (RNs) and licensed vocational nurses (LVNs). Client care activities carried out by parapro-

fessionals, such as home care aides (HCAs), are always directly supervised by the nurse conducting the home visit or the primary care nurse. It is the responsibility of the nurse in charge of the case in the specific nursing model outlined to develop the care plan and supervise all HCA care given to a client. HCA supervision is covered more extensively in Chapter 2.

Primary Care Nursing

Primary nursing combines the concepts of total client care and all-professional nursing staff. In primary nursing, a RN (the primary nurse) assumes total responsibility for planning the care of one or more clients from admission to the agency to discharge. The primary nurse establishes the care plan and provides direct care for clients assigned to her. If someone else provides care in her absence, those providers follow the care plan established by the primary nurse and report back to her. It is also the responsibility of the primary nurse to coordinate communication between all members of the health care team and the client and family. Good communication and feedback are essential when primary nursing is the model used in a home health agency.

In home care, the primary care nursing model has been used extensively, but increasing costs have made this model difficult to implement in an environment that regulates costs so strictly. Often the model is used in combination with the team approach, in which RNs are seen as the individual primary nurses and LVNs are supervised as part of the team and work under the direction of the RNs.

Team Nursing

In team nursing, small groups of nurses work together under the direction of a professional nurse called a team leader. As coordinator of the team, the team leader is responsible for knowing about and planning the care of each client cared for by her team regardless of whether she directly cares for the client. In team nursing, communication between members is essential and can be achieved through formal methods, such as team conferences held on a periodic basis, or informal methods, such as having the team leader communicate frequently with team members.

Team nursing has been used successfully by many home health agencies. By using highly trained and experienced home care nurses to lead the team and make client assignments, RN and LVN team members can contribute their own special skills in caring for clients. For example, if a member of a team is especially apt at caring for clients with ostomies, then she might care for the majority of the team's clients with this condition. Some agencies that use team nursing have the team leader visit clients and perform supervisory functions for the members of her team. The team leader coordinates the care given to all clients, and other members of the team are kept up to date on the progress of the team's clients at team meetings and conferences. It is important to remember that in team nursing, all team members share the responsibility and accountability for the nursing care delivered.

Functional Nursing

Functional nursing, historically seen as the most economical means of providing care, is the model that assigns specific tasks to the nurse, rather than one that delegates total care of specific clients to an individual nurse. For example, medication nurse, treatment nurse, and charge nurse are roles assumed by nurses in hospitals to perform certain functions, and on a unit all three nurses, each with a different role, could carry out the various tasks for the same client during a shift. Because it would be ineffective and inefficient to have various nurses see individual clients in their homes, functional nursing is not a model used to provide home care services.

Case Method

The case method model of nursing, or total client care, is the oldest model of organizing client care. This model was used at the turn of the 19th century by private duty nurses who delivered care primarily in the client's home. Today the model is used primarily in intensive care settings within an acute hospital. The true case method model of nursing is not used in home care agencies, although one could argue that it is used if a client has only a private duty nurse, which might be hired through another branch of the agency (Marquis & Huston, 1987).

Case Management

In the late 1980s, case management and managed care became the buzzwords of health care delivery. New case management models are evolving in institutional and outclient settings. Some home health agencies have organized their nursing units using a case management model; often this model varies somewhat among agencies and may be a combination of the models discussed so far. The following discussion of case management and managed care will help to clarify the different ways that case management can function in a home care nursing department and the roles that nurses can assume in the models.

Some home health agencies implement the case management model, in which the case manager (CM) functions as a team leader and directs the care given to a group of clients (team nursing). The CM may also provide direct care to a group of clients (primary care) and assume supervisory responsibilities, such as the orientation of staff, development of management reports, and evaluation of staff members who work under the CM's supervision. In this model, the CM tracks the reimbursement of clients but may not formally evaluate and report the cost-effectiveness of the care given.

Knollmueller (1989) defines case management as a process that is more than a structure or outcome. She goes on to discuss the American Nurses Association (ANA) description of nursing case management as "a health-care delivery process whose goals are to provide quality health care, decrease fragmentation, enhance the client's quality of life, and contain costs." This coordination of care and communication with all care providers is what public health and home care nurses have been doing for years.

The preceding discussion of nursing models addresses case management as a model to organize nursing services in a home health agency. There are other definitions and models of case management, which exclusively involve the coordination, monitoring, and evaluation of options and services to promote quality, cost-effective client outcomes. Case management as an area of practice is discussed in Chapter 8.

Case Management and Managed Care

Although managed care and case management are often used synonymously, they are very different. In most situations, the term *case management* describes the coordination of care a client receives within the context of the benefit system, but not directly linked to the payer of services. In other words, CMs consider the care a person needs but are not totally responsible for finding all the payment for the needed care. In some instances, CMs and case management systems are set up independently of direct care providers so that the risk of conflict of interest is minimized. Managed care, on the other hand, is the coordination of client services administered by the payer of services, such as an insurance company. Managed care is always tied to reimbursement, and the systems developed to oversee the care provided are linked to payment and utilization of services. For example, an insurance company may have a managed care department that looks for cost-effective ways of caring for clients with certain diseases. That department, then, authorizes the care given in light of the client's insurance benefits and the least expensive services needed to reach the client's goals.

PRODUCTIVITY

Increasing concern about health care costs and the need to control factors that improve efficiency have increased the focus on productivity in home health agencies. The discussion of productivity and visit standards need not conjure up negative responses from staff members within an agency if everyone understands the reasons why productivity and visit standards are so important to a home health agency. First, no agency can survive without at least breaking even on expenses and income, and, to do that, personnel must be efficient. Second, the agency wants to ensure quality, and monitoring productivity can increase the likelihood that staff members are providing high-quality care.

Although productivity is difficult to measure in health care, it is not impossible, and many home health agencies have developed ways to reach this goal. Before the home care nurse can become familiar with the productivity standards used in an agency and understand how they are applied, she must understand the following productivity concepts summarized here from Benefield's (1988) work:

- Productivity is the relationship between the use of resources and the results of that use.
- Efficiency is not necessarily how fast work is done, but how well time is used.
- Quality can improve at the same time that productivity increases.

Improving productivity involves all departments in a home health agency, never just one department or staff member. Productivity is a "people issue," and because approximately 80% of a home health agency's budget is spent on personnel, all agency personnel contribute to productivity. Hands-on skills are very important, but so also is the home care nurse's ability to think critically, solve problems, and make decisions that impact on the total care the client receives. These attributes must be factored into productivity issues.

Visit standards should be developed that consider the intensity of service provided to the client (complexity level of the client) and the case mix (types of clients) of the population served by the agency. The agency should also take into consideration the efficiency of the paper flow in the total organization.

Effectiveness of the service is an important productivity component and a crucial aspect of the agency's quality assurance program. The expectations of the outcomes of the home visit and the standards set for what is to go on in a home visit are important parts of understanding productivity in home care.

FACTORS THAT AFFECT PRODUCTIVITY

A staff nurse should be looking constantly for ways to work smarter, not harder. Studies of professional productivity conclude that the focus should not be on working faster (rushing through visits) but on using time efficiently and spending time doing those skills that the nurse was trained to do (Benefield, 1988). This is an important concept for all employees of the agency to remember, and it can be helpful when finding ways to help others be more efficient. There are several factors that can be considered to increase productivity.

Caseload Management

The caseload is a group of clients assigned. For a primary nurse, CM, or team leader, the caseload will be the clients whose care she must direct. For a member of a team, the caseload will be the case(s) assigned for a given time period, such as a day, week, or whatever the length of time the client is on service. The way that the work relating to these clients is organized is termed *caseload management*. There are many factors that affect the nurse's ability to manage a caseload, including the following:

- the frequency (number of times a week) and length (visit time) of visits to the caseload clients
- the specific needs of the clients in the caseload (e.g., teaching, direct care, coordinating multiagency involvement, and psychosocial involvement). This can be visit- or nonvisit-related time.
- the level of difficulty of the clients in the caseload. This is usually determined by a client classification system used in the agency that categorizes the level of acuity experienced by clients by using several different variables.

Each agency should have systems in place to help the nurse to learn skills of caseload management. The best resources for learning caseload management are scheduling conferences with a supervisor about client issues and working with experienced nurses who can share the ways they have found to be more efficient.

Also, by using the strategies outlined in the home visiting section of Chapter 3 and the suggestions listed in the following pages about contracting and client teaching, the nurse will be able to develop her caseload management skills.

Workload Management

Workload is a summary of all the activities of a home care nurse, including caseload management. Each agency should have a process for analyzing a nurse's workload, often through the use of forms to be completed or interactions with the nursing supervisor. In addition to the material collected for measuring the caseload management activities, the nurse will be recording the time spent on activities other than home visiting. These can include agency activities, such as in-service programs, staff meetings, and conferences; community activities, such as clinics or committee work; work in off-site areas, such as schools; and personal time, such as lunch, holidays, and vacations.

The new staff nurse may not be familiar with keeping track of her daily time in this manner. She should be assured that she is asked to do this, not because of agency distrust, but because the nature of home care is independent and the agency needs to collect this information to justify costs to regulatory bodies and for budgeting purposes. Federal agencies, such as the Internal Revenue Service and the Social Security Administration, also require that this information be recorded. It is important that this information be accurate and up to date to be fair to the nurse and the agency.

Time Management

The only manager of a home care nurse's time is the nurse. To be effective and efficient in professional practice, the nurse must be insightful concerning her use of time. The new home care nurse will identify many items that are time-wasters or time-savers, adding to the list that may have been started earlier in her career. Home care is a very independent practice, and the nurse must use self-discipline and motivation to stay efficient. The use of contracting, outlined in Chapter 8, is the best time-saver a home care nurse can use in clinical practice working directly with clients. There are other ways to manage time effectively, including the following:

- Schedule clients who live in close proximity to each other together to minimize travel time.
- Keep a daily file to identify clients who need to be seen and other activities planned for certain days. A tickler card file or a calendar appointment book

can be used to keep information from becoming misplaced. This is important so that planned visits are kept track of and clients are seen on time.

- If you use a tickler card file, identify the monthly or periodic tasks (e.g., filling out Health Care Financing Administration [HCFA] Form 485) and the date due on the card. When you have completed the task, cross it out or change the due date. File the card at the next new date.
- Tickler cards that are color coded are helpful in alerting you to tasks that need to be done. You may want to use blue cards for supervisory visits, red cards for clients whose physician orders are due, and yellow cards for daily visits.
- Look at your calendar or tickler file daily. Update it as soon as you have new information.
- Find a quiet place to do your recording. This is not always easy in a small office that has a lot of distracting activity going on. If possible, documentation should be completed in the client's home during the visit or immediately after the visit. Many nurses find restaurants in their visiting area that offer enough space and privacy to do their paperwork while the nurse has a soft drink or cup of coffee. If most of the nurse's visit recording is completed before her return to the office, she will be better prepared for the other work activities that await her, and the quality of the recording will improve because the information will have been recorded when it was clear in her memory.
- Charting should be done so well that few additional notes are needed. The recording should be complete enough that if there must be communication with others, such as social workers or physical therapists, the client's record should include the bulk of the required information. Nurses are notorious for repeating orally what they have written (or should have written) in the record—a carryover from the change-of-shift report. This is a waste of time, especially in home care.
- Limit socializing. Most of the workday is spent with clients not colleagues, so it is important to make time to socialize with coworkers. The nurse must determine when that will be and for how long. Meeting with other nurses for lunch can often be a positive use of time while it frees up the time in the office for work-related issues.
- Keep phone time to a minimum. As much as possible, make all telephone calls in one block of time and always have something to work on (e.g., a client record) while on hold. Prepare an agenda for phone conversations to avoid forgetting any pieces of information.

- Delegate work to others. The agency employs support staff that are available to free the nurse for nursing-related functions. The staff nurse should look for ways to improve the quality of interaction among agency staff members, through constructive feedback to the supervisor and in staff meetings. Remember, when a nurse identifies a problem area, it is also up to her to develop ways to solve it and then become committed to making the approach work.
- Always call clients and give them an approximate time for the home visit (e.g., late morning, early afternoon). Do not predict a precise arrival time because scheduling is based on estimated time spent on earlier visits, and the nurse does not want to set up a situation in which the client is worried needlessly about the nurse because she is 15 minutes late.
- Always put specific directions to the client's home on the record so that finding the way will be easier for the nurse and other staff members who may visit the client.

STRESS MANAGEMENT

Home care nurses, who are expected to be highly skilled in assessing and providing care to a diverse group of clients, often develop additional skills as therapists, nutritionists, counselors, and social workers when these specialists are not available. The home care nurse is probably the only person who can change a dressing; prepare a sterile solution; order medical supplies and explain how they will be paid for; recommend a podiatrist who makes home visits; teach a specialized diet; and arrange services for home meal delivery, grocery shopping, homemaking, and transportation for a client with a disability, all during a routine half-hour visit. It is no wonder that clients and families develop a real dependence on home care nurses, because very few professionals in the community can provide as much skill, care, and information.

Most nurses who are new to home care bring some specialized skills, but they usually realize immediately that they have a lot to learn. Even nurses who have worked in home care for years usually feel they are still learning. Community resources are always changing, and the unique dynamics of each home care case continue to provide many challenges.

In order to feel prepared to handle the stress in home care nursing, it is helpful to know what specific issues in home care can be particularly stressful. How does the stress compare with stress in the hospital environment?

Cestari (1989) did a study comparing the stress of hospital nurses and home care nurses. Stressful situations described by home care nurses are interesting and often quite surprising. Nurses working in urban, suburban, and rural areas all described similar stressful situations related to client noncompliance, which was the issue most often mentioned as a recent stressful situation. The stressful situations described by home care nurses included many comments such as, "I keep getting referrals on the same clients. No matter how many ways I try to establish a regime and help them become independent, they always drift back to their noncompliant behaviors. When they are readmitted, the ER wants to blame the home care agency for poor management of the client." Home care nurses also described stress related to aggressive behaviors by clients. "Several of my clients get verbally abusive when I try to explain that their demands for my agency to provide 24-hour care at home are unrealistic." Other nurses seemed frustrated by poorly coordinated efforts by other care providers. "If the aide doesn't show up the client calls me to complain and I get tired of apologizing. Some clients have even gotten my home phone number. They seem to think I'm on duty 24 hours a day!"

Most of the concerns that home care nurses mention regarding physicians are frustrations when physicians do not call back or were unconcerned or uninformed regarding client care management in the home. One nurse described a particular physician who refused to change treatment orders for wound care even though he had not seen the client in several weeks. Several others described physicians who made unrealistic promises to clients about the services that the home care agency could provide. "The doctor told the family that whatever he ordered Medicare would pay for." Situations like these often put the home care nurse in the position of trying to explain to families that the physician did not provide accurate information, something that families may not easily accept.

Stressful situations involving work overload are often described by home care nurses. When asked to describe the two most stressful work situations, the general issue of work overload is a frequent response. "Paperwork" is mentioned most often, with more in-depth descriptions usually referring to cumbersome documentation, HCFA forms, and poorly coordinated office support. Other nurses describe work overload in terms of their daily visit expectations and managing large caseloads. As one nurse commented, "I have a heavy caseload of very sick clients. I can't visit them as often as I should, because I'm so busy trying to coordinate care for too many clients and there is no one to help."

Political and bureaucratic problems that are identified as stressful usually involve regulatory guidelines and paperwork. Nurses often described difficulties in trying to explain to clients why Medicare does not fund certain services or why services have to be discontinued at a certain point. Nurses are often uncomfortable discharging clients who still need care. These comments are echoed by many community health nurses. "Once the Medicare benefits run out we have to discharge most of our elderly clients. They still need the help, but there is no one to pay for it. I hate having to explain the system to people because I don't believe in it myself." The documentation required for Medicare and other insurance claims is also mentioned by many community health nurses as being very stressful. "I don't mind paperwork, but the documentation required by Medicare is ridiculous and they keep adding more!"

Problems with communication in the work unit also concern home care nurses. These concerns focus on the inherent problems nurses in home care face by working primarily outside of the office. "It's hard to get to the staff meetings. I feel like I'm constantly back and forth to the office." Home care nurses often miss the peer support they have in the hospital with nurses on a particular unit. Staff in home care may come and go from the office at different times from day to day. Certainly there is more autonomy in this situation, but it is important to make time to communicate with coworkers.

STRESS MANAGEMENT STRATEGIES

There are several strategies the home care nurse can use to handle the stress she encounters in her work setting. These strategies center around issues of managing conflicting demands, feeling comfortable with the amount of knowledge she is expected to have, and dealing with her increased autonomy and independence.

The biggest overall issue that home care nurses identify as stressful is the broad issue of work overload. Certainly this issue is familiar to nurses in all settings, but the work overload in home care is somewhat different and is based primarily on the volume of clients that the nurse manages, the heavy volume of paperwork, and the subtle stress associated with managing difficult cases without the structure of the hospital or other institution.

Nurses in home care need to anticipate that they will be managing many more cases than they would have in the hospital, initially without much firsthand knowledge of individual clients. New staff nurses should not be expected to assume a large caseload immediately. The most successful approach involves gradually as-

suming a caseload, perhaps over the period of a month. Unfortunately, with recent trends toward staff turnover, the luxury of time may not always be available. Uncovered cases may have been shuffled around among other staff members in the absence of a new primary nurse. All too often the new nurse is greeted with a large file of clients, a barrage of phone calls, and paperwork on clients about whom she knows nothing. In any case, it is best not to expect to be familiar with all of the clients and understand their individual problems right away. The difficult and demanding clients are likely to make themselves known soon enough, and other staff members will surely be familiar with them. Do not be pressured into making decisions and taking action without the initial support of a supervisor or preceptor.

The volume of paperwork in home care takes every new nurse by surprise to some extent. The best advice regarding paperwork is to realize from the outset that it will never be all caught up. The new staff member who works late every evening and takes work home every night to catch up will likely find those solutions to be addictions; she will never be able to manage without taking work home on a regular basis. To some extent, the paperwork becomes more manageable once all of the forms are familiar, but it can still be overwhelming at times. Recently, many agencies have developed committees dedicated to revising paperwork and paper flow, and input from new staff members can be helpful. Committee work can provide an outlet and, in the long run, lead to some creative solutions.

Becoming an expert on all of the reimbursement issues and community resources, in addition to having hands-on nursing skills, is an ongoing learning process. Most nurses new to home care find they are immediately more aware of current events and their impact on the community, especially legislative issues. Becoming active in the community is a natural inclination as the significance of social, political, and bureaucratic issues takes on a new dimension. For the nurse doing home care in her own community, this role may be even more rewarding.

Many new nurses in home care look forward to increased autonomy and independence, and these are certainly welcome changes from working in an institutional setting. Very often, however, the autonomy can lead to a sense of isolation, especially for new staff members. If other nurses are being oriented at the same time, this may not be a problem. The new nurse can try to plan office time when most of the nurses seem to be in the office, either early in the morning or in the late afternoon. New staff nurses can learn much by observing how other nurses manage their caseloads, paperwork, and phone calls. It may be helpful to find out whether people have a meeting spot for lunch, or whether there is another nurse seeing clients in an area convenient for meeting. Many home care nurses admit to eating many of their meals in their cars, but it is a good idea not to get into that routine every day.

Recognizing the stress in home care nursing is probably the biggest issue to confront in beginning to develop strategies to identify and deal with the stress better. In order to improve collaboration within the profession, nurses in all work settings need to develop a more contemporary view of home care nursing practice. This recognition can begin with nursing faculty in community health programs, who should be helping nursing students develop a more realistic perception of community health nursing—the good, the bad, and the difficult issues. Providing this foundation for all nurses, whatever their eventual work setting, will have many benefits. Exposure to the work stressors of home care nurses may begin to diminish the current sense that nurses in other settings are unaware that home care nursing can be stressful.

Nurses in work settings outside of home care would also benefit from additional inservice and exchange programs to put them in touch with the contemporary practice environment of home care nursing. Firsthand knowledge of the home situations, the chronic non-compliant clients, and the voluminous paperwork and case management expectations of the home care nurse is largely unknown by other nurses. As discharge planners and hospital nurses understand these demands, there may be better discharge planning and referrals to home care agencies. Nurses considering positions in home care should recognize that all nurses deal with stress in the workplace. Certainly there are many attractions to home care nursing and highly skilled, sensitive, hard-working staff nurses are always needed. The types of stress faced by home care nurses are different, but so are the rewards. The combination of these challenges is what keeps many of the profession's best nurses where they are happiest, in home care nursing.

SUPERVISION IN HOME CARE

Successful performance of staff nurse functions in a home care agency depends on philosophical harmony between the mission of the agency and the beliefs of all the staff. Most agencies have a mission statement that guides organizational planning and purpose. It is not enough to believe that staff supervision is a mutual educational and administrative effort. This belief must be demonstrated through practice in professional relationships. The staff nurse is the agency's primary rep-

resentative to the community and conveys the agency message of its mission and standards of care by the way nursing in the home is practiced. It is the staff nurse who brings life to the agency's goals and mission.

The method by which the nurse relates and carries out the clinical work through practice is a dynamic process, and, as with any experience, maturing in the role does much to enhance success. Bringing together the primary roles of staff development and administrative management is the function and process of supervision that guides and directs nursing practice. The staff nurse has the most contact with and is most influenced and affected by the supervisor. Early in a staff nurse's experience, a discussion about the purpose and expectations of supervision is very important.

The terms *nurse manager* and *client care manager* are replacing the older term of *supervisor* in many home care agencies. Essentially, the role is identical or very similar. One difference in current practice from the traditional supervisory role is the increasing focus on the supervisor being involved with and an expert in clinical practice rather than only administrative issues. Just as the assignments of activities may have differences for the traditional supervisory role, there may be variations of nurse manager responsibilities depending upon the home care agency's needs. For the purpose of this section, the more traditional term of *supervisor* is used.

Defining Supervision

The word *supervision* brings to the minds of many an image of an overbearing, order-giving authority demanding certain behavior and checking up on the work of the staff member. Although it is hard for the supervisor to avoid some of that description, for the staff nurse, supervision can be positive, enabling her to feel good about the work done and know that advice is available if and when it is needed, and does not only consist of having one's work scrutinized. Unfortunately, supervision is often thought about in negative rather than in positive terms.

One definition of a supervisor that should be primary to the home care nurse is that of an enabling person through which staff are helped to make the best use of their knowledge and skills, to improve them, and to do the job better. Supervision should emphasize the helping and nurturing aspect of relationships. The ultimate goal is to fulfill the agency's mission through more effective efforts on the part of its workers. The supervisor is the person in the middle who represents the agency and its administration to the staff and the staff to the administration.

The Purposes of Supervision

The first purpose of supervision is to facilitate and accomplish work through the staff. This involves carefully planned and timely participatory exchanges between the staff nurse and the supervisor. Communication should be candid and, at times, critical, with emphasis placed on how the supervisor can help make the staff member's work more successful.

A second purpose of supervision is to see that the care rendered to the client and the family by the staff nurse or other worker is safe and appropriate. Concern for public safety is of prime importance for both the home care nurse and the supervisor. Should there be any evidence of a threat to safe nursing practice, the supervisor must immediately take steps to see that it is corrected. Corrective steps include counseling, observing the care as it is being given, and being certain that the needed educational opportunities are made available for the nurse.

A third purpose of supervision is to facilitate staff development. This should include both an individualized plan and an agency commitment to guide the staff member toward improved clinical practice and build for greater growth in the nursing profession. Facilitating staff is important, but all too often it is not seen as requiring major effort. Developing leadership from within the staff ranks is important, but many supervisors may not have a planned approach for achieving this goal with staff members. The supervisor and staff member should discuss goals as an integral part of the relationship between them and lay out a plan for progressive experience based on demonstrated success in earlier work. Developing staff can lead to the staff nurse's growth in more responsible positions within the organization. Supervisors of talented staff nurses will want to reap the benefits of work done. It is right for the supervisor to take pride in observing a staff worker making progress and contributing to the profession, regardless of whether the nurse stays with the home care agency or moves to another work situation.

Many nurses now working in home care have had years of experience in acute care settings and, with the changes because of health care delivery reform, find they can secure home care staff nurse positions. The role of the supervisor is shaped differently in hospitals because there is more support and there is the immediate capability for consultation with a colleague concerning clinical problems. Intervention in a clinical crisis is readily available.

In home care, the nurse is alone in the home where astute clinical assessments and decisions must be made accurately. The key person for the nurse is the supervisor who serves as consultant and advisor in clinical decision making. Telephone or in-person discussion at the office is common. The staff nurse quickly realizes the value of a competent and sensitive supervisor who is a colleague, coach, and compassionate critic.

Expectations

Growth and development in clinical practice as a staff nurse parallel some of the stages used to describe human development. Many changes can take place within each stage, but a person moves from one to the next as new skills and tasks are accomplished and builds toward increasingly more difficult skills and more defined use of clinical judgment. Therefore, the pace of acquiring clinical practice expertise is not the same for each nurse. Accordingly, each has needs and expectations that require individual planning and implementation.

Expectations of the Staff

New staff nurses will expect the supervisor to explain and describe the background of the agency and the role and tradition it has filled in the community over the years it has been in business. They will need specific instruction about techniques, procedures, community resources, caseload management, time management, and organizational skills. A staff nurse will want the supervisor to explain the appropriate channels of communication and to provide information on how and why a policy or procedure was developed.

An experienced staff member will want freedom to develop ideas, to be creative, and to take on increasing independence. Further, the nurse should expect opportunities to broaden her clinical practice and look to the supervisor for ways to achieve this. Finally, a home care nurse will expect assistance in increasing her clinical competence and will have a good measure of job satisfaction as a result of that increased competence.

The supervisor is a role model for the staff nurse who focuses on clinical decision-making skills that are basic to competent staff nurse home care practice. The staff nurse should be encouraged to buy selected reference books and subscribe to journals that will enhance her base of clinical knowledge.

Expectations of the Supervisor

The supervisor is expected to have a positive influence on the quality of home care services provided by the agency and to provide leadership that results in efficiency and job satisfaction for the staff member. Of course, the supervisor is influenced by previous work experiences and by the size and scope of the agency's services. Again, expectations are shaped by what the supervisor feels comfortable and competent doing. New and unfamiliar aspects of supervision require more concentration and time to develop a level of confidence.

The nurse's supervisor wants the nurse to feel free to seek and to accept direction in new experiences and to have the support of the agency to guide and foster competence in the role. A constant flow of new information must be assimilated and used in caring for the home care client. It is the supervisor who is most likely to make this information available to staff nurses. The agency will purchase books and reference materials, subscribe to special resources, and find ways to facilitate the use of other provider specialists so that pertinent clinical information is made available for staff. As the staff nurse builds a clinical library, the supervisor, too, expands subscription lists and builds a personal professional library that can be shared with staff.

Expectations of the Administrator

The administrator is usually involved in the outside affairs of the home care agency, whereas the supervisor and staff nurse are focused on the day-to-day activities. In the same way that supervisors get their work done through staff members, administrators get a measure of their work done through the supervisor. Administrators will expect the staff to be knowledgeable and continue to learn about the role of the agency, the scope of safe clinical practice in the home, and, to some extent, the larger health care system. The administrator expects the work unit to be managed effectively and to be efficient in providing services and enhancing staff productivity. Whenever it is necessary, interpretation of agency policy and services to others in the community is expected to be done by the supervisor or staff nurse. It is an integral part of the staff role to offer to participate in clinical development of peers as a role model and to demonstrate teamwork among colleagues. The administrator expects support from both supervisors and staff nurses as well as a partnership in providing the best home care available.

Balancing Supervisory Roles and Functions

The home care nurse must become acquainted with the breadth and functions of the supervisory roles.

There are many responsibilities that fall to the supervisor and that are not often recognized by staff nurses as being essential. These responsibilities can be divided into three categories: administrative, educational and staff development, and communications linkages. The staff nurse is the primary beneficiary of all of these. It is possible to identify certain duties for each category that will highlight the broad practice scope of the nursing supervisor in a home care agency. Some of the supervisor's administrative duties include the following:

- managing the work flow of all workers in a designated unit
- participating in planning, developing, and evaluating agency programs
- participating in planning, developing, and evaluating agency policies that affect the delivery of home care services
- hiring and terminating professional staff
- managing the quality assurance program for the work unit
- assisting in the budget process for the work unit
- collecting and analyzing service, statistical, and fiscal data
- monitoring the workers' productivity and fiscal activities of the work unit
- facilitating and participating in research activities

Selected educational and staff development responsibilities include the following:

- helping staff members, individually and as a group, to learn and to build on that learning as an orientation experience or, later on, as experienced staff nurses
- developing and implementing recording formats so that necessary and current information is provided for more informed clinical practice
- encouraging and facilitating staff participation in agency and professional activities
- preparing formal and informal performance evaluations to aid in growth of staff members
- fostering formal and informal educational efforts and facilitating staff participation in continuing education, inservice education, and academic educational programs

Some functions in enhancing communications include the following:

- providing a forum for open communication between upper-level management and staff nurses

- representing the agency to the community in formal and informal ways
- collaborating with other home care providers in planning and providing services to the ill at home
- informing staff about regulatory changes or policies that influence the home care services being provided

These lists highlight the scope of responsibilities that a clinical supervisor has in a home care agency. Although the staff nurse is the direct recipient of the performance of these duties, all who relate with the home care agency benefit from them. The staff nurse and the supervisor work so closely together that it goes unnoticed that the supervisor influences so many aspects of the home care agency service. By understanding the supervisor's activities, the staff nurse becomes a potential supervisor.

Limits of Supervision

There are limitations to what can be provided by the supervisor. Identifying the boundaries of supervisory practice is essential; it is easy for the nurse to expect too much from her supervisor and then be disappointed when the expectations are not met. One limitation is that the supervisor and the nurse do not work in the same setting. The supervisor cannot be present at every move and action of the staff nurse. This is especially true in home care where the clinical activities are performed in a home without other advisors available except by telephone. The supervisor should function much like a coach on a playing field. The coach does not play a position or cover a base but expects the player to do that. Similarly, in home care the work is delegated to the staff nurse, and it is expected that the care will be done appropriately.

Another aspect of supervision that may be viewed as a limitation is that while the relationship between staff and supervisor is close, it should be an independent relationship. The supervisor should not be seen as a counselor for personal problems, although it may be necessary for the supervisor to advise and refer a worker for assistance if outside problems interfere with work.

Key Supervisory Roles

Orientation

When a new staff nurse begins work at a home care agency, it is the supervisor who arranges for and provides a large part of the orientation that is necessary for learning the work. This is one of the most important functions of the supervisor, next to the ongoing day-to-day clinical supervision that is in place for staff. The initial orientation includes basic information concerning the client care record, selected agency client care policies and procedures, and other information provided in this text. Spending a day with other nurses acquaints the new nurse with the typical visiting day and associated activities.

As mentioned in Chapter 1, discussion about the philosophy and mission of the agency should be included in the orientation so that the new nurse can begin to think and "feel" what they mean in practice. They should be reviewed during a job interview, but become relevant during the orientation period when the nurse puts them into practice. Orientation is intense, and although the new nurse may not be out making visits and working hard in caring for a client in the home, the nurse will be tired by the end of the day because of all the information that must be remembered.

After this initial time of learning about home care, the agency, and some of the usual activities, the orientation moves toward more clinical work. For instance, the scope of home care nursing practice begins to help the nurse think about and do some caseload management before she is introduced to community resources and related content. This is one of the most important times in any staff worker's life, and it is also one of the most difficult times because it seems so distant from the real work. Home care, for some, is medical-surgical nursing moved from the hospital to the home. Although home care nursing can include medical-surgical work, the scope is much broader because family and community are important aspects to include in a plan of care, as discussed in Chapter 2.

Staff Motivation

Often one hears administrators or supervisors say that a certain staff member "is such a pleasure" to have on the agency staff. Just what is it that makes that person so special? When it comes down to it, often it is that the nurse is highly motivated and excited about the work, shows initiative, and finds professional and intellectual stimulation through supervisory contact. This can be a problem for the supervisor who has many people to supervise and not all are equally motivated in their work. The staff member who is resistant and demonstrates little or no individual initiative is difficult, but not impossible, to deal with. Such people can cause particular problems if they complain frequently and influence other staff members in the work unit by using a divide and conquer tactic.

Studies have identified some common factors that predict an increase in motivation on the job. These include a sense of achievement, recognition, and responsibility, with salary being near the end of the list of items. The use of tangible rewards, usually money, is one way to recognize and motivate a staff worker. Placing too high a value on money can be risky because, in some ways, money is the easiest reward to give, but it may be offered at the expense of other rewards that do more to promote professional growth. A staff member also can be rewarded through attendance or participation at a professional conference, subscription to a professional journal of choice, or the purchase of a clinically appropriate book.

Productivity

Productivity is a reflection of motivation. If staff members feel a sense of "ownership" of their product (clinical service), they will show a measurable level of achievement. Productivity is viewed by some as one type of management control. Measuring actual output or work done by staff and comparing it with budgeted expectations is increasingly common in home care agencies, and it can influence the revenue that can be assigned to support staff activities, including staff salaries. This may be viewed by staff as a punishing approach, but the fact is that when chargeable visits are made and accounted for, there is a direct impact on the income side of the agency ledger. The escalating cost of health care, including home care, is a total agency concern, not just one for the board of directors and the administrators. Improving the efficiency of staff is an essential part of the productivity strategy. There may well be ways that the staff nurse can focus on the clinical assessment and intervention of a home visit and not have to attend to the many other important details pertaining to admission and billing. Perhaps a time has been reached when a nonclinical person can complete these parts of the admission process, beginning with securing data by phone and possibly following up with a home visit to secure financial information. Hospitals have nonclinical staff handling the admissions process, and many home care agencies are considering the same thing. This reduces the burden on the staff nurse of nonclinical work with the result of greater productivity in substance and numbers of home visits to clients. Staff members, especially nurses, have much material to keep in mind when recording a visit. There are many details to put onto the clinical record and onto various forms that must be submitted for accounting purposes. Agency administrators can come up with a variety of system changes to facilitate the nurses' work, but the effective use of these systems depends on the nurse.

All of this work is necessary as a part of demonstrating productivity levels. This responsibility is shared by the supervisor and the staff member.

Staff Development

Development activities with the new employee initially will focus on proficiency in the day-to-day work. As the staff nurse gains experience, efforts can be directed toward other issues involving home care. In the beginning of a staff nurse's work experience, the supervisor should establish a system of regular conferences for the purposes of coaching and planning caseload management. Aside from working with an individual staff nurse toward early independence in clinical practice, staff development is aimed at increasing the clinical competence of a staff group. Staff development is a process rather than a structured program, and, as such, it is a dynamic and ongoing event in the life of the staff member that should be shared and planned with the clinical nursing supervisor.

Clinical Conference

Clinical conferences are not a new concept, but often they are undervalued because of the time needed to focus a group discussion on a given client situation or a clinical condition for purposes of clinical management. One of the best ways to learn from one another is to share clinical situations and discuss appropriate interventions and care plans. It is always useful to have access to a clinician (a nurse, physical therapist, or physician) during these discussions as a way to expand knowledge and to consider additional clinical planning on behalf of the client. Although one may think that the case presented at such a clinical conference must be unusual, the best learning happens in those situations that are common in any caseload of the home care nurse.

Individual Conference

Years ago, it was expected by both the staff member and the supervisor that weekly conferences would be scheduled and that these appointments were kept. It was during these discussions that coaching in the ways of clinical practice were formulated and plans for implementation were made. Until the staff nurse feels comfortable in these sessions, there may be some tension, although this feeling should not last beyond the first month. The format of individual conferences is usually a tutorial in case management and caseload planning, as well as an opportunity to ask questions and explore methods of clinical practice pertinent to the responsibilities of the community and client home care needs. It is regrettable that individual conferencing has been dropped in many agencies and replaced with group teaching or, worse, no opportunity for coaching at all. The new staff nurse can encourage individual conferencing in her agency if clinical conferences are not currently being held.

Caseload Planning

Educating staff members in caseload management is a supervisory function that was once discussed primarily in individual conferences and now has shifted to group or team conferences. Managing client care requires identifying the needs of clients served by the home care agency and establishing an appropriate and timely plan of care. This is achieved most successfully in individual discussion between the supervisor and the staff member. It is not necessary to do this every day, but given that the average length of stay on the home care caseload is a scant two to four weeks, it is essential to discuss and review care plans when the client is first admitted to the agency for care and every few days thereafter. Caseload planning includes consideration of care by other home care providers, such as the medical social worker; physical, occupational, or speech therapist; and HCA. Too often the staff nurse will discharge the client when nursing services are completed but other providers need to continue. Because the nurse is usually the coordinator of the client's care, it is essential in case planning to account for these providers and their work on behalf of the client.

Field Observation

Field observation is the tried and true method of assisting a staff nurse in the practice of home care nursing. When it is carried out well, it can be a most useful tool for teaching and for evaluating clinical performance. Often observation can affect the comfort and spontaneity of both the staff member and the family in their interaction. This can be avoided by having the staff nurse, in preparing for the visit, outline its purpose and expected outcome and discuss the extent to which the supervisor will participate in the visit.

A shared home visit is a variation of this supervisory method. In this case, the staff nurse and supervisor negotiate ahead of time about which parts of the visit will be performed by whom. Generally it is appropriate to plan field observations from time to time. Periodic field visiting with the staff nurse keeps the supervisor informed about the level of practice at which the staff nurse performs. As new technology is implemented in the home, it is useful for the supervisor to visit with the staff nurse and to learn about or teach

the client about the new procedure. Conducting field visits with the staff nurse is the best way to initiate demonstration and return-demonstration of procedures or techniques of a skill and to observe the staff member's interaction with the client and the family. Most supervisors work weekends and holidays and must be able to describe a new technique or technology to staff members working with them. This is a good way for all parties involved to keep current on new and changed methods of care for the home care client.

Performance Evaluation

There are few activities that strike terror in the hearts of the staff more than when it is time for the performance evaluation. This need not be the feeling if the evaluation is developed as an instructive process during which plans are made jointly for facilitating the professional development of the staff member. Evaluation is perceived as a managerial activity more than an educational activity because it is often tied to merit or annual salary increments. A primary purpose of evaluation is to encourage each staff member to improve performance in the current job and to provide opportunities for workers to grow within the job. Too often, evaluation can be a litany of criticism and fault finding regarding past performance, or it is a glowing report of perfect performance. Neither approach is appropriate. The evaluation process should move beyond the past, which is a point from which to start but not at which to stop. Goal setting is the key to a future-oriented approach that stimulates improvement and growth. These goals should be developed by the staff member, and the supervisor should respond with ideas about ways to assist the worker in keeping the goals realistic and in achieving the stated goals. In the Test Yourself section at the end of this chapter, the agency's schedule and process for performance evaluations can be examined with your supervisor.

Problem Solving

Problem solving is often discussed as though it were a simple matter of coming up with the right answers. Actually, problem solving involves analyzing a problem and using factual information as a basis for examining it. The nurse must consider alternatives and implement the one that best suits the individual, the work unit, and the agency. Much supervisory time is spent in problem solving with staff, whether it is regarding assigning clients to staff workers, rearranging work activities, settling conflicts, thinking through a plan for clinical intervention for the home care client, or planning and implementing changes in the work unit. The staff member acquires problem-solving skills for routine day-to-day activities in a fairly short period of time. The more complex situations, especially those of a clinical nature, take longer to grasp and the staff member will often require the expertise of others.

What Makes Supervision Fun

The part of the supervision that is exciting for the staff nurse and the supervisor is the noticeable growth that occurs professionally. This growth is expected. It happens in different ways and in different time frames, depending upon where the staff nurse is in her clinical development. It is rewarding to feel some evidence of clinical growth and leadership when the staff nurse realizes her potential and reaches for the next rung on the ladder of professional advancement. It may not be possible for the home care agency to recognize the achievement made except to approve the recommendation of the supervisor at evaluation time for a merit increase in salary. There are other ways of recognizing good clinical judgment and practice among nurses and paraprofessionals. One is to develop an in-house ceremony for presenting a certificate or statement recognizing a particular situation where exemplary clinical nursing or HCA practice made a difference. Another way is to nominate a staff nurse with an excellent practice record for a state nurses' association award or recognition for expertise in home care. Too often, the time is not taken to recognize, however informally, a nurse or paraprofessional colleague's work for a special intervention from which others can learn and for which all can applaud.

Clinical Exercises Common in Home Care

The Complex Clinical Condition

As a staff nurse of eight months, you are visiting a client who is homebound, in fact, confined to bed unless there are two people to assist her to the chair with the help of a lift. The son with whom she lives is unable to manage the increasing personal care needs for his mother. For this reason, contact with her primary physician is irregular, and medical care usually takes place in the emergency department of the local hospital without this physician seeing her. Your clinical assessment determines that this client is physically compromised and headed for serious trouble. The primary physician agrees, in response to your call, that the client belongs in a long-term care facility. The physician states further that continuing home visits and requesting more help in the home (e.g., more aides, more equip-

ment) only helps the son to postpone making the necessary plans. The physician then says, "I will not sign any more orders for home care services." You had not discussed this situation with your supervisor because she was new in the job (about four months), and you now need help. What do you do now? How? When?

Supervising HCAs

The district where you are assigned a home care caseload has a large need for the services of HCAs. In fact, you realize that your HCA supervision is increasingly hard to do in a timely way. You calculate that in a month's time, on the average, you must make about 20 supervisory visits. Scheduling them for when the aide is in the home and doing them every two weeks is becoming a problem in planning. This, of course, is in addition to new admissions of clients, new HCA orientations, and continuing visits for clients for clinical nursing care. You discuss your problem with your supervisor. What plans for supervising aides might you consider?

The "Special" Assignment Nurse

Your staff nurse caseload is focused in the specialty area of high-risk maternal-child health care. You came to the home care agency with hospital experience in newborn intensive care, your area of expertise. This agency has not sought this client population in recent years, so it was necessary to build a reputation in the care of high-risk maternal-child health clients with providers who might refer clients to the agency. The intent was to improve discharge planning and to facilitate care in the home. After a year, this program was evaluated and showed minimal growth in numbers of referrals among infants and virtually no referrals of high-risk mothers. This is puzzling, and you wonder what you should do differently to secure appropriate home care referrals for these high-risk clients. Meanwhile, because your caseload is very small and you continue to attend meetings at different hospitals on the average of two per week, your daily productivity is minimal. You know your supervisor is concerned, and you decide to discuss this with her. What ideas do you offer?

Team Leader and Leadership

You have worked for this home health agency for 10 years and you know your way around well. You have seen many staff nurses (and supervisors for that matter) come and go. Your supervisor rotates team leadership on a weekly basis among the nurses and other home care staff on your team. The supervisor remarks that this is really not team leadership, but rather a necessary practical move for distributing the work for the day and planning among the staff nurses which home care visits the LVN might make that day. You are tired of this team leader business and resent having to take your turn. When you see your name on the list, you seem to forget to assume the task for the week, leaving everyone confused and angry with you. You decide to discuss the need to continue to take your turn inasmuch as you have seniority and should be able to be dropped from the list. Just as you think about this, the supervisor calls you into her office for a conference and she begins with. "I'm troubled about the way you conduct yourself on the team. During the time you are assigned to lead the daily planning you don't show up." Where do you begin?

Consulting a Clinician

As a staff nurse covering a district for home care clients, you find that the cases are becoming increasingly more clinically complex. Several reasons explain this. Clients are discharged earlier from the acute care hospital, the people are older and more vulnerable as a result, and conditions that clients present with and now survive with seem to increase in number. You discuss your cases regularly with your supervisor, and one day she solicits your ideas about the need for some more clinical nursing consultation that might help staff nurses become better informed. You are not sure what this means and how it would be implemented. What you are certain of, though, is that this might be a reflection on how your nursing practice is viewed and you don't feel good about it. How do you proceed?

Time Management and Caseload Management

In any given week, your caseload is expanded by at least six new cases. Of course, during this time, some discharges exist because of rehospitalization, recovery, or death. You find that much of your time during the first, and often the second, visit is spent securing the necessary client signatures for various forms, reviewing the client bill of rights, and checking the insurance, Medicaid, or the Medicare card for the spelling of the name and number that goes with it. Each signature requires explanation. You feel frustrated because you notice that so much of your visit time is spent on these necessary tasks that you worry you might be skimping on getting a thorough enough clinical assessment on which to base your plan of care. At your next supervisory conference, you mention this to your supervisor and the two of you think about how this might be addressed and remedied. What are your ideas?

Productivity: Is It Only Numbers of Visits?

You are seated in the office with your supervisor who lays out the previous month's productivity report. Your eyes fall to the bottom line and note that your monthly visit numbers and the year-to-date numbers seem to be inconsistent with the other staff; you have too few visits. The discussion begins with that bottom line and immediately you feel yourself getting defensive and you decide to be careful what you say. As a result, you seek an explanation of the various columns (travel time, nondirect service time, preparation and postvisit time, etc.) to determine what all the numbers mean. What do you do next?

Finishing the Paperwork

Your desk is a mess. Papers are stacked, records have piled up, and a note from your supervisor on the top record says "Can't find the 485 for Mr. Jones . . . the request from the intermediary for more information is due today for Mrs. Brown . . . the visit made three days ago for Mrs. Black is not charted." You go to your supervisor and say that you need help to get all the paperwork done and submitted. You realize that no one can do this work for you and that, with each day, you can easily get further behind, especially if you have to do paperwork for an admission client. Now what?

The Motivated Staff Nurse

You just love your work and the variety of clinical situations you must attend to during your day with the home care agency. There is so much to learn and so many new procedures to do that your brain feels full. You decided earlier this year that you would subscribe to two nursing journals, and you pledged to read them as well. You are reading an article one evening at home about a procedure for drawing blood from a Port-A-Cath, and you remember having heard a nurse colleague discuss this a few days earlier. You bring in the article and share it with the nurses (including the one who had been discussing it) and then post it for the entire unit to read. Your supervisor is pleased that you did this and comments about it to the group of nurses. A couple of days later, you overhear a staff nurse say, "Yeah, you know she's trying to be smart and make us look bad because she gets those journals." You decide to discuss this with your supervisor at your next conference. How do you begin?

PROFESSIONAL DEVELOPMENT OF THE HOME CARE NURSE

Unlike other areas of nursing, the home care nurse spends much of her time independently, visiting clients in their homes. This means that there is little time or opportunity for discussion, informal socializing, or sharing clinical issues with peers. If a nurse is accustomed to hospital-based practice, this partial isolation may take some adjustment. There are strategies that the home care nurse can employ to avoid the feelings of isolation and to foster professional development in home care nursing.

In many health care organizations, there are sufficient numbers of nurses working together to allow for informal socialization or collaboration. In home care nursing, the nurses may come into the agency for an hour in the morning and may or may not return to the office at the end of the day. Because the rest of the day is spent conducting independent home visits, there is little time for socialization or discussion of clinical issues with peers. The home care nurse should try to carve some time out of the schedule on a regular basis to meet colleagues for coffee or lunch. This is probably impossible on a daily basis, but once or twice a week is a good goal. If the agency has a regular coffee break time for staff before they leave for home visits, the nurse should try to attend. Interaction with all agency staff members can go a long way toward helping the nurse feel part of the whole home care agency.

It is also important for the home care nurse to continue to develop her knowledge and skills in the area of home care nursing. In hospital settings, many opportunities exist for impromptu discussions of clinical issues or informal inservice demonstrations of a new procedure. In home care nursing, these opportunities are not available and must be scheduled into the daily routine. The agency will likely have regularly scheduled inservice programs for nurses. The nurse should attend these programs, even if they cover a topic with which she is very familiar, because they can provide her with the opportunity to refresh and update her knowledge and interact with peers. Home care nurses should try to take advantage of the many continuing education programs offered by home care agencies and colleges in the community.

Publications on Home Health Care

In addition to inservice and continuing education programs, the nurse can remain abreast of current issues in the field through a review of the literature coming from the state nurses' association, the state home care association, and home care journals. The agency may have a central location where newsletters from various associations are posted. The nurse can ask her supervisor where those are kept and plan to spend a few minutes each week catching up on the current is-

sues facing home care. The following are some journals, newsletters, and videos to which the home care nurse may have access:

- *Caring* is a monthly home care journal published by the National Association for Home Care (NAHC). Each issue has a theme and includes articles on trends and clinical services of interest to home care agencies.
- *Journal of Home Health Care Practice* is published quarterly by Aspen Publishers. This journal chooses a home care topic and then has several articles that apply to that topic. For example, issues have focused on case management, aging, pediatric/private duty services, and continuum of care.
- *Journal of Nursing Administration* (JONA) has a home care section. It is a good overall journal for managers and administrators, and the home care section makes it especially useful. This journal is published by Lippincott.
- *Homecare Direction* is a monthly newsletter from Beacon Health Corporation. The stated purpose of the newsletter is to provide "homecare tested solutions to the tough challenges you face every day." This aid is focused on delivering quality care under Medicare regulations. It is a newsletter especially helpful for the staff nurse and home care manager. Beacon Health can be reached at 1-800-553-2041.
- *Home Health Care Nurse*, published by Lippincott, is a monthly journal that covers the clinical and general aspects of home care nursing. It is especially directed to the needs of the staff nurse and clinical manager.
- *Home Health Digest* is published by Aspen Publishers. This monthly newsletter gives a synopsis of current significant home care articles recently published in more than 100 journals. It is a time-saving resource to keep up to date without taking the time to read and subscribe to several journals.
- *Home Health Focus* is a monthly newsletter from Mosby. The objective is to "assist and confirm the home care nurse's practice as well as challenge the nurse to think about new possibilities wherever she lives or works."
- *Home Health Line* is a weekly newsletter that focuses on all aspects of home care and is especially useful for administrators.
- *NAHC Report* is a weekly newsletter that comes to members of the NAHC. It covers the events in Washington that affect home care, trends occur-

ring across the country, and news of the association.

- State newsletters are published by state home care associations and come out in various time frames. They have news about state laws and regulations as well as information about state trends, continuing education, and meeting news. Many also have excellent coverage of national issues.
- *Ostomy/Wound Management: The Journal for Extended Client Care Management.* This is a journal published nine times a year by Health Management Publications. It focuses on the clinical aspect of wound care management.

If your agency does not subscribe to a home care nurse journal, it would be helpful for you to have an individual subscription to keep informed about the current issues in home care. It is important that the home care nurse have educational resources available to her as she practices. Because the home care nurse sees a variety of clients with different diagnoses in the course of the day, she will need to have several books available to her as references. Some home care nurses keep their books in a small box in the trunk of the car. The home care nurse should have access to:

- A nursing drug reference: Although the agency may have the *Physicians Desk Reference* (PDR), a drug book aimed especially at nurses is critical. This book should include a detailed description of medication indications, actions, contraindications, and side effects.
- A standard medical-surgical text: A medical surgical nursing text that describes the physiologic basis of disease, medical treatment and procedures, and suggested nursing care is essential.
- Clinical reference guides: There are several easy-to-read, small, compact books that detail the specifics of home care practice. An example of a clinical reference guide is Humphrey's *Home Care Nursing Handbook,* published by Aspen Publishers. This book is a quick reference guide to situations the nurse would find in the home.

Professional Goal Setting

Professional development requires that home care nurses determine their career goals and the strategies to achieve those goals. When a nurse is new to home care, her professional goals will most likely include getting used to a new practice environment with a new body of knowledge. As she becomes accustomed to home care practice, goals will shift from maintenance of the professional role to professional growth.

Many home care agencies are large enough to allow the home care nurse to professionally develop within the existing organizational structure. As the home care nurse practices, she should be aware of the areas of practice that she finds most rewarding. This will give her direction to her professional goals and help determine strategies to achieve those goals. For example, if a home care nurse finds that she enjoys coordinating other providers of care, supervising HCAs, and providing resources for the professional development of her peers, she may find that the role of clinical supervisor may be attractive. On the other hand, if the home care nurse really enjoys caring for the most complex clients, researching new and innovative care strategies, and evaluating the effects of that care, perhaps the home care nurse should consider becoming a clinical specialist or a nurse practitioner in home care. Whatever the desired direction of her professional career, there are many opportunities for growth in home care nursing.

Home care nurses interested in advanced education have many opportunities available to them. For those home care nurses who aspire to a career in home care administration, master's level preparation in nursing administration, business, public health, or health services administration is available at many colleges and universities. Any one of these programs of study would prepare the home care nurse with the necessary knowledge and skills to move into a management or administrative role. For those home care nurses who want to develop as expert clinicians, graduate education can focus on a specific area of clinical practice, such as pediatric nursing, psychiatric-mental health nursing, or oncology nursing. Some home care nurses choose to become family nurse practitioners because they see the value of having advanced assessment and clinical management skills in the home care setting.

The explosive growth in the home health care delivery system has resulted in a wealth of opportunities for home care nurses. The home care nurse must determine her professional goals and develop strategies to achieve those goals. Whatever the direction of her professional practice, the home care nurse may seek advanced education to prepare her for new challenges in home health care.

TEST YOURSELF

1. What model of home care nursing delivery do you use in your agency? How does that affect the way you practice?

2. What tools are available in your agency to assist you in caseload management?

3. How does your agency ensure that clients don't "fall through the cracks" and that visits are not missed?

4. List five time-wasters and five time-savers you anticipate will affect your practice. Think again about these time-wasters and time-savers three and six months after your initial employment date.

5. What are the three major expectations you have of your supervisor? What are the three major expectations you think your supervisor has of you?

6. Review your agency's schedule and process for performance evaluations. Discuss them with your supervisor.

7. Ask a home care nurse who has been employed by your agency for more than one year what she identifies as the major stressors in her job. Discuss methods she uses to relieve those stressors.

8. What strategies do you think you will use to develop your professional role in the agency?

REFERENCES

Benefield, L. (1988). *Home health care management.* Englewood Cliffs, NJ: Prentice Hall.

Cestari, L.R. (1989). *A comparison of stress among hospital and community health nurses.* Unpublished master's thesis, Southern Connecticut State University, New Haven, CT.

Knollmueller, R. (1989). Case management: What's in a name? *Nursing Management, 20,* 38–40.

Marquis, B. & Huston, C. (1987). *Management decision making for nurses.* Philadelphia: J.B. Lippincott.

Legal and Ethical Aspects of Home Care Nursing Practice

chapter
10

OBJECTIVES

Upon completion of this chapter, the reader will be able to identify:

1. Major client issues related to confidentiality and access to home care records
2. How home care nurses are accountable for their practice
3. Risk management participation
4. Issues in insurance and health care fraud and abuse
5. Liability issues related to home care nursing practice
6. The process involved in a home care liability case
7. Various roles of the home care nurse in litigation
8. Several legal situations that can involve a home health agency
9. The American Nurses Association's *A Statement for the Scope of Home Health Nursing Practice* relative to ethics
10. Definition of the advance medical directive

KEY CONCEPTS

- **Defensive strategies for home care nursing practice**
- **How to maintain a high level of professional accountability**
- **Various ways professionals are called upon to testify**
- **Legal implications of the home care nursing role**
- **What to do when served a summons or subpoena**
- **Ethical issues in home care**
- **Advance medical directive**

AGENCY-SPECIFIC MATERIAL NEEDED

- Confidentiality policy
- Procedure for client to obtain home care record
- Policy regarding professional practice liability insurance
- Procedure for discharging a client
- Standards of care
- Policy or procedure for employees served with legal papers
- Agency policies, procedures, and committees that deal with ethical issues
- A copy of advance medical directive policies and procedures

INTRODUCTION

This chapter is included in the home care nurse's orientation to teach the ways that home care nursing practice is affected by legal considerations. All nurses, wherever they practice, should be familiar with the legal ramifications of their acts in order to develop a way of practicing that is based on sound clinical judgment and consideration of the legal aspects of practice. Most nurses become anxious when approaching the legal aspects of practice, feeling that they would rather not know the possibilities of legal problems so that they will not have to worry. This text is based on the premise that the only way to prepare a professional home care nurse is to educate her to the many aspects of the field so she will be prepared to practice at a high level.

This chapter first describes briefly the many legal issues that are basic to the home care nurse's knowledge. The issues of confidentiality, the nurse's relationship to the agency, risk management concerns (such as incident reports and insurance coverage), and health care fraud and abuse are basic to nurses at all levels of practice. This helps the nurse see how these issues specifically relate to home care. This material should be covered in the initial orientation to the agency.

Next, there is a more detailed discussion of home care legal issues, using as examples situations home care nurses have encountered. These situations focus around negligence, liability, and the role home care nurses may be asked to assume in testifying in a case. This discussion is included not to intimidate the nurse or make her fearful of home care practice. Rather, thorough discussion of these situations (not so rare in home care nursing practice) can assist the nurse in understanding her role if these situations arise and help her to practice defensively every day. This section should be used later in the orientation period and can serve as a reference for future situations. Appendix N is a legal glossary that clarifies concepts used throughout this chapter and serves as a continuing reference guide for home care practice.

Lastly, the chapter covers both the basic ethical dilemmas the home care nurse may encounter in practice and the advance medical directive.

BASIC LEGAL CONSIDERATIONS IN HOME CARE NURSING PRACTICE

Confidentiality

The client has a right to privacy that is protected through various sources. One of these is the American Nurses Association (ANA) *Code for Nurses with Interpretive Statements*, which states, "The Nurse safeguards the client's right to privacy by judiciously protecting information of a confidential nature" (ANA, 1985). Exceptions to the rule against disclosure include the right and obligation of the nurse to discuss client situations for purposes of providing client care within the organization, participating in quality management activities in which client situations are discussed, and providing information relative to a client situation in a court of law when a client waives or lacks nurse-client privilege of communication.

Various state and federal laws also protect confidentiality of client information and records. For example, Medicare regulations require the client's written consent for sharing any information about his or her care or diagnosis not authorized by law. The client may waive his or her privilege to maintaining confidential information by signing a consent form, although most agency consent forms are very specific regarding the purpose of sharing client information and with whom it may be shared. Every home health agency should have written policies concerning the release of information in client's health care records and the home care nurse should be thoroughly familiar with these procedures.

Unauthorized disclosure of client information could put the nurse at risk for liability under the torts (legal wrong) of defamation of character or invasion of privacy. Defamation of character would involve publishing or disclosing untrue information that harmed the client's reputation. Invasion of privacy is an unwarranted exploitation of one's affairs and, usually, must be of a sufficient nature to cause shame, outrage, or humiliation for a client.

Every home care agency needs to have a policy concerning documenting the presence of human immunodeficiency virus (HIV) and acquired immune deficiency syndrome (AIDS) status in clients. The agency's policy can be affected by state laws concerning testing for HIV and AIDS. If this type of information is included in a part of the record that may be accessible to third parties, such as insurers, its confidentiality must be considered and any applicable legal requirements must be taken into account. Strict confidentiality of this information is the general rule, and release of this information without consent of the client (even to family members) could subject the nurse to legal actions by the client. Release of the information to others can have serious legal, social, employment, housing, and financial consequences. The nurse should check her agency's policies regarding caring for AIDS and HIV-positive clients.

Although the various ways to ensure confidentiality discussed here may seem complex to the nurse, they really are very simple. In all situations, the nurse must always think about the confidentiality of client information. The nurse must use a great deal of common sense as well as have knowledge of the law and the professional standards previously discussed. Because all information about the client is to be kept confidential, the nurse should keep this thought paramount in and outside the agency. Do not talk about clients in public to either nonagency or agency personnel. Typically, home care nurses meet for lunch and may need to discuss client care or may do so to relate interesting incidents. Be very aware that others may overhear these conversations, which could compromise the confidentiality of the client. Additionally, anecdotes about the client and family that may be intriguing to others are not appropriate to be shared, and client names never should be used. Even if professionals are presenting client situations in case conferences, quality management reports, or professional research that positively impacts on the client's care, strict rules of confidentiality must apply.

Client Access to Health Care Records

Although the agency has ownership rights in the client's health care record, the client has a legal right to the information contained in the record. In most states there are statutes concerning client access to health records that should be reviewed, because there may be exceptions to the general rule of access (Killion, 1985). The right of the client's ownership of the information in the record has been articulated clearly in court opinions as part of the common law. There should be a written agency policy regarding particulars of access for clients. For example, the agency does not usually have to provide immediate access, and the client usually may be charged a reasonable fee for duplication. The home care nurse should be mindful of the fact that the client may have an opportunity to read the documentation, and recording should always be done in an objective and professional manner.

Clients should be asked to submit a written request, signed by them, as a prerequisite to releasing medical information to others, such as insurance companies, who may have a legitimate interest in their health care. State law may provide what information must be in the request. In any event, as an extra precaution, such written authorization should include the name and address of a witness to the authorization, and it should be a part of the client's permanent record. In some instances, no permission is required to allow third parties access to the health care record. Examples could be for state licensing agencies, Medicare and Medicaid authorities, or to comply with reporting statutes, such as for communicable diseases or subpoenas issued as part of a legal proceeding. If the client is incompetent, a guardian may be appointed in a legal proceeding to authorize release of the record. If the client is deceased, the administrator of the client's estate usually can authorize release.

Access to the medical records of minors also presents a recurring problem. The agency should have a policy regarding this matter, but as a general rule if minors can consent to their own care under state law, then the parents will not have a right of access to the record. Examples could be if the minor was receiving services related to pregnancy, venereal disease, or substance abuse. Sometimes, if the minor is relying on parents for payment of the services, the parent may have a right to access. The administrator of the agency would need to check the circumstances in the particular situation and follow through. Once again, your state may have a law addressing minors' access to their medical records.

If a client were to ask to see what the nurse was writing in the record, the nurse should talk to the client about the information rather than show the record immediately. Most often, the data will need to be interpreted in order to make them comprehensible. The nurse should use this opportunity to provide client education and information rather than hand over a copy of the chart to be read. Because requests to view the record are handled formally at the administrative level, the home care nurse would most often be informing her supervisor of the client's request. Usually when the client requests to see the record, it is a signal that communication should be strengthened with the client regarding his or her care.

Witnessing Documents

A home care nurse may be asked by clients to witness documents. First, the agency's guidelines regarding this situation should be consulted so that the nurse can follow them. A notation should always be made in the client's record listing any documents that were signed by the client and nurse. Second, the nurse should record a brief statement on the client's orientation, state of mind, or any special circumstances. The nurse may be asked to represent the agency in having a client sign an agreement or contract for service. When this is the case, the nurse should ask a family member or another person to witness the document between the parties. This same procedure should be followed in other situations, such as when the client receives official information provided by the nurse when she is following guidelines set forth by regulatory agencies.

Occasionally, a home care nurse may be asked to witness documents that are not related to her role as a nurse (i.e., those related to the client's personal business needs). When a nurse does witness these documents, she does so as an individual. Therefore, a nurse should not then use the title "RN" with her name. A further suggestion is to limit participation by including the phrase "Witness to signature only" after the nurse's name (Connaway, 1985, p. 45).

It should be noted that the nurse or anyone who witnesses a document could be called upon to testify about the execution of the document. As a general rule, it is best to ask a family member or a friend to witness any service or nonservice-related document.

LEGAL IMPLICATIONS OF EMPLOYER/ EMPLOYEE RELATIONSHIPS

An employment contract setting out rights and responsibilities of both the employee-nurse and the employer-agency is a legally binding agreement between the parties. As such, this employment contract is enforceable in a court of law. To be valid, the contract need not be in writing and may be based on oral statements, but it is easier to prove once it is in writing and signed by the parties. Expected areas to be covered in the contract relate to working hours and conditions, salary, raises, length of the contract including notice of and grounds for termination, and benefits such as sick leave, overtime, and vacation time. The position for which the nurse is employed, job expectations and duties, and types and frequency of evaluations should be covered. If any area is not covered in the contract that the nurse-employee feels should be included, it is wise to maintain some personal notes that reflect discussion on the issue.

If a problem should arise where either party feels the contract provisions are not being upheld, the first step would be to explain this to the other party. Written facts and specific instances should be used to support such an allegation. In the case of the employee, this may be in the form of a written performance evaluation based on criteria specified in the job description. Most nursing employment contracts are terminated by giving proper notice of termination usually within the length of a pay period or two weeks.

A second means of obtaining rights and responsibilities as related to a job can be through collective bargaining or unionization. This allows employees to

negotiate provisions collectively, such as salary and benefits. Typically, if there is a labor dispute, a formal grievance procedure is initiated, with specifics outlined in the collective bargaining agreement. Certain rights and responsibilities attach to these types of agreements as provided by state and federal labor laws.

Unless the nurse has either an employment contract or a collective bargaining agreement, the employer may have the right to "terminate at will." The concept of "employment at will" means that either the employer or the employee has the right to terminate employment at any time, for any reason, or for no reason at all. Of course, even when employment is "at will," it still cannot be terminated for reasons prohibited by law, such as unlawful discrimination based on race or sex. The employment at will concept is a matter of state law, and its application and exceptions can vary greatly from state to state. Recently, there have been important exceptions carved out by the courts and state legislatures in several states to limit this right of the employer to dismiss an employee without notice and without cause.

Employee Rights and Duties Owed to Agency, Supervisors, and Board

Generally speaking, nurses have a duty to uphold the employer's expectations with regard to job performance. In home care nursing this usually means that the staff nurse should expect to be evaluated at regular intervals by supervisors. The nurse should expect these evaluations to be factual, objective, well-documented, and substantiated by appropriate data. For example, if it is alleged by the supervisor that a nurse designs inadequate care plans, examples should be included. Employee evaluation data should not come as a surprise if the employee is kept informed at regular intervals. Employees have a right to evaluations that are made in good faith without intent to discredit or harm them.

Another duty the nurse has to the agency is to have standards consistent with the state nurse practice act and to maintain these standards through continued self-assessment and continuing education. The agency or employer needs to know if the staff nurse is unprepared to undertake an expected task. The agency has a duty to make reasonable assignments consistent with the employee's education and skill. The agency, and ultimately the board of directors of the agency, has a right to expect notice from the employee of anything that is adversely affecting his or her ability to carry out the job. Examples would be if the nurse had concerns about personal safety or had knowledge of serious threats to the agency's reputation. Thus, even though there is no direct liability from the staff nurse to the board, the staff nurse provides information to the agency's administrative officers who channel the information to the board as necessary.

Another consideration given to the nurse-employee is the right to view information contained in her personnel file. This usually includes any performance evaluations by peers or supervisors, letters of recommendation, forms from previous employers or educational institutions, or any disciplinary actions against the employee. Usually the nurse can review this personnel file in the presence of another agency employee, and she may have a right to copy the documents contained therein. Supervisors may have their own anecdotal notes to support statements in the file that the nurse would not necessarily have a right to review, unless official action was taken and they became part of the nurse's record. The extent to which a nurse-employee has the right to view the information contained in her personnel file is usually determined by the agency, at its discretion, but some states have a law requiring employees to be given access to at least some of the information in their personnel files.

Evaluating Other Employees

The home care nurse may be asked to provide written evaluations of peers for quality management purposes or of employees under the nurse's supervision, such as home care aides. In the case of peer review, it should be clear whether the evaluation is solely for improvement of the individual's practice or whether it has implications for job status.

The same principles would apply in regard to a supervisor's evaluation of a staff nurse's performance. In the case of the home care aide, the nurse is acting in a supervisory role and thus has the responsibility to judge the performance of the individual. Objective, up-to-date, well-documented, and ongoing data need to be recorded to substantiate such evaluations. Included in the nurse's notes should be any corrective action (e.g., teaching a procedure again) that has been taken. As long as these evaluations or any subsequent letters of recommendation are done in good faith, the nurse need not fear liability for these statements. Even if there are negative or potentially defamatory (i.e., injurious to one's reputation) statements made, they are protected. However, one is not allowed to make statements known to be untrue, to act in reckless disregard of their accuracy, or to act with malicious intent to harm someone by these statements.

Occupational Safety and Health

Legal requirements to protect the health and safety of health care workers have increased greatly. These protections usually are established by either the federal Occupational Safety and Health Administration (OSHA) or a comparable state department, but other agencies can become involved (e.g., the Environmental Protection Agency [EPA] for infectious waste) and legislatures may enact statutes dealing with specific subjects, such as universal precautions.

OSHA has been particularly active in this regard, establishing standards concerning occupational exposure to bloodborne pathogens, tuberculosis (TB), and hazardous substances. In various ways, these standards require exercise of universal precautions, use of personal protective equipment, use of appropriate procedures for handling contaminated waste and sharps, availability of vaccinations against hepatitis B for at-risk employees, access to information concerning hazardous substances, and employee training, to name only a few of the criteria covered. Further discussion of these standards is found in Chapter 3.

Consequently, many safety and health measures an employer requires of its employees not only are good employment practices but are mandated by law. Although the employer must abide by these regulations, compliance also requires each employee to understand and observe the requirements. If an employee does not follow the legal requirements, it can result in substantial penalties against the employer and lead to the employee's discharge.

RISK MANAGEMENT PARTICIPATION

Risk management is a method of identifying, evaluating, and treating the agency's risk of financial loss. Most agencies are required by Medicare, accrediting agencies, or insurance liability carriers to maintain such programs. A well-managed program serves the interests of clients, employees, the agency, and the public.

Central to the operation of the program is a reporting system of incidents or unusual occurrences with respect to any aspect of the operation of the agency. An example would be reports of frequent equipment failures that pose a potential risk. After a trend is established, an appropriate intervention could be carried out to solve the problem.

Staff nurses have an important function in reporting any incidents in order to ensure that risks are documented and identified. The home health agency will have a procedure for reporting incidents and specific forms to be completed. Another level of participation by the nurse could be as part of an agency committee, sometimes a multidisciplinary committee, that reviews, monitors, and acts on risks. Individual participation in this process will continue to become an important area of concern by home care nurses in the future.

Incident or Occurrence Reports

Incident reports, sometimes called occurrence reports, are a means to report any unusual occurrences with regard to care of a client and serve as a valuable record made at the time of the event, when memories are clear. An incident report is usually an internal document for the agency's use as a risk management tool. Through identification of areas of risk for clients, the agency can take preventive steps to avoid reoccurrence. For example, if there were several incident reports related to complications developing in intravenous administration devices for home care clients, inservice education for staff members and a better means of instructing clients could be instituted.

It is important that nurses recognize their valuable contribution in reporting incidents to help evaluate risks and potential liability for the agency. However, completing an incident report consistent with agency policy does not substitute for documenting the event in the client's record. For example, if a client falls while the nurse is ambulating him or her in the home, a brief factual account of what happened should be made in the record. Assessments and follow-up instructions care should be included. There is no need to state "incident report filed." Doing so could lead a court to decide to incorporate the incident report by reference into the chart.

An incident report may be discoverable by the plaintiff should litigation arise over the incident. Incident reports should, therefore, be carefully worded so that they contain factual statements without admission of liability, fault, or how the incident could have been prevented. It is better to write the report in a manner that assumes it could be used for litigation. Some courts have taken the view that these reports are prepared for litigation and are, therefore, "privileged communication" or "attorney work product." Access to incident reports could help to substantiate a claim that the standard of care was not met. It is essential that all agencies have a clear policy for reporting unusual occurrences and that the nurse be aware of it.

Suggestions by Connaway (1985) to help achieve privileged status for incident reports include:

- having only one copy of the report
- providing a checklist on the form to limit narrative comments
- addressing the report to the agency's attorney or to the insurance claim manager
- not using the incident report as a disciplinary tool
- not providing a copy for the client

All of these measures are designed to protect the confidentiality of these documents and to encourage the reporting of incidents as a risk management tool. Whether or not these measures are helpful to your agency will depend upon your state's law. It is best for your agency's attorney to assist in developing its incident reporting procedures and for the nurse to be aware of agency policy regarding this.

Abandonment

Abandonment generally means a unilateral severance of the professional relationship between a health care provider and a client without reasonable notice at a time when there is still a need for continuing health care. Generally, the issue of client abandonment occurs in home care when the home health agency decides it must discontinue service and there is a continuing need for care.

From time to time, a home health agency may need to unilaterally terminate service to a client for any of the following reasons:

- The client refuses to cooperate with the agency and its staff in the provision of home health care.
- The client will not pay the bill.
- The client is unruly, obnoxious, or difficult to treat to the point that it is in the best interests of all concerned that the agency discontinue service.
- Reimbursement for services has been denied, or the agency has ceased to be a Medicaid or Medicare provider.
- Certain environmental factors exist that endanger agency staff, such as physical threats, a dangerous dog, or sexual harassment.

Avoiding Abandonment

The key to avoiding client abandonment and any liability for injury that might occur in such a situation is to make sure that reasonable notice of the termination of service is given to the client. The reasonable notice element is critically important because with such notice the client could presumably be able to secure alternative care and then could not be abandoned. The *reasonableness of notice* (i.e., the length of time involved from client notification to termination of service) varies depending on the particular circumstances of the client. Considerations include the availability of substitute service, the client's condition, the ramifications if alternative care is not secured, and the urgency of the need to terminate service.

For example, if the majority of care the client is receiving, such as that from a home care aide, can be performed by family members, the notice may be shorter than for the situation of a client who needs IV therapy every day. Also, if the agency staff faces abuse from the client to the extent that they are physically threatened, the need to terminate may be more urgent. Home health agency administrators and managers work with the staff nurse within the internal policies of the agency and external state and federal laws to make these decisions. You will not have to make them on your own.

If you find yourself in situations where abandonment is an issue, you should discuss the matter with your supervisor and refer to agency policies relative to discharging clients from service. Throughout the entire process, the client's physician should be consulted, and all problems and decisions should be communicated in writing to everyone involved, including the client, family, physician, and any other providers or reimbursement sources working on the case.

INSURANCE ISSUES

Individual versus Agency Coverage

Considering the purchase of an individual professional liability policy is a personal decision for each nurse. The numbers of lawsuits against health professionals have increased dramatically over the last decade, with nurses being named as individual defendants in some cases. There are several reasons why it is advisable for the nurse to maintain such an individual policy.

Many nurses believe that their employer is responsible for any of their acts while the nurse is performing duties within the scope of her employment. Although this is generally true, there can be exceptional circumstances. For example, institutions often have limitations in their policies. The new staff nurse can ask to see the agency policy and review it carefully, noting any exclusions or limitations to the policy coverage.

In some cases, a nurse named as a defendant may have to provide and pay for her own defense. In one

such case, a registered nurse (RN) anesthetist was named in a lawsuit along with her hospital (Sandroff, 1983). The hospital settled the case in exchange for a covenant or promise not to sue, a common right outlined in most insurance agreements. However, the nurse did not have her own insurance policy, and she had to pay for her own defense. Even though the jury returned a decision in her favor, she had to pay her own legal expenses.

If an agency pays a claim because of negligence of one of its nurse-employees, the agency has the right to sue the nurse for indemnification or reimbursement. Although not often used, the legal right does exist, and having one's own coverage would provide protection against such a claim.

Some nurses mistakenly believe that having one's own policy will increase the likelihood of being sued or will automatically trigger an indemnity suit, but there is no evidence to support this belief. In fact, it does not matter to the client bringing the suit whether the nurse has insurance. The fact of insurance coverage or its amount is not disclosed at trial so as not to prejudice the jury.

Types of Coverage

Another limitation to the employer's policy could be the type of coverage. Many employers carry a claims-made type policy, which covers events that happen only when the policy is in effect. Thus, if the nurse has left the agency and a claim is made after her period of employment, the nurse will, most likely, not be covered. The home care nurse can protect herself from this situation by having an individual occurrence policy that provides for broader coverage. An occurrence policy covers incidents that occurred during any time period for which premiums were paid, even if the claim is made some time later. Another way to cover gaps in insurance policies is to purchase "tail" coverage. This could cover a gap created when a claims-made policy is canceled. Another factor to consider in deciding to purchase individual coverage is whether the nurse engages in nursing activities outside of her agency employment. For example, volunteer activities on a professional board or as a camp nurse would not be covered by the agency's policy but are usually covered by individual policies.

Nurses are being exposed to greater risks of liability. As a professional, the home care nurse is performing a wider variety of highly skilled and specialized services. As an individual, the nurse can be personally liable for any judgment rendered against her. This means that if the nurse does not have personal liability protection, a judgment can be satisfied against her with her personal assets. Even if there are no current personal assets, future wages can be used to satisfy a judgment. With these risks at stake, it is unwise for a nurse to practice without individual coverage, especially considering the relatively low cost of such coverage.

It is still important to be knowledgeable about the agency-employer's policy even if the nurse decides not to purchase an individual professional liability policy. The amount of coverage, whether it is a claims-made or occurrence policy, and what exclusions or limitations of coverage are specified must be determined. For a thorough discussion of liability and insurance issues, see an informative pamphlet on *Liability and You—What Registered Nurses Need To Know* published by the ANA in 1987.

HEALTH CARE FRAUD AND ABUSE

Efforts to combat fraud and abuse in health care have increased dramatically over the past few years. Today, all health care providers must be sensitive to what constitutes health care fraud and the kinds of arrangements that are prohibited. Failure to do so can result in substantial criminal and civil penalties as well as prohibition from participating in the Medicare or Medicaid programs.

A complete discussion of health care fraud and abuse is far beyond the scope of this text. The prohibitions go beyond the blatant submission of false claims to a payer or paying kickbacks or bribes for referrals. What must be recognized is that an activity that is completely lawful for other businesses can be a felony in the health care setting. For example, your local bank may give away toasters to encourage new accounts, but a home health agency may not do the same thing to encourage Medicare or Medicaid business.

Combatting fraud and abuse are not limited to federal laws concerning efforts to induce referrals of Medicare and Medicaid business. Prohibitions exist for making false statements to obtain payment of Medicare or Medicaid benefits as well as for making physician referrals to entities in which the physicians have a financial interest. Furthermore, many states are adapting antikickback laws to prohibit remuneration in return for any type of health care referral, not just Medicare and Medicaid business.

Illegal Remuneration

The federal Medicare and Medicaid fraud and abuse law prohibits much more than obvious kickbacks and bribes. It provides criminal penalties for individuals

or entities that knowingly and willfully offer, pay, solicit, or receive any remuneration (including any kickback, bribe, or rebate) in order to induce business reimbursed under the Medicare or Medicaid programs. It applies to remuneration made directly or indirectly, overtly or covertly, in cash or in kind. In addition, prohibited conduct includes not only remuneration intended to induce referrals of clients, but remuneration intended to induce the purchasing, leasing, ordering, or arranging for any goods, facility, service, or item paid for by either Medicare or Medicaid.

This prohibition has been interpreted by the courts very broadly. If just one purpose of the remuneration is to induce referrals, the law has been violated. It does not matter that there may have been other legitimate purposes. This was established in a federal court of appeals case involving a physician who operated a Holter monitoring service (*United States v. Greber*, 1985). The physician paid the physicians (who referred clients to his Holter monitoring service) to interpret the test results for their clients. The government charged the physician with violation of the federal Medicare and Medicaid fraud and abuse law, saying his payments to referring physicians were actually kickbacks to obtain their referrals. The physician argued that the payments were legitimate compensation for their time in interpreting the results. The court held that, even though it may not have been the only purpose, because one purpose of the payments was to induce referrals to the physician's Holter monitoring service, the federal fraud and abuse law was violated.

Questions To Ask Yourself

If you become involved in efforts to improperly obtain payment for services or to increase client referrals or others approach you in that regard, ask yourself four questions:

1. Are you being asked to certify something that is not true, such as saying services were provided when they were not, or backdating a record?
2. Is one purpose of the proposed arrangement to induce referral to either your agency or to another provider?
3. Is something being offered, directly or indirectly, to induce referrals?
4. Is what is being offered or its amount dependent in any way on the number of clients referred or the volume of business generated?

If you answer yes to any of these questions, there is a *possibility* that the arrangement implicates federal and/

or state fraud and abuse prohibitions, and you should obtain knowledgeable legal advice before proceeding. Remember, if claims are submitted based upon false information or if just one purpose of remuneration given or offered is to induce referrals, the law may be violated.

Your state professional nursing and home health associations or the state attorney general's office should be able to provide more complete information concerning the health care fraud and abuse laws that apply in your state.

LIABILITY ISSUES IN HOME CARE NURSING

Negligence

Home care nurses, like all professional nurses, are liable for any harm to clients that is due to their negligence. Nurses are held legally accountable to a standard of care that is expected of reasonably competent nurses. The home care nursing standards of care are discussed in Chapter 2. The essential elements that must each be proved in a professional negligence or malpractice suit are:

1. a duty to the client or a standard of care
2. a breach of that duty or a breach of the standard of care
3. causation, including the fact that the breach of the duty proximately (directly) caused the injury
4. harm or damage, usually in the form of actual physical damage, to the client

If an injury to a client occurs that is alleged to be caused by a nurse's negligence, the client, as the plaintiff, may sue the nurse, who becomes the defendant. A major focus in the trial is to establish what the duty or standard of care was in relationship to the client's injury.

Sources of the Standard of Care

Nurse Practice Act

The basic starting point to define the standard of care for any nurse is the Nurse Practice Act or state statute on nursing in the jurisdiction where the nurse is a registered practitioner. Although practice acts vary from state to state, they usually contain broad language to permit a variety of activities by nurses. Many states have advanced practitioner statutes for nurses that apply if one assumes this role. It is important for the nurse to be familiar with the individual nurse practice act in her state.

Professional Organizations

Professional organizations or associations are another important source for the standard of care. For example, the ANA has established general standards of practice and a code for nurses that outline ethical duties. A Missouri case illustrates how the nurse's ethical duty is brought forth in a lawsuit (Cushing, 1982). The incident occurred in the operating room where it was alleged that the nurses should have stopped the surgeon before such extensive damage was done to the client. In finding in favor of the injured party, the court accepted the evidence presented by the plaintiff that professional ethics mandated that nurses countermand a doctor's action if they feel it is incorrect. The duty of the nurses was to take whatever action was necessary to protect the client.

Home care nurses must be particularly alert to the standards set forth in the ANA *Standards of Community Health Nursing Practice* (1986a) and *Standards for Home Health Nursing Practice* (1986b). For example, if a home care nurse fails to perform a thorough skin assessment (breach of duty), and the client subsequently develops a decubitus ulcer that does not respond to treatment (proximate causation and injury), the nurse's duty may be partially established through presenting evidence of standards II through V. These standards relate to the nurse's duty to collect data, diagnose, plan, and intervene, and they could be used to support a finding of liability for malpractice or professional negligence.

Other groups involved in setting and outlining standards for home care nurses include the American Public Health Association (APHA), public health nursing section; the Association of Graduate Faculty in Community and Public Health Nursing; and the National League for Nursing (NLN) (Northrop & Kelly, 1987). Regulations or guidelines established by these organizations could be relevant to the issue of what specific duty is owed to a client. It is imperative that nurses keep current as to standards set forth by these organizations.

Agency Manuals and Policies

Another source for the standard of care is agency manuals or policies. A home care nurse has a duty to follow agency policies and procedures that are consistent with accepted nursing practice. Two cases illustrate how failure to follow hospital policies has been used to find negligence on the part of hospital nurses. The same principles would apply by analogy to the home care situation. In the first case, *Czubinsky v. Doctor's Hospital* (1983), an operating room nurse left the first client to begin assisting the surgeon for a second operation. This left only a scrub technician and anesthesiologist to manage the first client, who was subsequently left paralyzed and comatose. The court held that these injuries resulted from failure of the circulating nurse and scrub nurse to monitor the client properly and render essential aid. Part of the evidence presented by the plaintiff was the hospital procedure manual, which stated that the circulating nurse's duty was "to assist the anesthesiologist during the entire procedure." Thus, the policy set forth the standard of care.

In the second case, *Utter v. United Hospital Center* (1977), the plaintiff also prevailed on his claim of negligence against nurses who did not take any further action beyond informing the physician of the client's obvious untoward symptoms and documenting their observations in the clinical record. A policy in the nursing manual outlined a procedure for calling questionable care to the attention of the department chair if the matter could not be resolved with the physician. The court found that the nurses had failed to comply with the policy in the manual and, therefore, were negligent and the hospital was liable.

Implications for home care nurses are that they should be aware of agency policies regarding how to deal with questionable care on the part of the physician or others in order to protect themselves and clients if a problem should arise. In all situations that the nurse may find in home care practice, she must also be familiar with procedures and practices specific to her own agency. Because the site of practice is in the client's home, the agency has procedures for nurses to follow to receive guidance and support in questionable situations. It is the home care nurse's responsibility to be knowledgeable about them.

Publications and Current Literature

Texts and current literature in the field are other examples of sources to establish the standard of care for nurses. In *Guigino v. Harvard Community Health Plan et al.* (1980), the plaintiff submitted a number of professional publications and newspaper clippings warning practitioners of the harmful effects of a Dalkon shield (an intrauterine device), relating to the time of the incident in 1975. The case was eventually settled out of court, but it alerts health care practitioners to the duty to review professional literature in their field. A further illustration is the case of *Pisel v. Stamford Hospital* (1980), in which well-recognized textbooks and professional literature at the time of the alleged incident were used to help establish the standard of care for nurses. Expert witnesses, who were nurses qualified to testify on the accepted standard, stated how often the client should have been assessed and what interventions were

necessary to ensure the client's safety. These experts used literature in the psychiatric field to formulate their opinions. In the absence of any written hospital policy, the court accepted the opinion of plaintiff's expert witnesses as the prevailing professional standard.

Expert Witness

In a malpractice case, the plaintiff must show the standard of care to be applied to the case. The usual method of introducing this evidence is to have an expert witness testify as to the prevailing standard. In fact, it is crucial that a witness who is familiar with the area of practice present an opinion. Both plaintiff and defendant will have expert witnesses render opinions when there is a question of professional negligence. In formulating an opinion, an expert relies on his or her experience, education, credentials, professional involvement, and any of the aforementioned sources for the standard of care. An appropriate expert witness to give testimony on a question of negligence in the home care setting would be a nurse who is experienced with the particular type of client situation, caseload, and intervention that is brought into question in the lawsuit.

Testifying As a Nurse Expert Witness

A home care nurse may be asked to provide expert testimony as proof of the standard of care in a nursing malpractice case. In most jurisdictions, a nurse would testify on the proper standard of nursing care, although some jurisdictions would allow a physician to do so (Northrop & Kelly, 1987). Some states provide access to a panel of nurse experts through the state nurses' organization.

The ability or competency of the expert witness to render an opinion is tested by the sufficiency of the expert's knowledge of the subject matter at hand. Expert testimony is admissible and, in fact, necessary, when conclusions by the jury depend on facts or scientific information that is not common knowledge. Lawyers will seek the most qualified expert witnesses. Josberger and Ries (1985) suggest that the following criteria be recognized in evaluating potential witnesses:

1. graduate education in nursing
2. clinical expertise
3. research
4. continuing education

The nurse expert would review all written records, policies, environmental issues, and supportive management criteria (such as nurse-caseload ratios) and pertinent literature to determine if the proper nursing process was followed. The nurse expert would be asked to interpret these data and render an opinion as to the actions of the nurse in the particular incident as alleged in the lawsuit, usually involving a question of nursing negligence.

A home care nurse may be called as a nurse expert to give testimony related to issues of child custody, termination of parental rights, child abuse, or criminal cases. Specific information regarding how to testify is provided in a later section on providing a deposition. The nurse can also refer to the documentation section in Chapter 5 for guidelines involving recording these sensitive areas of practice.

Case Illustration—Negligence in a Home Care Situation

The following case example illustrates several important areas of practice for home care nurses. In *Bass v. Barksdale et al.* (1984), allegations of negligence were claimed by the plaintiff, an elderly woman whose treatment for TB was being monitored by nurses employed by the health department. The client was given a month's supply of medication to treat her TB by the defendant nurse. Thereafter, other nurses from the public health department made home visits and delivered monthly medications to the client over the next five months. The defendant nurse made the initial home visit and testified that she discussed the client's medical history, informed her of the possible side effect of decreased visual acuity, and checked her vision with a 10-foot eye chart and recorded the readings. However, the client denied this. Interestingly, the eye chart the nurse said she used did not have a 10/100 line, which is what she recorded for the right eye.

The client and her sister, who was present at the initial home visit, testified that the nurse had forgotten to bring an eye chart and then checked her vision by asking her to point out certain objects in the room. The client also claimed she was informed only to watch for color changes in her eyes. The nurse who delivered the second month's supply of medication testified she checked the client's vision at that time. It was undisputed at trial that the health department nurses who delivered the medication over the next three months did not check the client's vision.

The client testified that she informed her private physician at her regular checkup of her abrupt vision decline. The physician denied she told him this. It was not until eight weeks after this acute vision loss that the client went to an ophthalmologist who, through consultation with a neurologist, concluded that one of the medications she had been taking for treatment of the TB was the cause of her vision loss. There was uncontradicted expert testimony at the trial that if vision checks had been performed, her loss of vision could have been detected, the drug stopped, and her vision loss possibly could have been reversed.

In addition to questions of negligence arising in the nursing assessment and documentation for the client in her home, the case further illustrates the need for clear communication among all health professionals responsible for an individual client's care and for clear documentation of these responsibilities. Initially, the client's private physician telephoned the health department and talked with the defendant nurse, who was charge nurse of the TB health clinic, about the care of the client. The content of the conversation was disputed at trial. The private physician believed that he had turned the care of the client over to the health department and at trial denied prescribing her drugs.

The nurse, on the other hand, testified that the private physician had ordered the drugs after she discussed the protocol with him. She further stated that then she asked the health department physician to sign the prescriptions, with the phrase "per telephone order" of the doctor at the top (*Bass v. Barksdale et al.*, 1984). The health department physician stated he never agreed to take care of the client and that signing a prescription form does not amount to assuming the responsibility of taking care of a client. The court agreed that even if the signing of the forms by another doctor was negligent, it did not create this relationship with the client.

The standard of care for a doctor prescribing the drug involved in this case, ethambutol, was established as including vision testing before prescribing the drug, giving warnings about the possible side effects, and what course of action to take if side effects occur. Based on the facts of this case, it is clear that a home care nurse should not ask a physician other than the one who prescribed the medication to sign a prescription form. Doing so can create confusion as to who is responsible for supervising the client while on the medication, and it can lead to serious consequences.

Another point revealed at trial in this case was that when the defendant nurse had the health department physician sign the prescriptions, there were no markings on the "refill" line. However, plaintiff's counsel had been furnished copies of these prescriptions with "PRN" circled on each. Neither the defendant nurse nor the health department physician could explain the apparent alteration on these forms. Routinely utilizing PRN refill for medications should be discouraged, because periodic rewriting by a physician would clarify accountability for supervision and monitoring of the client.

Another issue discussed in the case was whether the health department physician, as the defendant nurse's supervisor, had a duty to ensure that she was acting competently with regard to the care of the client, that is, checking for side effects from the medications and checking her visual acuity. Although the issue was not resolved in the case, the court stated that the jury could find negligence on the part of the nurse and negligence on the part of the health department physician for failure to supervise her acts. Although the court did not make a finding in this regard, the trial court's outcome was reversed and a new trial was ordered to decide these and other issues.

Particularly in home care, there are areas of shared responsibility and accountability for physicians prescribing medications and for nurses monitoring their administration in the home setting. Documentation of telephone conversations and their content, relaying prescriptions for physicians to sign after telephone orders are received, and documentation of client teaching and assessments will help prevent problems illustrated by this case.

Defending a Claim of Negligence

Pretrial Discovery

Before a trial on the issues related to liability goes forward, most states permit a period of pretrial discovery. This period of time allows for investigation of the plaintiff's claim and involves an information-gathering process. Through various processes, the plaintiff or client seeks to establish that he or she has a valid claim. On the other hand, the defendant, usually the agency or nurse against whom the complaint is made, wants to gather facts to demonstrate failure of the plaintiff's claim. This discovery process helps the parties evaluate the case and can facilitate settlement of meritorious claims.

The first step in the discovery process often is to request all records pertinent to the incident, such as the health care records of the client. Through review of these records, nurses who have knowledge of the incident are identified, usually through their documentation. A nurse is then identified as a potential witness for the trial. The right of discovery permits opposing parties to question witnesses before the trial.

Interrogatories. One way to seek statements from witnesses is to have them answer written questions called interrogatories. A nurse-witness should consult with the agency administrator and her private counsel or the agency's attorney about providing answers, because they are given under oath and need to be true as stated. Attorneys help their clients complete interroga-

tories to ensure that objectionable questions are properly objected to and that the wording of answers does not suggest liability.

Providing a Deposition. A second means of obtaining information from a potential witness is through a deposition. A deposition is a witness's sworn statement, taken under oath, that is admissible later in a court of law. The witness who is being deposed is questioned by the opposing side's attorney. Also present are a court reporter, who records all questions and answers verbatim, and the witness's attorney, who is there to object to irrelevant questions and to protect the rights of the witness. Occasionally, depositions are videotaped and can be used later at trial.

Being asked to give a deposition does not automatically mean that the nurse will be called as a witness at trial. It may be that the deposition reveals that a nurse has no significant knowledge of the matter, and this would end her involvement in the case. However, if a nurse is a named defendant, an expert witness, or a significant witness, the nurse's involvement will continue. The deposition is used to fix testimony for the trial, and it can be used to impeach the nurse's credibility, should there be differences between testimony at trial and that which was provided at a deposition.

At the time of deposition a nurse may be asked to discuss what she remembers about a particular incident. Copies of the medical record and other documents are provided for reference and review. Also, hypothetical questions may be asked. An example could be, "What should a home care nurse do if she observes that a cardiac client is cyanotic?"

Guidelines for a Deponent or Witness

There are several guidelines that a nurse should follow when providing a deposition or appearing as a witness at trial. It is important to be prepared for the deposition or testimony. This usually involves meeting with the attorney representing the nurse to review the process, discuss anticipated questions, and review notations in the plaintiff's health care record. During the deposition, information must be provided in a truthful and honest manner. A nurse should not guess at answers; just state simply "I don't know." Only information that is requested should be provided. The nurse as the defendant or as the deponent (one who is being deposed) is not expected to search for information that is not readily available. One should not volunteer information.

A nurse-witness or deponent is usually asked to comment or state opinions based on the clinical record. Because it is often years later that one is called as a witness, this underscores the importance of clear documentation at the time of care. The client's record, containing information recorded at the time of the incident, may be the only evidence of what was observed or what happened, because it would be difficult to recall solely on the basis of memory. This in turn reminds caregivers that documentation should contain facts related to what is observable and measurable. For example, "client looked better" or "wound improving" are nonspecific, evaluative statements only. It would be better to describe observable signs of improvement, such as skin color, vital signs, a measurable decrease in the size of the wound or decreased measured amounts of drainage, and what it looks like.

Sometimes the opposing attorney will try to intimidate a witness or deponent or try to put words in the witness's mouth. One should provide well-thought-out answers in a calm manner and avoid showing anger, defensiveness, or excitement. Questions should be repeated or clarified if they are not understood. A deponent will have the opportunity to review the transcript of the deposition after it is completed and will be able to correct any errors or misstated answers. Throughout the deposition, the opposing attorney will be evaluating the nurse as a potential witness at trial, paying attention to the nurse's facial expressions, manner, and appearance.

COMPETENCY HEARING TESTIMONY

All competent adults have the right to make decisions affecting their health care and other aspects of their lives. This right includes whether or not they choose a recommended test or treatment and general control over their affairs, such as whether to enter into contracts. Generally, state law defines a competent adult as one who has reached a certain chronological age, usually 18 or 21 years of age. Exceptions to this rule include minors (under the age of competency); who may consent to certain health care services, such as drug abuse treatment and contraceptive services, and to marriage; when they are deemed competent to make their own decisions.

Thus, unless a person is found legally incompetent by a court, he or she is presumed to be competent to make his or her own decisions. The burden of proof to declare a person incompetent usually involves a showing of clear and convincing evidence, which is a higher burden than required by some other legal proceedings. When a person is declared incompetent, there are serious consequences concerning personal autonomy and the right of privacy. Judges rely heavily on the opinions of nurses and other health care workers in rendering a decision regarding the person's competency status. If a person is declared incompetent, the court would appoint a guardian who would then make decisions for the individual. Nurses are frequently asked to testify at competency hearings and would be asked to provide factual information, not opinions, as to the competency of the individual.

Will Contest

Another situation that the nurse could be asked to testify in with regard to the client's competency is a will contest. In this instance, someone, usually a family member, is contesting the ability of the deceased to have made a proper and legally valid will. One of the issues that needs to be resolved at the will contest hearing is whether the deceased had the capacity to make the will at the time the document was executed. Thus, the individual's competency during the time in question is at issue.

The home care nurse may be asked to testify regarding her knowledge of the client at the time the will was made or changed. Relevant statements by the nurse include how the individual managed dressing and eating habits, household activities, and health care. If the client had problems in many of these areas, it could be determined that the client was unable to care for his or her person or property. By presenting this type of evidence, the one who is challenging the will hopes to prove that the deceased lacked the capacity to understand what the effect of the will would be at the time it was executed so that the will would be declared invalid.

In order to assess the deceased's state of mind, the testimony of nurses and others who had frequent contact with the client is invaluable. This can occur even if the nurse did not sign the actual will as a witness. Once again, documentation in the home care record assists the testimony. The nurse can usually refer to the record to refresh her memory, so detailed notes made on the condition of the home and the personal hygiene and decision-making capacity of the client are important. Any direct statements by the client concerning the will or business affairs should be included in the nursing notes because they could be helpful in any later proceeding.

Witnessing a Document

If a nurse is asked to witness a will in the client's home, it is usually better to ask that someone else do this. Having witnesses sign a document helps ensure its validity and with some types of documents, such as wills, may be necessary to be legally enforceable. Taken at its face value, signing as a witness means that a nurse has seen another (the client), sign his or her name. This serves to substantiate that the person signing the document or will intended to be bound by what was signed. Witnesses serve a valuable function in any dispute that arises later regarding the will. The witness can give valuable testimony surrounding the circumstances of signing the will or document. Such proof may address issues related to forgery, duress, or coercion in obtaining the signature or the mental capacity of the one who executed the will (Connaway, 1985). Because a witness could be called at any time to testify or give information on these issues, it is considered prudent to have someone else sign as a witness. Some agencies have policies against home care nurses signing as a witness to a will executed by a client. However, this does not mean that a nurse may not be called upon to testify on her knowledge of the issues as based on the nurse-client relationship.

Guardianship

Guardianship hearings would be another example of a proceeding where a home care nurse could be called upon to testify on the issue of competency of a client. This usually arises when the ability of an elderly person to handle his or her own affairs comes into question. Again, testimony would center around the individual's physical and mental condition, care, and safety. It may be that the home care nurse notifies the family of the individual or a protective agency when there is sufficient information for concern. The court proceeding will then attempt to determine whether the person lacks sufficient understanding to communicate responsible decisions concerning his or her person, including provisions for health care, food, clothing, and shelter, because of any mental disability, disease, senility, or chemical dependence (Northrop & Kelly, 1987). Petitions to declare a person incompetent come from any number of sources, including friends, relatives, or health care workers. A finding of legal incompetence and subsequent guardianship can be made only by a court and should be distinguished from a physician's diagnosis that a client is incompetent. Sometimes, legally incompetent clients have been able to participate in decisions involving their health care.

In a New York state case, the right of involuntarily committed (incompetent) mentally ill clients to refuse antipsychotic medications was upheld (*Rivers v. Katz*, 1986). Wide latitude should be given to the client in participating in health care decisions. One cannot assume that mental or physical impairment makes an individual decisionally incapable. The right of the client to make informed choices is fundamental to the nursing care that he or she receives.

ACTIVITIES SURROUNDING A LAWSUIT

Initiation of a Suit

The first step in a lawsuit is for a party who believes that he or she may have a cause of action against another person to initiate the suit, usually through an attorney. The person who has the cause of action becomes the plaintiff and is sometimes referred to as the injured party. The defendant is the answering party and is the person against whom the action is sought.

In most cases there is more than one defendant named in the suit. A nursing negligence case would typically name the agency as a defendant as well as members of the nursing staff. Also included could be manufacturers of products or companies that supply products used by the nurse. There is usually a time period within which the suit can be brought in cases of personal injury. This time period, called the statute of limitations, is generally two years, with some exceptions, as in the case of minors. It is important that any malpractice insurance policy cover the statutory time limit period even if the nurse changes jobs or no longer practices as a nurse.

Summons

The next step is for the defendant to be served with a summons to appear before the court at a specified time. This process is known as service and functions to notify officially a named defendant that a lawsuit is pending. If a nurse receives a summons as a named defendant, she should notify her supervisor, her attorney or the agency's attorney, and, if appropriate, her liability insurance carrier. This is especially important because the defendant must answer the complaint within a certain time period or risk forfeiting the right to defend the suit. If a nurse has an individual liability insurance policy, the insurance company may provide her with an attorney to defend the suit. This is a usual feature of most liability policies, and the nurse can review hers to check for this right. If not, the nurse should arrange to have an attorney of her own, because it could be that the agency's interest in the matter may be adverse to the nurse's.

Notice should also be given to the employing agency, usually through the supervisor, so that the agency's attorney can be prepared to represent any interest that the agency may have in the matter. Once the legal process has begun, the nurse-defendant should discuss the suit only with her attorney or the agency's attorneys or persons designated by them. Statements made to others may be introduced as evidence at trial and could be used against the nurse-defendant.

Subpoena

A subpoena is a document issued by a court requiring one to appear to give testimony on a particular matter. This may be in a competency hearing at probate court, child custody dispute, or a matter involving an allegation of negligence. A *subpoena duces tecum* is a subpoena that not only compels the witness to appear in court but also requires him or her to provide books, documents, or other tangible items in his or her possession that may tend to clarify the subject matter at trial. The nurse-witness should always check with her supervisor before supplying any such agency documents or client records. Usually when these requests are made, the person to whom the subpoena is served can request a fee for administrative costs or photocopying the materials. The person accepting the subpoena should promptly telephone the attorney requesting these records, so that payment can be arranged before any records are released. The same procedural step as to payment could apply when records are released to a client upon his or her valid written request, whether connected with a lawsuit or not.

It is important to remember that a subpoena must be complied with because it is a court order. Failure to do so may subject a person to being held in contempt of court. This is the reason for a subpoena; it is a formal process with a written statement delivered personally to an individual. In addition, the individual is required to sign that it was received, as proof of service. This helps ensure that the proper procedural steps are complied with as required by law.

ETHICAL ISSUES IN HOME CARE

The growth of the home health care system is due in part to the increased number of elderly individuals, cost-containment policies in hospital care, and limited numbers of nursing home beds. Most important, home care has grown because it is the care option of choice for most people. As home care has grown, the ethical dilemmas that the home care nurse faces become more numerous and complex.

Home care has, as its mission, the support of individuals without loss of autonomy in the community

(Collopy, Dabler, & Zuckerman, 1990). Yet, constraints upon the home care nurse's practice by regulatory bodies, third-party payers, and hospitals often place the nurse in the position of having to make difficult ethical decisions. At times, home care nurses are required to discontinue service to clients who no longer meet the criteria for reimbursement even though they still have a health care need. The subject of abandonment is discussed earlier in this chapter.

ANA Scope of Practice

The ANA has outlined the ethical considerations for the home health nurse in its document entitled *A Statement of the Scope of Home Health Nursing Practice* (ANA, 1992). It states:

The importance of ethics in health care has dramatically increased as society grapples with the allocation of health care resources and the use of advanced technology. Advances in research and development have greatly enhanced the tools available to health care providers to extend the length, though not necessarily the quality, of life. Not only does the home health nurse deal with issues of allocation, but also with principles of autonomy, beneficence, nonmaleficence, justice, confidentiality, and truth telling.

Guided by the *Code for Nurses with Interpretive Statements* (ANA, 1985), the home health nurse pursues or creates a forum to deal with the myriad ethical issues confronted in practice. Such a forum allows nurses, clients, and caregivers to identify, differentiate, and clarify ethical and legal dilemmas and begin the process of negotiating solutions that accommodate the often conflicting needs and goals that emerge.

The basic conceptualization of home health sets the tone for the nature, allocation and range of services accessible to clients. Home health care is not merely a change in delivery site or a version of acute care delivered at home. Home health requires a change in the definitions and structures of care so that there is a broad array of services and caregivers available to clients experiencing enduring frailty, multidimensional problems and services outside the realm of normal or standard medical treatment (Collopy et al., 1990).

Due to the complex nature of home health services and the predominately elderly population home health serves, the ethical issues that arise pose dilemmas that will benefit from identification, discussion, and reflection by all parties. Premature discharge of clients based on exhausted or diminished reimbursement sources can influence the decision to provide home care. Clients who are underserved and families who are unable to successfully meet the demands of care can pose difficult problems for the health care organization and the nurse. Clients, families, and caregivers may demand services that are not required or covered by insurance sources, reject reasonable and beneficial treatment and planning activities, refuse to improve environmental conditions essential to a nursing care plan, or avoid reporting abuse or neglect. Many situations in home health involve the autonomous concerns of different parties: the agency and nurse provider, the client, the family caregivers, the community, and the third-party payer.

The types of ethical dilemmas encountered in home health care are illustrated by, but not limited, to the following situations:

- The home setting may diminish formal caregiver authority while encouraging client autonomy. Competing perceptions of autonomy from the professional, client, family, and informal caregivers can develop.
- Decreased autonomy can occur as the frailty of the client diminishes his or her ability to act on decisions, even though the ability to make decisions about care has not been impaired. Increasing dependency on others for a desired quality of life may require accommodation of competing interests.
- Balancing beneficence requires acknowledgement of the benefits and burdens of the care options, caregivers, and choices of services. The assumption that home health is innately appropriate and good for clients as a substitute for other types of care is open to challenge. Specific situations and individual values influence the benefits of home health nursing practice for clients.
- Justice demands that all health care recipients receive adequate information concerning both the burdens and benefits of home health care as a service option. Denial of access, overutilization of services, and the selection of vulnerable populations for inappropriate or limited services challenges the ethic of justice in home health practice. All clients and caregivers have the right to expect that their human rights will be duly observed during the course of service.
- Confidentiality demands that disclosed or observed information entrusted to a formal caregiver remain undisclosed to unauthorized individuals. Because there may be several parties entrusting the nurse and home health staff with confidential information, the potential for ethical conflict can occur from the multiple demands for disclosure posed by various parties. The home health nurse may be the recipient of the most intimate and private information about the client, family, and caregivers. In the informal environment of home health, confidentiality of client disclosure is to be protected without compromise.
- The nature of home health care demands the mediation of values, obligations, and interests of formal and informal care providers. Home health nursing practice must include the use of formal and informal ethical structures or committees that can assist in educating, counseling, and supporting all concerned in mediating the ethical dilemmas that arise in home health nursing practice. On the health policy level, scarce resources, societal values, and allocation proposals will continue to provide difficult challenges to the practice of home health nursing.

The home care nurse will encounter various ethical dilemmas in her practice. The consideration of the above-mentioned issues, the review of agency policies and procedures that deal with the handling of ethical issues, and the ongoing communication with other agency personnel, physicians, and the profession will continue to assist the nurse in dealing with these issues.

Advance Medical Directive

In 1990, the federal government passed legislation called The Patient Self-Determination Act. This act, which was part of the Omnibus Reconciliation Act of 1990, required that hospitals, skilled nursing facilities, home health agencies, health maintenance organizations, and hospices provide written information to patients about their option to accept or refuse medical or surgical treatment and formulate advance directives in compliance with state law. This act also mandates that the health care provider document in the medical record whether or not clients have executed advance directives (The Patient Self-Determination Act, 1990).

There is growing evidence that clients should have a voice in decision making regarding treatment options and the refusal of medical care (Annas & Glantz, 1986; ANA, 1986a; Markson & Steel, 1990). This is not a problem when people are alert and can make their wishes known to their primary care providers. In January 1993, the advance medical directive was initiated to clearly identify a course of medical action in a situation in which the client would be unable to make decisions and communicate those decisions to the primary care provider. The advance medical directive is a document that indicates the wishes of the client regarding various types of medical treatment in representative situations (Markson & Steel, 1990). There are two types of advance medical directives, living wills and health care proxies, sometimes called durable power of attorney. Either type of directive would come into effect only if the client became incapacitated and unable to make decisions, and both directives are subject to change at any time.

Living wills are usually used by people to record their decisions to decline life-prolonging treatment should they become hopelessly ill. The living will indicates the circumstances in which it would be implemented and the care that should be provided should those circumstances arise. Durable power of attorney or a health care proxy focuses on naming a decision maker who would make health care decisions for the client if he or she became unable to make them. The proxy would have knowledge of the client's wishes regarding care.

In response to the legislation, home care agencies have provided education regarding advance directives to their direct care staff. As part of the admission process to a home care agency, the home care nurse must discuss advance directives with the client, their meaning and their use. In this discussion, the nurse must be careful not to influence the clients in any way with regard to their choices and decisions. Each time clients enter a health care system (hospital, nursing home, home care agency), they will be confronted with questions regarding whether they have completed an advance medical directive. Collaboration between providers will reduce the frequency with which clients will have to communicate their wishes about their care. When a client is transferred to another health care agency, the home care nurse is responsible for informing that agency that the client has an advance medical directive.

The regulations concerning the implementation of the Omnibus Reconciliation Act of 1990 differ from state to state. An example of a form used in Connecticut to provide information on advance medical directives, health care agents, conservatorship, and gift donation is included in Appendix G. Many agencies provide this form for clients if they want to execute an advance medical directive. Once completed, a copy of the advance medical directive must be maintained in the client record.

TEST YOURSELF

1. Outline your agency's procedure for releasing information from a client's home care record.

2. You are on a visit to Mrs. Smith. In the home are her two sons and a notary public. They ask that you witness the signing of her power of attorney to the one son. What would you do?

3. Discuss your responsibilities in complying with the agency's exposure control plan.

4. What determines that an incident or occurrence report is filed in your agency? Fill out a report, making up a client situation, then review the content of your report with your supervisor and track where the report goes.

5. At work this morning, you were served a subpoena to testify in a competency hearing for Mr. Jones. What are the steps you would take?

6. You are delivering services to Mr. Grant, whose insurance company has decided to no longer cover his service. You and the physician determine Mr. Grant still has a need for home care services. What would you do?

REFERENCES

American Nurses Association. (1985). *Code for nurses with interpretive statements.* Washington, DC: Author.

American Nurses Association. (1986a). *Standards of community health nursing practice.* Washington, DC: Author.

American Nurses Association. (1986b). *Standards for home health nursing practice.* Washington, DC: Author.

American Nurses Association. (1987). *Liability and you—What registered nurses need to know.* Washington, DC: Author.

American Nurses Association. (1992). *A statement of the scope of home health nursing practice.* Washington, DC: Author.

Annas, C., & Glantz, H. (1986). The right of elderly patients to refuse life sustaining medical treatment. *Milbank Quarterly, 64* (Suppl 2).

Bass v. Barksdale et al., 671 S.W. 2d 476 (Tenn. App. 1984).

Collopy, B., Dabler, N., & Zuckerman, C. (1990). The ethics of home care: Autonomy and accommodation. *Hastings Center Report, 20*(2), 1–16.

Connaway, N. (1985). Documenting patient care in the home—Legal issues for the home health nurse (pt. ii). *Home Health Care Nurse, 3,* 44–46.

Cushing, M. (1982). The legal side: A matter of judgment. *American Journal of Nursing,* 990–992.

Czubinsky v. Doctor's Hospital, 139 Cal. App. 3d 361, 188 Cal. 685 (1983).

Guigino v. Harvard Community Health Plan et al., 403 N.E. 2d 1166 (Mass., 1980).

Josberger, M.C., & Ries, D.T. (1985). Nurse experts—Selecting and preparing them for litigation. *Trial, 21,* 68–71.

Killion, S. (1985). Patients' rights to their medical records. *Health Span, 2,* 28–33.

Markson, L., & Steel, K. (1990). Using advance directives in the home setting. *Generations, 14,* 25–28.

Northrop, C., & Kelly, M. (1987). *Legal issues in nursing.* St. Louis, MO: Mosby.

The Patient Self-Determination Act, Omnibus Reconciliation Act of 1990, Pub. L. No. 101-508, § 4206 Medicare, § 4751 Medicaid (1990).

Pisel v. Stamford Hospital, 180 Conn. 314, 430 A. 2d (1980).

Rivers v. Katz, 504 N.Y.S. 2d 74, 495 N.E. 2d 337 (1986).

Sandroff, R. (1983). Why you really ought to have your own malpractice policy. *RN, 46,* 29–33.

United States v. Greber, 760 F. 2d 68 (1985). Cert. Denied 474 U.S. 988, 1985.

Utter v. United Hospital Center, 236 S.E. 2d 213 (W.Va., 1977).

Special Home Care Programs and Services

OBJECTIVES

Upon completion of this chapter, the reader will be able to identify:

1. Four areas to consider in the hospital versus home care decision for high-tech care
2. Three main types of high-tech care provided in the home
3. Strategies for implementing the nursing process in high-tech home care
4. Working within the framework of the high-tech home care team
5. Teaching and documentation strategies for high-tech home care clients
6. Organizations that issue regulations or standards for home infusion therapy
7. Four reasons why there has been significant growth in pediatric home care
8. Factors to consider before discharging a pediatric client needing high-tech home care
9. Home care services required to care for pediatric clients with specific illnesses in the home
10. Adjustments and issues to consider as families transition from hospital care to high-tech pediatric home care
11. The philosophical foundation of hospice care
12. The Medicare hospice benefit
13. Differences between traditional Medicare home care and the Medicare hospice benefit
14. Purposes of early newborn discharge and psychiatric home care programs

KEY CONCEPTS

- **Nursing considerations for high-tech home care clients**
- **Ways of implementing enteral and intravenous therapy in the home**
- **Home ventilator care**
- **Preparing for the pediatric home care client**
- **Guidelines for high-tech pediatric clients**
- **The philosophy of hospice**
- **The Medicare hospice benefit**
- **Specialty home care programs**

AGENCY-SPECIFIC MATERIAL NEEDED

- Policies and procedures for high-tech home care clients
- Teaching tools for high-tech home care clients
- Client record and care plans specific to the high-tech client
- Policies, procedures, assessment forms, and care plans that incorporate child health issues
- Hospice policy, procedures, and referral mechanisms
- Information about internal and external early newborn discharge and psychiatric home care programs

INTRODUCTION

The rapid changes in the provision of home care outlined previously in this text have opened new specialty areas of practice for the home care nurse. The provision of high-technology care, such as enteral and intravenous (IV) therapy and care to clients on ventilators, has created the new field called *high-tech home care.* This chapter discusses high-tech home care provided to adult and pediatric populations. Other specialty areas and programs are being created and refined to meet the changing health care needs of our population through the home care system. Although these are too numerous to describe in this chapter, the authors have chosen the specialty areas of hospice care, psychiatric home care, and early newborn discharge programs as the other specialty programs currently most seen in home care.

These programs are presented in this text to introduce the new nurse to this information. All nurses in home care need to be aware of the various home care services available in their own agencies, as well as throughout their communities. Just as the nurse might be called upon to refer a client or family member to a community resource, the home care nurse will need to know the types of home care specialty programs that are available for referral. Additionally, the general home care nurse will work with several specialty practitioners and programs while caring for her caseload of clients and needs to know at least the basics about these services. As the growth in home care continues, specialty programs offer the nurse opportunities for advancement in both the clinical and managerial aspects of home care.

HIGH-TECH HOME CARE

Historical Perspective

Home care has changed dramatically since the 1970s, and several factors have played a role in creating the differences seen in home health care today. In the late 1970s, when the Social Security system was scrutinized closely, one thing was apparent. The current method of health care delivery, centered in acute care settings, such as hospitals, was costly, inefficient, and, many times, ineffective. More recently, the focus on revamping the national health care system has placed a demand on the home health care industry to provide comprehensive care for all clients. The initial changes in the late 1970s spurred the manufacturing, health care, and insurance communities to began preparing to po-

sition themselves favorably and safely in the face of new rules and regulations.

The pharmaceutical and durable medical equipment (DME) industries in particular were the first to respond to the challenges and have continued to be leaders in the provision of this specialized home care.

Although national companies have been very active and successful in high-tech home care, with the movement toward managed care, all home care agencies are looking to provide comprehensive home care in an integrated model. A successful home care agency that wants to vie for managed care contracts and strong relationships with insurers must be prepared to include the provision of sophisticated, technical services. Home health care is a business, and, like any other, it will continue to change in response to market demands.

Market Changes

What were these changes in the market, and how has home care responded to them? The first change was the formulation and introduction of the diagnosis-related group (DRG) system. In an effort to make hospitals care for clients more efficiently and effectively and thus reduce costs, diagnoses were assigned a number, a reimbursement amount and a predetermined length of stay. This concept is known as prospective payment. The principle was that if clients were cared for well, they could be released on or before the predetermined time, and the hospital would be reimbursed adequately. If the client went home early the hospital made money; however, if the client overstayed the DRG time limit, the hospital was financially responsible. Thus, efforts were made to have clients released sooner. No longer could someone recover at a leisurely pace as an inpatient. More emphasis was placed on families, friends, and health care agencies to manage the recovery period. The hospital has become a truly "acute" setting.

Therapies that had in the past prolonged an inpatient stay, such as IV antibiotics, pain control, chemotherapy, hyperalimentation, enteral feedings, and ventilator care, became a costly burden for the hospitals. Recognizing this, the pharmaceutical and health care products industries shifted their attention to providing these services in the home. Rapid advances in technology led to the development of lightweight, user-friendly electronic pumps for delivery of IV drugs by the layperson and portable ventilator units. Third-generation antibiotics were developed that could be given every 12 or 24 hours, which made home antibiotic therapy more feasible. Insurance companies, recognizing that the daily cost of hospitalization, ranging from

$500 to $1,000 a day, was reduced by approximately one third with home care therapy, began revamping their health policies to include these services.

The development of high-tech home care did not occur in a vacuum. A need was recognized, and many industries and home care agencies worked simultaneously to answer the need. As more and more clients experience these types of therapies in the home, there has been greater acceptance among clients, families, and the community. Home care nursing has now become more specialized, and the nurse who works in home care needs greater training and expertise, especially in using highly technical equipment and in performing comprehensive assessment and monitoring of acute care in the home.

This section focuses on what separates high-tech from less acute home care. Whether the nurse provides high-tech home care directly, works in cooperation with a high-tech provider, or refers a client to another agency, she will need to be familiar with the aspects of high-tech home care nursing presented in this section. In an effort to prepare the nurse at all levels of experience, a step-by-step approach is taken. The home care nurse is the axis of total client care in all areas of home care. The responsibilities of providing high-tech home care can seem staggering, but by following well-established policies and procedures and using an organized approach, the nurse can perform her role safely and effectively.

Models for the Provision of High-Tech Home Care

There have been many models for the provision of home infusion and respiratory therapy. Initially, clients receiving infusion and enteral therapies were trained in the hospital, picked up their supplies and equipment at the hospital pharmacy, and compounded their own drugs at home. The therapies used were usually antibiotics or simple hydration, making this method of service delivery feasible. Soon outside pharmaceutical vendors took over this responsibility, and although training was still provided in the hospital, the vendors compounded and delivered the medication the client required. Nurses were employed by these companies to visit the client, often in conjunction with the home health care nurse, to manage the infusion therapy portion of the care. Although this model is still very prevalent in home care today, more agencies are assuming the total responsibility for the client's care, which means that the home care nurse must possess infusion skills in addition to medical-surgical nursing knowledge and home care skills.

This recent change to comprehensive service delivery has been created, in part, by the movement to a managed care model of care and reimbursement. This model requires that total, comprehensive care be delivered to the client either through contract or directly with one entity responsible for the total coordination of care. The goal is to eliminate duplicated, fragmented services.

The Decision for High-Tech Home Care Services

It is essential to determine if high-tech services are feasible for a client prior to discharge from the hospital. In most situations, the client, family, physician, nurse on the unit, and the hospital discharge planner determine, in conjunction with the home health agency, if a client is appropriate for referral and make plans accordingly. If a client is discharged without this planning, or the client is currently receiving services from the agency, the primary home care nurse is responsible for the initial assessment of the client and evaluation of the appropriateness and suitability of the proposed therapy.

There are four areas to be evaluated when determining whether a client is suitable for high-tech home care services:

1. the client and family involvement with, commitment to, and understanding of the therapy
2. the safety and efficacy of the therapy itself
3. the availability of equipment, supplies, and expertise
4. the availability of financial resources

These evaluations are as important as the physical assessment of the client and should be completed early in the client's hospitalization so that any concerns may be addressed before high-tech home care is considered a serious option.

Client and Family Involvement

The first area for evaluation is the client and family involvement with, commitment to, and understanding of the therapy. This will likely be the most important evaluation and is foundational for success of high-tech home care. The decision to send a client home with infusion, enteral, or respiratory therapy should be made with thought to all the people involved. The physician faces almost constant pressure from hospital administrators to discharge clients as soon as possible, especially those who have overstayed their DRG time. The client also may be weary of hospital routine and wish to go home "at any cost." Or it may simply be that the discharge planning department views home therapy as routine for this diagnosis and has set the discharge wheels in motion. Whatever the reason, home care is often ordered and provided with little advance notice. The success of providing highly technological care at home resides in the initial evaluation and planning.

The Three "Rs" in the Evaluation Process

It is the primary home care nurse's responsibility to assess the client's and family's understanding of three areas we'll call the three "Rs," that is, the *results*, the *responsibilities*, and the expected *risks* of therapy. Ideally, a family conference with client, family, physician, and primary care nurse should be scheduled prior to discharge to discuss these areas. In reality, this is often not possible, and it becomes the home care nurse's responsibility to make this evaluation through individual discussions, often at the time of the initial in-home assessment. However it is accomplished, this assessment should be completed prior to implementation of therapy.

First, the client and family will need to have a realistic understanding of the expected *results* of the therapy, be it curative, palliative, or unknown. For example, a client must be able to distinguish between chemotherapy received in the past in the hope of a cure and the palliative chemotherapy that may be proposed at the present. It is equally important when the expected results are unknown or unclear, as in the case of pain control, human growth hormones, or some antibiotics. Any false hopes or expectations should be brought to light and discussed. By using simple, direct questions, the nurse can evaluate the client and family understanding of the expected results. Some sample questions are:

- Can you tell me what this therapy is supposed to do for you?
- Have you had any medications or solutions similar to these in the past?
- What was the result of that therapy?
- What is your understanding of this new medication or therapy as compared with others like it that you have received in the past?
- Are you comfortable/happy/pleased with what your physician has proposed as a course of treatment?
- If not, what are your concerns?
- Are there any terms, such as *palliative* or *hyperalimentation*, that you need explained in more detail?

- What do the words *palliative/curative* mean to you?

The client and family must also have a clear understanding of the *responsibilities* involved with the provision of the therapy. All too often, physicians and other health care workers in the hospital leave the client with brief, surface assurances that the home care nurse will take care of everything and "it will take only a few minutes or hours a day." Those involved need to realize that the time commitment to high-tech home care can often be extensive and restrictive. They must also recognize and be prepared for the client's shift in dependence from hospital staff to family, friends, and home health agency personnel.

The most effective way to help clients realize these responsibilities is to outline for the client and family what a typical 24-hour period will be like with therapy. It is important to tie aspects of the therapy into their individual daily lives and routines. For example, the nurse may explain, "Mrs. Jones, you will be giving your mother the antibiotic at 8:00 A.M. and 8:00 P.M. daily. You will need to begin preparing your supplies at 7:30 so that you can start on time. The infusion takes 30 minutes so that at 8:15 you will have to assemble all your disconnection supplies. You will need to plan to be involved with this whole process from 7:30 A.M. to 8:45 A.M. Knowing this will allow you to plan enough time to get ready for work. The therapy is scheduled for a month and one-half (six weeks)." By giving those involved time frames as they relate to their own daily routines and schedules, there is less chance for feelings of disillusionment and frustration with the therapy.

The final R involves the *risks* of therapy, and this is both an important and delicate subject. The risks of each type of therapy should first be discussed with the physician and home health manager responsible for this function prior to detailed discussion with the client and family. A word of caution: All clients are entitled to be informed of all risks involved in their therapy. It is also important to indicate the risks inherent in the delivery of therapy at home versus the hospital as well as side effects of the medications or therapy itself. A physician or family member may wish that certain risks be de-emphasized. This is not a decision that the primary nurse should make in isolation, but rather it should be first explored with the physician and nursing supervisor and, as indicated, other family members.

The home care nurse's responsibility in assessing the client and family understanding of the three Rs is imperative to successful therapy. The nurse must feel confident that all involved clearly understand what the therapy is for, how much they will be doing, and what risks they accept as part of the therapy.

Safety and Efficacy of the Therapy

The second evaluation area is the safety and efficacy of the therapy itself. This is independent of the client's understanding of risk factors. Safety factors include the environment in which the therapy will be provided (both physical and emotional), side effects and effects of the medications or solutions, and the functional ability of the client or caregiver who will be performing the procedures.

For example, in pain control therapy, there must be a caregiver who is physically and emotionally able to deliver the medication. The client, under the influence of a narcotic, is often neither physically nor mentally able to safely perform the necessary procedures. A close family relative, such as a spouse, may be emotionally incapable of safely adjusting narcotic doses or accepting the client's response to narcotic therapy.

Another safety factor involves the expected effects or side effects of the medications or equipment. For example, the side effects of many chemotherapeutic agents, such as cisplatin, are often severe. In the case of a severely debilitated client, it may be difficult to safely provide this therapy within the home setting. The nurse's evaluation of possible alternatives or the use of support personnel will be required. With regard to equipment, caring for a ventilator-dependent client on a home respirator in a house with old or unsafe wiring or a home in a remote location that is difficult to reach by emergency personnel may be inappropriate.

Finally, a more subtle and often overlooked safety factor is the ease with which a therapy can be delivered in the home. The goal in home care is to teach the client and family to eventually be independent in the client's care. Because mechanical and electronic equipment is often required, it is imperative that the client and family are able to learn how to use and troubleshoot the equipment. For example, hyperalimentation therapy with concomitant pain control and chemotherapy requires the use of several pumps and numerous solution changes daily. The complexity of this therapy regime may be far beyond the ability of most family members. When the demands of the therapy are so complex as to convert the home to a hospital, it may be that the hospital is, in reality, a safer and more economical choice. The provision of supportive services, including nursing visits or shifts to manage the care, is an alternative and requires investigation. Insurance coverage for extensive nursing support in the home has dwindled dramatically over the last few years.

To summarize, the safety and efficacy of the therapy must be evaluated based on the equipment being used; the mental, emotional, and physical abilities of those involved; and risk factors of the therapy, medication, or equipment.

Availability of Equipment and Clinical Expertise

The third major evaluation area is the availability of equipment and expertise. When the therapy is initially mapped out, the primary nurse will need to determine whether it is possible to deliver the therapy as ordered. Specifically, in reviewing the therapy orders the nurse must determine what equipment and how much support personnel at what skill level will be necessary. There are still limitations to current technology. For example, the client may not be capable of manipulating the programming buttons on a mechanical pump and may require a nonmechanical elastomeric pump for therapy. The questions then become, is a disposable pump reimbursable by the payer and is the medication stable in this type of device? The type of pump, stability of the drug, and dosage requirements must all be considered in the selection of equipment.

The availability of clinical and technological expertise is as important as the availability of equipment. When the client is unable to assume responsibility, there must be a caregiver or outside support personnel able to perform the necessary procedures or provide backup. With relation to personnel, the nurse must assess:

1. Does this case require additional specialized professional help, such as oncology or pediatric nursing?
2. Are these specialists available at the times of the day and night when the client needs them?
3. Does the family need full or partial support?
4. Are the outside personnel available in the client's geographic area?

All of these questions must be answered before a determination can be made about the feasibility of providing the therapy in the home. It is, again, the primary nurse's responsibility to assess whether this therapy can be safely and effectively provided with the equipment and personnel available.

Financial Resources

The fourth and final area to be evaluated, financial coverage, is an important factor. When nurses call the insurance company directly, they find dealing with insurance companies, clients, and government agencies regarding finances difficult. The home care nurse, however, can be the critical link that determines whether a therapy will be covered. Consider what goes into the coverage decision. Insurance companies have rigid coverage guidelines, and the representatives making coverage decisions will often be nonclinical employees. In the initial stage of determining coverage it is best to ask broad questions and listen well.

When calling the insurance company, the nurse or someone else designated by the home care organization should identify the agency, his or her position, and information about the client's coverage for home care. Before calling, have all pertinent information readily available. The following information is essential:

1. client's name
2. subscriber's name (in whose name the insurance is carried)
3. policy number
4. Social Security number of client and subscriber
5. subscriber's employer
6. client diagnosis
7. type of therapy
8. expected duration of therapy
9. equipment needed
10. support personnel needed (e.g., nursing visits, shifts)

Questions should be similar to the following:

• Does Mrs. Smith have home care coverage in her policy?
• Does this policy include intravenous/enteral/ respiratory therapy?
• Are registered nurses (RNs), licensed practical nurses (LPNs), and other therapists covered under this policy?
• What, if any, are the restrictions to this coverage?
• What information does the insurance company require to make a coverage decision?
• What information does the insurance company require to ensure reimbursement?

All answers should be carefully documented. Answers will come in various forms, such as "intravenous therapy is covered only when it is deemed medically necessary." Ask for their definition of medically necessary and inquire as to what proof they require (e.g., physician's letter, a hospital document, or a determination by their own medical review board).

When determining coverage for nursing service, the answer, for example, may be "the client is allowed 40 visits per calendar year." Ask how the insurance provider defines a visit (an hour or a four- to eight-hour block of time). Can there be more than one visit per day? Does the insurer pay for visits exceeding the 40? Has the client used any visits within the current calendar year?

Should the nurse find the representative's answers incomplete or unsatisfactory, she can ask to speak with an RN case manager or reviewer. Many insurance companies have created such positions to review the appropriateness of care. At this point, talking with a professional peer, the home care nurse can discuss and clarify the coverage issues. With the advent of managed care, these decisions are most often made by the case manager or managed care coordinator. Recognize that clients have a right to use their benefits to the fullest, and home care can be a cost-effective alternative. It is often the nurse's responsibility to "sell" this concept and the proposed care plan to the insurer. The nurse will need to be familiar with governmental requirements and restrictions, such as for Medicare and Medicaid.

Clarification of coverage can be determined by restating the information provided: "Based on Mrs. Smith's coverage, it is safe to assume that her four-week course of antibiotic therapy is covered. She will require daily visits by an RN, equaling 28 days this calendar year, out of her allowed 40. In addition, it is my understanding that only a portable, electronic pump is covered and that all drugs and biologicals will be covered at 100%." The discussion is concluded by clarifying what paperwork the insurance company requires, which is usually physician's orders, nurse's notes, a letter of medical necessity, and any forms specific to the insurance company. It is imperative that all information provided by the insurance company be carefully documented, including the date and time of the conversation and the full names of all personnel providing information. With the coverage information in hand, the nurse can discuss with the client, family, and physician how and to what extent to proceed with home therapy.

The decision to provide therapy in the home in lieu of hospitalization is often not a simple one. Depending on the model of service delivery in an agency, the responsibilities of the staff nurse in each of these areas may vary. Whether done alone or as part of a team, completing a step-by-step assessment of the feasibility of home care before the client goes home will ensure a more successful course of therapy.

Types of High-Tech Home Care

The definition of what constitutes high-tech home care is changing daily. For the purposes of this section, the focus is on three broad areas: enteral therapy, IV therapy, and home ventilation.

Enteral Therapy

Enteral therapy involves the provision of nutrients through a tube resting in the gut. This can be a nasogastric, gastric, or jejunostomy tube. Feedings consist of highly concentrated solutions containing the carbohydrates, proteins, vitamins, minerals, and electrolytes necessary to sustain life. Enteral therapy is most commonly used for clients with partial obstructions, malabsorption syndromes, or increased nutritional needs. The placement of the tube is dependent on the length of therapy and the condition of the intestinal tract. With advances in the provision of partial and total parenteral nutrition (TPN), the frequency of home enteral therapy has diminished.

Enteral therapy is provided by bolus method, continuous drip, or a modified combination of the two. Nursing considerations relate to:

- the placement and integrity of the tube
- the client's tolerance of the solution
- the client's acceptance of the diagnosis and enteral therapy routine
- the client's fluid and electrolyte balance

This therapy is perhaps the easiest to provide in the home because the procedure itself is simple and easily taught to both client and family. In addition, it is usually covered by insurance carriers, including Medicare. It is important to remember that to ensure coverage, the primary diagnosis must justify the need for enteral feedings. For example, although the client's primary diagnosis may be cancer, the home care diagnosis must describe the condition creating the need for enteral feedings, such as partial bowel obstruction or malabsorption syndrome.

Table 11-1 summarizes the common complications of enteral therapy. Teaching the client and family is the nurse's primary focus of care for the client with enteral therapy. The home care nurse's teaching tools should clearly show the client and family how to assess for possible complications and what actions to take to manage these complications. Documentation must reflect this teaching, the client/family response to instruction, and the nurse's own skilled observation of the client as they relate to these possible complications. Periodic reassessments should be made, as a client may initially tolerate enteral therapy and not display signs of complication until several weeks or months have passed. Continued monitoring will include periodic

weights, blood values, and progress toward client goals to determine the continued need for therapy.

IV Therapy

IV therapy is the broadest category in high-tech home care. Home infusion therapy (HIT) includes:

- anti-infective therapy (antibiotics, antifungals, and antivirals)
- antineoplastic therapy (chemotherapy)
- antithrombolytic therapy
- blood products and derivative (hemotherapy)
- biologic response modifiers (acquired immune deficiency syndrome [AIDS] therapies)
- colony stimulating factor therapy
- fluid and electrolyte replacement (hydration)
- ionotropic drug therapy (dopamine, dobutamine, amrinone)
- iron overload therapy
- pain management therapy
- parenteral nutrition
- post-transplant antirejection therapy
- tocolytic drug therapy (preterm labor management)

IV therapy is provided either peripherally or via a central line access. The myriad types of peripheral accesses cannot be reviewed individually in this text; however, the following are common devices used.

Peripheral Access. The common HepLock is currently the most widely used access. Various peripheral catheters are used, including Landmark and Streamline catheters designed for longer dwell times (3 to 14 or more days). For longer peripheral placement, the peripherally inserted central catheter (PICC) line is currently being used although it is not approved for home placement by nurses in all states. The PICC line, inserted through the antecubital vein, can be threaded to the subclavian vein (peripheral placement) or into the superior vena cava (central placement). All three specialized catheters require additional training to prepare the nurse in proper placement technique. The home care nurse should become familiar with the devices used in the area hospitals where client referrals are generated.

Central Access. Central access lines are of two main types: Hickman/Broviac and Port-A-Cath. Like peripheral lines, the variety of central lines can be classified into these two main types. The Hickman/Broviac is a cuffed central line that is placed in the chest or abdominal wall by blunt dissection. The tip is threaded through a major vessel, usually the brachial artery, into the su-

Table 11–1 Gastrointestinal Complications of Enteral Nutrition Support

Signs and Symptoms	Possible Causes	Management
Diarrhea	Dumping syndrome	1. Dilute nutrient 2. Reduce rate of administration 3. Consider continuous infusion rather than bolus 4. Consider use of antidiarrheal drugs
Nausea Vomiting	Nutrient source too concentrated Rate of administration too rapid	1. Dilute nutrient 2. Reduce rate of administration 3. Consider continuous infusion rather than bolus 4. Consider alternate enteral formula (lactose free, medium chain triglycerides) 5. Consider supplemental use of IV support
Bloating Cramping	Rate of administration of nutrient mixture too rapid Fat intolerance	1. Reduce rate of administration 2. Consider continuous infusion rather than bolus
Hypermotility Distention	Malabsorption Fat intolerance Nutrient source too concentrated Rate of administration too rapid	1. Reduce rate of administration 2. Consider alternate enteral formula 3. Dilute nutrient concentration
Flatulence Borborygmus	Fat intolerance Lactose deficiency	1. Consider alternate enteral formula 2. Reduce concentration

perior vena cava where it rests just outside the atrium. The external end of the Hickman/Broviac protrudes approximately 6 to 12 inches from the exit wound. Within the first three to ten postoperative days, wound healing occurs around the catheter cuff creating a "natural" barrier to infection. The Port-A-Cath is placed in the same manner but does not have an external apparatus. Instead, the "port" is placed under a skin flap in the chest wall, much like a pacemaker. The infusion line is accessed utilizing a special curved, nonboring Huber needle, which pierces the skin and face of the port. The needle is held in place by an occlusive dressing. The port is normally reaccessed once weekly or more frequently depending on the therapy. Each of these central catheters is placed by the surgeon in the hospital or outpatient setting.

Almost all therapies can now be administered through a peripheral line. It is still prudent, however, to provide many chemotherapy drugs, pain control, and hyperalimentation through a central access. It is important to consider the possible need for access to the venous system in the event of an emergency, such as anaphylaxis, narcotic toxicity, or other life-threatening events. The choice of venous access will often be made by the physician, but the nurse's understanding of alternative methods can increase the client's physical and emotional comfort with the process.

Pumps. Rapid advances in technical research and design have produced a large variety of small, lightweight pumps for use in all types of IV therapy. The primary care nurse must choose the most appropriate pump for the client and therapy. The pharmacist is often an excellent resource to assist in making this decision. As a general rule, pain control and chemotherapy should be given in a cassette-style pump with computerized locking mechanisms for the dose and rate. This ensures accurate dosage while preventing accidental or intentional tampering. Syringe, minibag-style pumps, and elastomeric nonmechanical infusers are all appropriate for use in peripheral antibiotic therapy. Stationary pumps are generally utilized for large-volume therapies, such as hyperalimentation, although the CADD TPN pump has been developed as a small portable alternative. Examples of syringe-style pumps include the Auto Syringe and Becton Dickinson. Examples of pumps that utilize a cassette-type reservoir are the CADD Plus, CADD PCA, and CADD TPN pumps. A third style of portable pumps allows for the use of 50-, 100-, and 250-cc minibags, such as the Pancreatic pump and the Parker Infuser. Nonmechanical pumps, such as the Travenol Infuser and the Intermate, are lightweight, disposable, and easy to use. The following six factors are considered when choosing the most appropriate device:

1. What is the volume of solution or medication to be delivered?
2. Over what time period will the medication be delivered? (hours, days)
3. How long, once reconstituted, is the medication stable? (hours, days, weeks)
4. Does the therapy require a constant rate and dosage or does the rate or dose vary?
5. What is the learning and functional ability of the client or caregiver who is going to be taught the use of the pump?
6. What types of pumps are covered by the client's insurance? (Many insurance companies require volumetric pumps for the delivery of drugs and biologicals.)

With this information, a comparison can be made of the pumps available. The correct pump should be appropriate for the learner, have the capacity for the volume of solution, and have features that provide the safe and efficient administration of the required medication.

Hyperalimentation is most often provided via a stationary pump, such as a HomePro, Travenol 6100, or Imed. Like the portable pumps, each of these was designed with specific features for safe, effective delivery of solutions. For example, the HomePro pump has a programmable tapering feature to establish a ramping up and ramping down delivery for TPN that is given on a rotating schedule (e.g., 12 hours on, 12 hours off). The HomePro's ramping feature automatically increases the rate at the beginning and decreases it at the end of the infusion time in an incremental fashion. This reduces the incidence of rapid blood sugar fluctuation in the client. In order to provide IV and enteral therapy in the home, the nurse must locate and familiarize herself with resources for the following:

1. compatibility and stability information for enteral and parenteral solutions commonly used in home care
2. acceptable diagnosis for each type of therapy (often a coverage requirement by insurance and Medicare)
3. pump specification and features for pumps used by the home health agency
4. policies and procedures for administration of each type of therapy

Home Ventilator Care

The final category of high-tech care discussed in this section is home ventilator care. Unlike the other types of home therapy for which the nurse will act as the primary coordinator, with home ventilator therapy the respiratory therapist will function in this capacity. Most respiratory therapy companies have very strict policies and procedures under which they operate. It is helpful for the nurse to obtain a copy of these and be familiar with them. The information outlined in this section is based on general guidelines common to many companies.

The initial assessment of the client to determine whether he or she is a candidate for home ventilator therapy will include physiological, sociological, mental, and emotional evaluations. The client must have 24-hour attendance at all times either by the family or qualified support personnel, and there must be a physician and registered respiratory therapist available oncall at all times. The home must meet all the electrical and structural requirements to support the respiratory equipment, as well as backup measures, such as a generator in case of power failure.

Training for ventilator therapy always occurs in the hospital setting. The hospital usually accepts responsibility for training the family in the elements of client care, including suctioning, tracheostomy tube cleaning and changing, cardiopulmonary resuscitation (CPR), and general management of complications. The care and functioning of the ventilator itself is most often taught by the company's respiratory therapist. If the model of ventilator that the client will use at home is different from the one that the client is using in the hospital, the home model is provided to the hospital at least one week before discharge. This allows the family to learn to use the equipment, and it allows the hospital team to evaluate the client's response to this new ventilator. The client and home support team will need to demonstrate, to the satisfaction of the company therapist at least 48 hours before discharge, proficiency in managing the equipment. This proficiency includes maintenance and troubleshooting procedures.

At the same time that this training is occurring in the hospital, the home is being readied for the client. A few days before discharge, a ventilator is placed in the client's home. A determination is made that all the electrical and structural requirements are adequate and that support systems are in place. In addition, the telephone, electrical, oil or gas companies, and fire and ambulance departments will be notified by phone and in writing that a ventilator-dependent client will be in this home. The same notification should be sent to the answering services for the physician, home care agency, and the respiratory equipment company. The primary care nurse needs to be familiar with these aspects and ensure that adequate planning has taken place prior to discharge.

On the day of discharge, the client should be seen by the pulmonologist. The client is then escorted home by an RN or credentialed respiratory therapy practitioner. All RNs scheduled to care for the client should have extensive experience in ventilator care and have current CPR certification. The home care nurse's role as primary care coordinator does not really begin until the client is home. As with any high-tech care, careful planning and anticipation of problems and emergencies with appropriate contingency plans will enhance the chances for success. The nurse should be proactive in becoming involved and being prepared long before the client arrives home.

Case Studies

The following case studies encompass the three main areas of high-tech home care discussed thus far. The first illustrates a client who received combination therapy that included hyperalimentation, pain control, and chemotherapy. The second client, the most complex case presented, required enteral, hydration, antibiotic, and heparin therapy. The final client required home ventilator therapy. These case studies are presented to emphasize the myriad areas the nurse needs to consider.

Client 1

Lynn was a 63-year-old woman with primary breast cancer with metastasis to the axilla. She was initially referred to the agency, following a radical mastectomy for chemotherapy and hyperalimentation. A single lumen Hickman catheter was placed for the provision of both hyperalimentation and chemotherapy. Lynn had experienced a 30-pound weight loss over a three-month period. Her initial TPN orders were for 500 cc of Travasol 8.5% with electrolytes in 500 cc D50W to be infused at 83 cc per hour for 12 hours. On Monday, Wednesday, Friday, and Saturday, an additional 500 cc of Intralipid 10% was to be added to the solution to be infused at 125 cc per hour. The hyperalimentation was infused using a HomePro stationary pump. Lynn's chemotherapy orders were for methotrexate 25 mg followed by 5-fluorouracil 500 mg IV push to be given every other Wednesday. The chemotherapy was utilized for curative purposes. Blood work was drawn peripherally once weekly to include a complete blood count (CBC), profile-13, platelet count, and sedimentation rate. Periodic carcinoembryonic antigen (CEA) levels were also obtained.

Lynn and her husband both learned the procedures for hooking up and disconnecting the equipment. The procedures were most often performed with Lynn and her husband in attendance sometimes sharing in the individual steps of the procedures. Lynn remained on the TPN regime for a total of 4 months, until she reached her weight goals and hyperalimentation was discontinued. The biweekly chemotherapy, however, continued for another 15 months. During this time, her blood level became more critical to monitor and chemotherapy injections were held if her CBC and platelet count fell below acceptable levels.

Lynn's body weight continued to fluctuate during this period as a result of inconsistent eating habits and a medical history that included a history of alcohol abuse. Despite careful teaching and close observation, it was suspected that she continued to abuse alcohol. She denied this and was never observed impaired while performing any procedures. It was noted, however, that her husband gradually assumed more responsibility for her care. She was able to gain some weight when she used nutritional supplements, such as Ensure, and did not return to the extreme weight loss that precipitated her need for hyperalimentation.

Nineteen months after admission to home care, her condition deteriorated and a lump was found on Lynn's upper arm. Computed tomography (CT) scans confirmed metastasis to bone and lung. Lynn again experienced a precipitous weight loss. Chemotherapy orders were changed to include Cytoxan 50 mg daily by mouth and nutritional supplements were increased. Lynn's condition continued to deteriorate, and she began to experience severe pain from the bone metastasis. At this time, two years after her initial admittance to home care, Lynn was placed on pain control therapy. A CADD PCA cassette-style pump was used to deliver a continuous infusion of 0.5 mg per hour of morphine. The concentration of the solution was 2 mg/mL in a total volume of 50 mL. Therefore, a 50 mL cassette lasted for a maximum of eight days with 12 mg (6 mL) delivered daily.

Over the next four weeks, the dosage was increased to a total of 1.5 mg/hour and thus the frequency of cassette changes increased. Her husband was able to continue to manage her care. The effects of the narcotic caused Lynn to become more sedated, her intake decreased, and, after one month the infusion was transferred to a volume of 2,000 cc D51/2 normal saline (NS) and she was placed on a FloGard 6100 pump to provide hydration as well as pain control. Lynn died at home 26 months after being admitted to home care.

Lynn presented with several problems, all complicated by her alcohol abuse. Although not an ideal situation, it did not preclude her from home IV therapy. To review the areas of assessment discussed earlier, both Lynn and her husband were very interested, committed, and able to learn the therapy. Her therapy was provided easily on a rotating schedule, allowing her the freedom to remain active during the daytime. The home chemotherapy weaned her from dependency on her oncologist and was more convenient. Her improved emotional state contributed to the quality of her last two years of life. Because of their familiarity over the two years with pumps and equipment, pain control was provided with relative ease and comfort. Lynn lived and died as she wished, at home.

Client 2

Michael was a 60-year-old man admitted with a primary diagnosis of cancer of the larynx and trachea, complicated by hypothyroidism and sepsis. He was discharged from the hospital on multiple therapies, including enteral feedings via a gastric tube and combination antibiotic, heparin, and hydration therapy via a Hickman catheter. Michael initially continued to receive inpatient chemotherapy treatments on a monthly basis. This client presented with many complex, interrelated needs.

Michael's hypothyroidism created frequent potentially life-threatening fluctuations in his blood calcium levels. To maintain an even level, his enteral feedings, which contained calcium, his vitamin D supplements, and his intravenous hydration had to be coordinated. Michael was intermittently noncompliant with his regime, either because of gastric distress or depression. Michael's antibiotic therapy was complicated by resistant organisms and superinfections. His general nutritional status contributed to poor healing at his G-tube and tracheal sites.

Michael's wife was a nurse and, therefore, well prepared for learning the techniques of these complex therapies. She, however, had to continue working in order to maintain the insurance benefits that covered this therapy. Nursing service was provided from 8 A.M. to 4 P.M. Monday through Friday to allow her to continue to work. Michael's 24-hour regime included:

- Oxacillin 2 g IV piggyback was given at 8 A.M., 12 noon, 4 P.M., 8 P.M., 12 midnight, and 4 A.M.
- Heparin 5000 u IV push was done at 8 A.M., 2 P.M., and 8 P.M.
- Ensure ½ strength and Enrich ½ strength 800 cc were given three times daily via the G-tube using the bolus method.
- Blood work was drawn on Monday, Wednesday, and Friday.
- Infusions of ½ strength NS were infused in amounts ranging from 1,000 to 2,000 cc, depending on blood calcium levels.

Once monthly, Michael was admitted to the hospital to receive an infusion of cisplatin. This was followed by a 96-hour continuous infusion of 5-fluorouracil 1,400 mg via a CADD 5100 pump given at home. The antibiotic therapy was interrupted during this time period, and enteral feedings were replaced by feedings of plain water to total 3,000 cc daily. This reduced his gastric distention, provided adequate hydration, and reduced the risk of aspiration from nausea and vomiting following the cisplatin. Chemotherapy was interrupted for the bolus injections of heparin. Due to the interruption in his enteral feedings, his vitamin D supplements were reduced and his calcium levels watched closely.

Four months after admittance to home care, Michael was readmitted to the hospital for revision of his laryngectomy. His Hickman catheter was replaced in an attempt to resolve his recurring infections. When he returned home, his antibiotic therapy was discontinued. Michael's enteral feedings were changed to Enrich full strength 500 cc with 500 cc water three times daily. The heparin and chemotherapy orders remained unchanged. Blood work was decreased to twice weekly. Michael became more involved in his own therapy and learned to give his own enteral therapy and heparin injections. Hydration was still used on an as-needed basis based on his blood calcium levels. With fewer restrictions from therapy, Michael was able to become more active, taking walks outside and car rides. One month after his second hospitalization, private duty nursing was discontinued. Michael's wife, a school nurse, was able to take the summer off and care for him.

The following autumn Michael was able to care for himself while his wife worked. This lasted until November when he again began to experience dramatic fluctuations in his calcium levels. A CT scan confirmed that the tumor had recurred. Private duty nurses were again scheduled to assist in providing hydration therapy. Michael was readmitted to the hospital on Christmas Eve. He was placed on a ventilator in January of the following year. His physician felt that he was not physiologically stable enough to return home on a ventilator.

Michael's was an extremely complex case with frequent potential for instability. Four things were essential to allow him to participate in home care: (1) his family member's (wife's) ability and commitment, (2) the availability of skilled nurses for both shifts and visits, (3) the availability of appropriate equipment, and most important, (4) a physician who believed it could all be done in the home. The appropriateness of his home care was reevaluated frequently to ensure that care was safe, effective, and provided within agency guidelines.

Client 3

Marion was a 54-year-old woman with chronic obstructive pulmonary disease (COPD) and respiratory failure who was ventilator dependent, complicated by multiple compression fractures of her dorsal spine. She was discharged to home on an LP 6 ventilator with suction equipment and a PulmoAide. Her husband and mother resided with her and, in conjunction with a nurse during the day, would provide her care.

Marion's blood gases at the time of her discharge were $PA(CO_2)$, 31, $PA(O_2)$, 87 and ambient oxygen was 38%. Her ventilator settings were for an assist control of 14 breaths per minute, tidal volume of 700 and 35% O_2. She was bedridden because of fractures of her spine and had multiple decubitus ulcers. Her orders were for PulmoAide treatments four times daily to decrease episodes of pneumonia. In addition, she was to be turned on a gel mattress every two hours daily through the evening to increase her mobilization and circulation and to heal and prevent decubitus ulcers. Her family, primary care nurse, and the day nurse were instructed in the use of the LP 6 ventilator in the hospital before her discharge. Daily, the nurse recorded the following information on her flowsheet:

- date and time
- volume setting
- pressure setting
- actual client pressures
- respiratory rate settings and actual respiratory rate
- FiO_2
- alarm settings
- temperature of inspired air
- if the circuits were changed and when

Each new nurse was instructed in Marion's care and the functioning of the ventilator by the respiratory therapist. Because of her constant back pain, Marion received narcotic pain control, which she continued to require in increasing amounts. In addition, two months after her discharge she began receiving antidepressant medication for posthospital depression. The combination of these medications complicated her care as they further depressed her respiratory function. It was felt that Marion had become overly dependent on her narcotic pain control, which she took in increasing amounts because of her depression. A weaning schedule to decrease her narcotic dependency was begun three months after her discharge.

This was a slow, difficult process that became cyclical. Her pain was real to her, and decreasing her pain medication made her both angry and depressed. The antidepressants caused mild fluid retention, which affected her respiratory capacity. The challenge for her nursing care was to secure her respiratory function, pull her out of depression, and manage her pain.

This goal was met eight months after discharge from the hospital. Marion was receiving two shifts of nurses. Her narcotic pain control needs had been reduced by 75% with her pain primarily controlled by non-narcotic methods. Social work services had been instituted, and a weaning schedule for her antidepressants had begun. Marion still remains at home, although because of her disease process, her respiratory status continues to decline slowly.

Ventilator therapy is perhaps the most difficult to plan, evaluate, and institute in the home. The determining factors in Marion's case were her determination to dictate her own lifestyle, the availability and commitment of her family, and the availability of appropriately trained personnel. Her total dependence, not only on a machine but also on the personnel around her, made home care a challenge.

These case studies have been presented for two reasons. First, they provide examples of what is possible outside a hospital setting, and, second, they provide a basis for the following section. In reading the steps outlined in the following section, the nurse can recreate the planning and implementation involved in each of these cases.

Planning High-Tech Therapy

Accepting the Client on Service

The very first step in providing care after the client has qualified for coverage is making the decision to accept the client on service. This process involves answering the following seven questions:

1. Do the client and family accept the proposed therapy? Will they be willing participants?
2. Does the physician accept their decision and is the physician a willing participant in managing the care of the client?
3. Is the home environment safe for the provision of this therapy?
4. Are the risks, responsibilities, and expected results of the therapy clearly understood by all involved?
5. What type of and how much support personnel will be required and is that support readily available?
6. What type of equipment is needed and is it readily available?
7. Is there adequate financial support for the personnel, equipment, drugs, and supplies that are required?

Once the client is accepted for home care, the primary nurse, in conjunction with the hospital and infusion or DME company, must perform discharge planning. In high-tech care, the home care nurse must remain as primary coordinator of discharge plans. In reality, this is often difficult. Hospital discharge planners and coordinators from equipment and pharmaceutical companies will also view themselves in this role, but, once the client is home, full responsibility will revert to the home health agency. It is essential that the nurse is directly involved in all the predischarge decisions and coordination of all events from hospital to home to ensure a safe and controlled transition.

Predischarge Planning from the Hospital

To accomplish the predischarge planning process the home care nurse will need to understand the steps involved and have the proper tools available. Predischarge planning includes the following eight steps:

1. preparing the home environment to receive the client
2. ordering and confirming the setup of all equipment
3. ordering and confirming delivery of all medications and supplies
4. establishing the teaching plans and time frame and completing preparations to accomplish them (This includes confirming what predischarge teaching has been completed and that personnel are scheduled for any teaching that will be done in the home.)
5. establishing the need for support personnel and the scheduling of those personnel
6. ensuring that emergency plans are in place
7. establishing a confirmed discharge date and time
8. planning for appropriate transportation from hospital to home with escort personnel as needed

Preparing the Home Care Environment. Preparation of the home environment includes setup of the sick room and ordering equipment, such as a hospital bed, commode, and ambulation equipment. This is often done a short while before the client arrives home. It is recommended that when several pieces of equipment are needed that the home care nurse make a predischarge visit to the client's home to assist the family in setting up the environment. The client is often anxious and tired postdischarge, and the ease of transition from hospital to home will be dependent on anticipation of the client's needs. A smooth transition will greatly enhance the success of the therapy. When a ventilator or stationary IV or enteral pump is being used, it also

should be set up and its functioning checked. Any necessary modifications to the plan can be identified at this time. For example, because ambulation was difficult for Michael, two stationary IV pumps were ordered for him. This allowed him the freedom of spending his days downstairs and evenings upstairs. The change of environment was essential for his mental and emotional well-being.

Ordering Equipment. Ordering equipment, supplies, and medications for these complex therapies becomes very difficult when many different vendors are involved. When ordering equipment, supplies, and medications, it is extremely helpful to have one vendor available to provide most or all of the client's supplies. For example, Michael's vendor was able to supply all his equipment, medications, enteral and IV solutions, and his tracheostomy care supplies. The time of delivery was set for 12 to 24 hours before discharge to allow review of the order for discrepancies and to enable last-minute changes, such as the extra pump. Remember, because of stability levels and shelf life, some medications may require a second delivery closer to the time of the client's discharge from the hospital. The primary care nurse is the staff member who can provide the most accurate evaluation of vendor companies regarding how comprehensive, accurate, timely, and efficient they are in providing care. In the start-up stage of implementing any new program such as high-tech home care, the nurse should keep supervisors well informed of these evaluative areas and recommend changes in vendors if necessary.

Initial Client Teaching. The decision to begin teaching before discharge or to wait until the client is home depends on several factors. The first is hospital policy regarding client contact by someone not employed by the hospital or a family member. It is well within the hospital's legal rights to restrict access to the client and the clinical record. If this is the case, the nurse will need to discuss alternate plans with her supervisor. A second factor is the teaching environment. The client can often be complacent in the hospital and, as a result, be a poor learner. The reality of actually performing the procedures may become apparent only at home. In addition, there are often numerous interruptions in the hospital environment that may make this a difficult place to conduct instruction. Liability is a third factor because the nurse, as an agent of the agency, is not covered under the hospital's insurance for teaching or performing any procedures for which the hospital may be liable. For example, if the home care nurse is teaching the heparin flush procedure to a client in the hospital and an air embolus occurs, the question arises of who is liable, the agency or hospital. The issue of whether the client can safely be discharged from the hospital without prior teaching is a fourth and important factor. In the case of home ventilator therapy, it is obvious that the client must be instructed in the hospital. With less complicated therapies, such as enteral or infusion therapy, teaching can begin at home as long as support personnel are available at the time of each procedure until the client and family are independent.

The Early Discharge Process. The final factor is the reality of the early discharge process. As the home care industry has become more familiar with high-tech home care, competition has increased at a tremendous rate. Often the decision to take a client home quickly is an operational choice, and to be seen as competitive an agency must be flexible and willing to accommodate the physician, hospital, and client. As a result, the client may be discharged without the home care nurse's input into the decision. The nurse must be able to respond quickly to make the transition home successful, often in less than ideal circumstances.

At all points in the process, the nurse needs to be a strong advocate for the client's safety and recommend whatever provisions are necessary to ensure this. Often this means increased visits to assist the client to safe partial or total independence. The advent of managed care means the nurse will continue to be challenged to provide safe care with decreasing resources.

Having good teaching tools and adequate support personnel is necessary to provide the safest care under any circumstances. Established infusion companies often have well-written teaching materials to provide clients upon discharge. The home care nurse should become familiar with these resources and develop or use other tools found in the literature to provide information regarding the equipment, procedure, and medications used. Because the amount of information is often too vast for the client to absorb if provided verbally, written materials left with the client provide a teaching guide for caregivers, serve as a reference in case of trouble, and can create a sense of security when the client is without one-on-one staff support.

Support Personnel. High-tech clients have special needs that require the professional skills that a nurse provides. Unlike the less acute client who can function just with family support for activities of daily living (ADLs), the high-tech client often requires skilled nursing care on a shift or continuous basis because of the complexity of the therapy. In high-tech home care, those who provide this type of care are called *support personnel* because they do just that, support the client and family on an ongoing basis, rather than with intermit-

tent visits. Support personnel may be provided by the home health agency, usually through a different section of the business known as private duty, or by contracting with an agency that provides shift nursing. If the client needs the services of support personnel, the primary care nurse from the home health agency will continue to see the client, conducting visits on an intermittent basis and working closely with the support personnel to reach the goals developed regarding the need for ongoing support and the overall care.

The need for support personnel must be evaluated to include the amount and frequency of skilled intervention needed and the special skills staff members must possess. It is important that the support personnel's skills and experience be reviewed prior to assignment to ensure that they are prepared to meet the needs of the individual client. For example, insertion of a PICC, Landmark, or Streamline catheter requires special training that few nurses possess. Administration of some medications, such as chemotherapeutic agents, requires knowledge of the short- and long-term effects and side effects of the chemotherapy, as they can be more serious than less toxic medications, such as antibiotics. In addition, the support staff should be trained and experienced in handling emergencies, such as anaphylactic reactions, extravasations, and central catheter emergencies, such as an air embolus. The primary care nurse may not have a large staff of support personnel and may be responsible for acquiring many of these skills. The nurse must understand this responsibility and evaluate her need for further training. If the nurse is uncomfortable providing certain types of therapy, even with additional training, this should be discussed with the supervisor.

Once the need for support personnel is established, a schedule should be developed for at least the first week following discharge. In many cases the client and family will be able to acquire the basic skills and be able to continue without support personnel in a week or less, although with very complex therapies the time may be longer. In either case the primary care nurse will need to keep agency staff who are responsible for scheduling well informed of the client's ongoing needs in time for staff to be scheduled. For example, Michael required a registered nurse for a full shift who could manage his infusion and G-tube and draw blood values. His need for ongoing support required several months of scheduling.

Final Preparations for Discharge to Home Care

Anticipation of and preparation for emergencies are best done at the time agency policies and protocols are established. Unexpected events can have a far more devastating effect in the home where emergency staff and equipment are unavailable. For example, support personnel can be delayed or unable to work, equipment can malfunction, power outages can occur rendering equipment unusable, or the client may panic while performing a procedure. The primary nurse needs to reevaluate frequently the ongoing needs of the client and anticipate changes in those needs as the therapy, client condition, and ability of the caregiver change. For example, as the client's condition deteriorates, the caregiver may not be able to continue performing procedures necessary for the delivery of therapy. In other cases, the client may lose family or caregiver support because of outside demands on the caregiver or family member.

Coordinating the Date of Discharge. Finally, coordinating the date and time of discharge is important. A quick phone call from the home health agency to the hospital on the morning of the client's discharge is recommended. Changes can occur overnight in the client's condition, and communication of a change in discharge plans may not occur in time. To plan for transportation from hospital to home, contact the hospital discharge planner, as this is often within the scope of their responsibilities. The discharge planner will need to know any special requirements, such as ventilator or IV equipment, that will be needed during transport.

The Day of Discharge. Even the most well-planned discharge day can be chaotic. The primary care nurse should plan to be at the client's home before he or she arrives. Once the client has arrived, take charge and get the client settled first; do not plan to do any extensive teaching at this time. The high-tech client is usually very ill, anxious at the sight of all the equipment, and very tired and weak because of the acute nature of the illness. The sight of the equipment in the home may be overwhelming, and a fatigued, anxious client is a poor learner.

Provide the client and family with a general overview of the first 24 to 48 hours. Guide them step by step through the expected events. For example, "Mrs. Jones, I am here now to begin your IV therapy. I will do the procedure today and ask you to watch. Tomorrow I will actually begin to teach you. I will stay with you now to show you what to do if any alarms ring or problems arise. Here are our phone numbers, where you can reach a nurse any time of the day or night. Jane will be here at 8 P.M. tonight to disconnect you from the pump. I will return at 8 A.M. tomorrow morning to begin teaching you the hookup procedure that you will be performing. After that there will be a nurse here each day at 8 A.M. and 8 P.M. until you are completely comfortable with the procedure and can perform it without assistance." Ask clients several times if they have any questions, but don't stop there. Ask them what they will "do if" for each problem that may occur (e.g., the infusion line is leaking or disconnects, or the alarms are going off). Post the agency number and the nurse's name in a highly visible place close to the phone.

The first 48 to 72 hours at home are critical. To make the transition from the hospital to home, the client must feel that support is readily and rapidly available. Included on the emergency list should be the client's therapy so that the information is readily available at the time of an emergency. The list provides assurance to the caregiver and can save precious minutes in an emergency. Be sure that agency on-call personnel are aware that a new client is on service and discuss how far the teaching has progressed.

As discussed earlier, client instructions can be obtained from any national or local pharmaceutical company providing home IV therapy. Instructions can be developed for each type of therapy and left in a prominent place in the home. Easily understood language and clear, concise, and abbreviated instructions should be used. The client should be provided with a loose-leaf–style home chart in which all instructions, care plans, and clinical notes can be kept. A standard format for this chart should be established and maintained so that all personnel can readily locate needed information. It is important that teaching be standardized so that the client does not become confused by many different staff members showing the client "their way" of performing the procedure.

Once the client has been settled at home, equipment checked, therapy started, and questions answered, the initial visit is completed. The nurse should follow the visit with a phone call one to three hours afterward; this assures the family that the nurse really is just a phone call away. The nurse should also contact any support personnel to update them on the client's condition, review what was taught, and relay any concerns or complaints expressed by the client. The initial visit can often take two to four hours, and sufficient time should be allowed to avoid being rushed. It is vitally important that all events during the visit be clearly and immediately documented.

Clinical Management

The primary nurse's role in the ongoing clinical management of the client includes the following: teaching, ongoing evaluation of the client and therapy, maintenance of adequate documentation, and acting as liaison between the client, family, physician, agency personnel, and drug and equipment vendors. Each of these is examined in this section.

Teaching High-Tech Care

Teaching high-tech home care can be both rewarding and frustrating. Unlike less acute home care, very complex material must be learned rapidly and thoroughly by the client and caregiver. It is far more difficult to teach a client to administer chemotherapy by means of a central catheter than it is to teach the basics of a low-salt diet. The principles delineated in Chapter 7, particularly Bloom's three learning domains, should be clearly understood and used as the basis for any teaching.

First, it is important to understand the six characteristics that make teaching high-tech care different from teaching general home care topics. By understanding the cognitive domain, these characteristics, and how they relate, an effective teaching plan can be prepared and implemented. These six characteristics that represent the difference between teaching high-tech home care and regular home care are:

1. The equipment and procedures taught are often highly technical.
2. Troubleshooting and emergency procedures must be taught first before important underlying concepts can be learned and understood by the client.
3. Learning very broad principles and theories, such as aseptic technique, must precede learning the technical procedures. These principles must be taught rapidly without sacrificing safety.
4. The client or caregiver must possess the functional ability and manual dexterity to perform the actual tasks.
5. The amount of information to be learned is vast. It must be reduced to a concise, logical, and clear package of information that the client can assimilate rapidly and thoroughly.
6. The procedures, equipment, and therapies themselves are often new to the home care nurse.

The Cognitive Domain. Understanding Bloom's concept of the cognitive domain, which includes knowledge, comprehension, application, analysis, synthesis, and evaluation, demonstrates the scope of teaching very complex procedures. The following example of teaching a new client how to operate an infusion pump will provide an application of these principles.

Knowledge: In order for the client to be left unattended with a functioning pump, he or she must know the mechanical parts of the pump and the function each part has in making the pump work (e.g., the rate/dose or on/off buttons).

Comprehension: To perform the "programming procedure" to set the dosage for the pump, the client must know the rate and dose of his or her medication or solution and how the rate and dose are programmed into the pump.

Application: The client must actually set the pump to deliver his or her medication at the prescribed rate and dose.

Analysis: If the "high pressure" alarm sounds, the client must know this means there is a blockage in the tubing and how to evaluate what is causing the blockage (e.g., kinked tubing, possible blood clot).

Synthesis: The client must then know how to eliminate the blockage.

Evaluation: The client will need to understand how to reset the pump and assess for the patency of the line following this procedure (e.g., evaluate whether the cause of the blockage has been eliminated).

The nurse must recognize that teaching high-tech care is not simply a matter of demonstrating a series of steps and explaining a few dos and don'ts. Without appropriate understanding of the rationale, the client can conduct a procedure and cause serious physical harm. For example, in evaluating the reason the infusion is sluggish or not running, the client will need to understand that there is a real possibility that a clot has formed and how to safely evaluate other reasons for the blockage (kinked tubing) without causing damage (dislodging a clot) by forcing the flush solution.

Examples of Teaching. The following exercises will illustrate the complexities of the high-tech subject matter to be taught by the home care nurse. Before proceeding with the teaching, the nurse should gather the teaching tools to be used. While reading this section, evaluate how effective the teaching tools used in the discussion are.

1. To begin, the nurse should list each step of the procedure that is being taught. The underlying principles the client needs to understand to be able to perform each task should be written in parentheses. For example, the procedure to draw up a syringe of heparin flush would be:
   a. gather supplies (identify technical names and recognize each item)
   b. wash hands (aseptic technique)
   c. open syringe package (aseptic technique)
   d. draw air into syringe (air pressure/fluid displacement)
   e. clean top of vial (aseptic technique)
   f. insert needle into vial (aseptic technique)
   g. inject air into vial and withdraw heparin (air pressure/fluid displacement)

h. withdraw 3 cc of heparin (medication dosage)
i. expel air bubbles from syringe (air embolus)
j. place syringe needle cap (universal precautions/prevention of needlestick injury)
2. Now continue this same exercise with the entire antibiotic procedure, including preparation, administration, and discontinuance of the dose via a peripheral heparin lock. In this exercise, the nurse must remember to include programming and troubleshooting the pump and equipment and assessing the patency of the IV line. The following activities should not be overlooked:
   a. checking the label for client name, dose, and solution
   b. checking the solution for discoloration and sediment
   c. disposing of the needles, syringes, and supplies properly
3. These teaching plans can now be broken down into teaching units. The nurse can sit down with a coworker and actually teach one section, including any demonstrations and return demonstrations. How long did it take to teach the section? Did the nurse find herself straying outside the prescribed contents of that section to make the material more understandable? Was there too little (or too much) information to absorb in one sitting?

These exercises can reveal how tedious, time consuming, and sometimes confusing teaching high-tech material to a layperson can be. It should soon become obvious to the nurse that teaching the technical aspects as well as the underlying principles can make the process extensive. Many of the underlying concepts are not included in written materials or can be overlooked by the nurse. Teaching high-tech care can be a reeducation for the nurse, but it should be remembered that a well-educated and well-prepared client is a safer client.

The Affective Domain. The second domain, the affective domain, is equally important in teaching high-tech home care. The client's or caregiver's involvement and commitment to learning the material may be different in the hospital than in the home. High-tech therapies can be frightening and overwhelming. Movement through the four affective levels is often far slower than when learning less complicated procedures, and the acuity of the client's condition can impair learning and create backslides to lower levels of comprehension.

The Psychomotor Domain. The final domain, the psychomotor domain, is frequently overlooked in high-

tech home care teaching. Many of the tasks that must be performed require a high level of manual dexterity. To understand this concept better, the nurse can review what physical abilities (manual dexterity) are required to perform the heparin flush procedure. Notice how the end of the heparin lock must be held free from contamination in one hand, while the syringe needle is uncapped with the other hand, without contaminating either the needle or injection port. Does the staff nurse remember how long it took to attain the manual dexterity and confidence to perform this task? Think of the time lay caregivers or anxious clients need to achieve this complex procedure. Often the actual physical process involved in performing intricate tasks can be more frustrating than learning technical terms and procedures. By using pictorial and video aids and actual demonstration, the nurse can help the client visualize what must be done.

Consistency in teaching is paramount to reducing anxiety, especially when teaching psychomotor activities. Working with unfamiliar equipment can feel less threatening if the client learns only one way to handle the materials. To understand the layperson's perspective better, the nurse should try this exercise. Have one nurse teach another how to use chopsticks. Do the chopsticks feel awkward? Is it difficult to translate the instructions into actions? The nurse may find herself a layperson in regard to this learning material just as the client might to the technical material presented.

As discussed earlier, preparation and organization will ensure the best possible outcome when teaching high-tech material. Through using care plans, checklists, and teaching outlines, the nurse will be able to teach competently and confidently. In addition, these tools will serve as the basis for accurate and complete documentation, including the principles and procedures taught and the learner's response to the material. Breaking material down to separate related components makes the task easier. For example, Lynn's (client 1) teaching was divided into three teaching topics: (1) her Hickman catheter and its care, (2) her chemotherapy and hyperalimentation and their effects and side effects, and (3) the equipment and its operation.

Another factor that the nurse must consider is how much detailed technical material to include. Some learners benefit from an in-depth explanation, whereas that same information may frighten or confuse another. It is important to tie related information together for the client. For instance, when teaching aseptic technique, the nurse must teach that it is important to observe aseptic technique when spiking the bag as well as when attaching the needle. All of these elements are part of the same "system," and bacteria in one area can cause the same harm that bacteria in another area can.

In addition to teaching tools, the nurse will use care plans to document plans for instructions. Prewritten care plans that can be personalized to the individual client's needs serve a twofold purpose; they ensure consistent care based on agency policies and procedures, and they serve as references for caregivers and agency personnel. Prewritten care plans guarantee that all procedures and information will be addressed consistently from client to client. An example of standardized care plans for high-tech home care clients can be found in Appendix H.

Care plans can be completed for specific disease processes, procedures, therapies, or nursing diagnoses. Only those that pertain to a specific client are chosen. A comprehensive care plan that ties the prewritten plans together can be tailored to each client. Some agencies use critical paths for some high-tech procedures; a discussion of critical paths is found in Chapter 8.

The goal for teaching the high-tech client is understanding the basic principles of how the equipment functions and the interactions between the medications and the client's body. The client must understand why procedures must be performed exactly as they are taught. The goal for the nurse-teacher is to make the client safely independent in the ordered procedures with a clear understanding of abnormal responses and what to do when a problem develops. As professionals, nurses often use shortcuts in technique in the client's presence. It is important to be aware of these and to caution the client never to try what the nurse is doing. It is always better for the nurse to perform the procedure just as it is being taught to the client and caregiver because watching the procedure being done correctly is an excellent form of learning. In addition to understanding the potential abnormalities that might occur, the client must have a clear understanding of the following:

1. when to call the nurse or the physician
2. what *never* to do
3. what *always* to do

The High-Tech Nurse-Teacher

The nurse-teacher is as critical to the teaching process as are the learner and the material. Regardless of previous experience, the high-tech teacher will continually be faced with having to supplement knowledge already attained with new information. As the name makes clear, high-tech care is very technical with rapid developments taking place daily. Keeping up with the

literature and new products and procedures is essential to allow the teacher to teach confidently and competently. The nurse's personal attitudes and values also affect the effectiveness of the teaching. Pain control, chemotherapy, and ventilator therapy can be controversial therapies, especially when used with terminal clients. The cost, complexity, and even the goals of many therapies can conflict with the nurse's personal values and beliefs. The nurse must examine feelings about the proposed plan of care before teaching a client. It is better to relinquish responsibility for teaching to another professional than to compromise the client's care and learning.

Ongoing Evaluation of the Client and Therapy

The ongoing evaluation and monitoring of the high-tech client involves the same process as any home care client and differs only in its intensity. The high-tech nurse works as a member of the health care team, which includes the physician, pharmacist, operations manager, and delivery person. In general home care, the nurse works as part of a team with the therapist and ideally keeps in close contact to monitor the client's progress. The difference in high-tech home care nursing is that, in many cases, the other team members are more dependent on the function of the high-tech nurse.

In high-tech care, the pharmacist does not have close contact with the client and must rely on the home care nurse's assessment to make critical decisions regarding the client's therapy. In most agencies the pharmacist becomes the liaison with the physician. This is usually in response to state pharmacy laws that require that the pharmacist receive medication orders directly from the physician. This creates the need for the nurse to keep the pharmacist well informed of any changes in the client's condition, including weight changes, response to the medication, and general findings, such as fluid retention, temperature, wound healing, and the status of venous access. To eliminate frequent phone calls to the physician, it is wise to notify the pharmacist when routine orders are needed to allow these to be obtained at the same time medication orders are being obtained. In the case of TPN therapy, it is critical to keep the pharmacist informed of client blood values to allow for appropriate changes in the solution.

The operations manager in a high-tech home health agency orders equipment and supplies and maintains the agency's inventory. The nurse works closely with the operations manager to determine what supplies are needed for each client, including special pumps, dressing supplies, and venous access devices. The nurse should become familiar with what items are usually stocked in order to recognize when a client requires items that must be specially ordered. Often agencies develop "pick lists," which are itemized lists of standard supplies used for each type of therapy. This list eliminates the need for the nurse to develop a new list for each individual client. These lists are used to choose the correct set of supplies to be sent to the client with each medication order.

The nurse will need to keep the operations manager well informed of changes in the client's usage of supplies to allow for appropriate order filling. In addition, the nurse will often work with the operations manager in evaluating new equipment and supplies, for example, a new type of dressing or IV tubing. The nurse may find these items of superior quality to currently used supplies and equipment, and, if so, the supervisor must be made aware of the differences. In the case of malfunction of equipment or failure of supplies (leaking tubes, breakage, or contamination), the manufacturer must be notified immediately.

High-tech home care agencies employ drivers who pick up and deliver supplies to the client's home. The driver must coordinate the delivery of supplies and equipment to all clients and is critical to the success of high-tech therapy. The nurse can best assist the driver by providing accurate and specific directions to the client's home, including the best times to make deliveries. In addition, if the client moves to a relative's home for any reason, this information will need to be communicated to the driver. In some cases, as when the client has a diagnosis such as AIDS, the client may not want the neighbors to know that therapy is being provided. If this is the case, the driver has to use methods so that deliveries can be made without the neighbors knowing that the items are from an infusion company.

In the case of respiratory therapy provided in the home, the nurse works closely with the respiratory therapist much in the same way as with the pharmacist. The nurse needs to communicate any changes in the client's condition and medications, as well as the client's response to respiratory treatments. As with the operations manager, the nurse needs to notify the respiratory therapy company immediately of malfunctioning equipment or problems with supplies.

Documentation of High-Tech Home Care

Documentation is of primary importance in high-tech care. To ensure that it is complete, one or both of the following methods should be employed. The first method is the clinical flowsheet, which is used to document the nursing visit. An example of the clinical flowsheet is found in Appendix I. This can be supplemented by flowsheets for lab work or flowsheets for recording daily weight, temperature, urine sugar, and acetone for the client on hyperalimentation. A second documentation method is called a documentation outline. This serves as a guideline for each professional to identify the parameters that must be addressed in each visit and documented on each note. Using a combination of both methods ensures that nothing is assumed, overlooked, or omitted in the documentation.

Documentation Outlines

The following are examples of documentation outlines that can be used for each clinical note. These are not complete listings but rather example guidelines specific to the therapies. These should be tailored to the specific client and for information required by the agency or payer source.

Enteral Therapy:

1. date and time of visit
2. solution, volume, rate, and method of delivery (bolus or drip)
3. placement of feeding tube and how evaluated (residual, auscultation of air injected)
4. the client's tolerance of the feeding since the last visit (reflux, bloating, diarrhea)
5. physical assessment, including weight and periodic temperatures, fluid and electrolyte balances (lab values)

IV Therapy:

1. date and time of visit
2. administration site appearance (color, odor, and discharge, if any)
3. method of site change or accessing and dressing change technique
4. name, dose, rate, and method of administration of all medications or solutions administered
5. type of pump and pump settings
6. topics taught and client response, including return demonstration (e.g., hookup or disconnect procedure); make specific reference to teaching tools (e.g., "Hookup procedure taught according to agency protocols as found in client care plan")

Ventilator Therapy:

1. date and time of visit
2. ventilator settings and readings at time of visit
3. physical assessment, including heart and lung sounds
4. summary of respiratory therapy notes since last visit

One of the responsibilities of the primary nurse is the ongoing evaluation of the client and therapy. Because of the severity of the client's condition, physical assessments are usually more involved and more frequent. The clinical flowsheet can provide an overview of the client's physical assessment and client complaints at a glance and allows the nurse to rapidly sort through a volume of information. For example, when reviewing Michael's flowsheet a pattern was readily visible that revealed a correlation between his intake and his calcium levels.

Discharging a Client

When it comes time to discharge a client from high-tech home care, the entire case must be reviewed carefully. The nurse's discharge summary and plan will need to be more detailed than a summary for a less acutely ill client. It will need to include the outcome of the therapy and whether it was considered successful. Coverage guidelines should always be reviewed before writing about the therapy's outcome. Many variables change with the high-tech client, and because the goal of therapy is often determined by insurance coverage, a misinterpreted discharge summary can have an adverse effect on coverage. Documentation must also be reviewed to make sure it is complete. Insurance companies are increasingly requiring complete copies of nurse's notes and physician's orders. If the photocopying is a clerical duty, it is the nurse's responsibility to make sure that the information is correct before it is sent to the insurance provider. Again, poor documentation can have an adverse effect on coverage. What might have appeared adequate on the day it was written may not look as complete in review.

High-Tech Nursing Policies and Procedures

Policies and procedures form the foundation for any well-run nursing program. This is not to suggest that it is the primary nurse's responsibility to develop them; however, the role she assumes functions within these guidelines. The high-tech home care agency's policies and procedures will both restrict and protect the home care nurse. Often the nurse will be asked to follow the contracted company's policies or the agency may develop its own. Whichever policies are used, the nurse will want to become thoroughly familiar with them. In practicing high-tech care, the nurse is judged on whether company polices and procedures were followed. To ensure that care is provided consistently and for her protection, the nurse should always work within policy guidelines. They should be a resource that outlines the correct way to perform a procedure and what is the standard of practice.

Policies and procedures can sometimes appear to be restrictive, but they protect the nurse by providing a basis from which to work. When they are incorporated into the home care nurse's daily functions and into documentation, there is no guesswork as to the quality of the care provided. When problems arise or the nurse is asked to provide what she thinks is unorthodox or unsafe care, policies and procedures and clinical standards protect both the nurse and the agency from liability. Outdated policies can be cumbersome and, at times, costly. For example, IV restart kits are fairly standard today and usually are cost-effective. If the agency's policies call for different solutions or supplies than those contained in the kit, ordering custom kits or ordering each item separately may be more costly to the agency or to the client. The nurse should review policies and procedures periodically to ensure that they reflect actual practice. In the event that they do not, it is the nurse's responsibility to inform the supervisor. It is always ultimately the agency's decision what standard practice will be.

In addition to policies, the nurse should be familiar with organizations that issue regulations or standards for home infusion therapy. These standards and regulations form the basis for policies and are a resource for the nurse. Copies of many of these regulations and standards should be available in the high-tech organization's office. The organizations that issue the regulations and standards are listed in Exhibit 11–1.

High-tech home care is becoming an integral part of the health care system of the present and future. It is complex, challenging, and exciting. The decision to provide high-tech care for any client is based on a thorough assessment of several critical factors. These include:

- client, family, and physician commitment and involvement
- safety factors, including the home environment, and the mental, emotional, and physical status of the client and family
- availability of equipment and personnel
- sufficient financial resources (This assessment must be completed and evaluated before high-tech home care is considered further.)

When high-tech home care is chosen as an option, careful planning must be done to ensure safe, consistent, quality care. Predischarge planning is done in the weeks and days before the client's actual discharge from the hospital. It is imperative that the designated

Exhibit 11–1
RESOURCE LIST FOR THE HIGH-TECHNOLOGY NURSE

Regulations:
Code of Federal Regulations
    Standard 209D—Sterile Products Complex
    NSF Standard Number 49—Biological Safety
        Cabinets
    Good Manufacturing Practices
Drug Enforcement Administration
Food and Drug Administration regulations
Environmental Protection Agency regulations
United States Pharmacopoeia
    Dispensing practices for home sterile drug
        products
Occupational Safety and Health Administration
    (OSHA)
    Handling of cytotoxic agents
    Disposal of biomedical waste
    Chemical hazard communication standard

Regulating Agencies:
State Board of Pharmacy
    Practice and facility regulations

State Board of Nursing
    Nurse Practice Act
State Board of Public Health
State licensing boards
    Home health agency licensure and certification
State Department of Environmental Quality Engineering
State Department of Transportation

Standards of Practice/Resources:
United States Pharmacopoeia
National Association of Boards of Pharmacy
    Home Care Pharmacy Guidelines
American Society for Parenteral and Enteral Nutrition
American Society of Hospital Pharmacists
Intravenous Nurses Society
Oncology Nurses Society
American Diabetic Association
National Alliance of Infusion Therapy
Community Health Accreditation Program (CHAP)
Joint Commission on Accreditation of Healthcare
    Organizations (Joint Commission)

home care professionals be intimately involved in all stages of the predischarge and discharge plans. The goals of high-tech home care are to ensure a safe transition from hospital to home and, once home, to establish a safe course of therapy. The day of discharge from the hospital is often the most critical. Sufficient time and personnel must be scheduled to cover both anticipated and unanticipated client needs.

Teaching is of equal importance to the assessment and discharge planning responsibilities in high-tech home care. There are several important characteristics that distinguish high-tech teaching. However, the basis, which involves integrating the cognitive, affective, and psychomotor domains, is the same for all home care teaching, and thorough planning will ensure successful learning. The nurse-teacher must continually keep abreast of developments in equipment, supplies, and the various therapies in order to provide accurate instruction. Resources for instruction are readily available from pharmacists, pharmaceutical and medical supply companies, and hospitals.

Clinical management of the client is more complex in high-tech home care than it is for most general home care. The nurse must have or develop the necessary assessment and technical skills to manage the

client's various needs. Client visits are generally more frequent and of greater length than for less acute care. Documentation must be explicit and must consistently include all information that is deemed necessary, as explained in this chapter. The goal of clinical management is to provide acute care in the home setting in a safe, efficient, and effective manner, and the client or caregiver must become independent in all aspects of care. The policies and procedures that govern the home care nurse's actions must be reviewed on a regular basis for appropriateness. All care must adhere strictly to these policies and procedures to ensure client safety and protect agency personnel from undue legal liability.

HIGH-TECH PEDIATRIC HOME CARE

Caring for children in their homes was pioneered by community health nurses in the United States in the late 1800s. In the past several years, caring for severely ill children has been moved from the hospital to home for various reasons that are discussed in this section. With this movement, the performance of more high-technology procedures in the home geared for the pediatric population has also increased significantly in the past few years. Children are now cared for on ventilators and are provided with short- and long-term IV therapy. Care is even being provided for the terminally ill children at home.

In this section, high-tech pediatric home care and major situations encountered by the home care nurse related to caring for ill children in the home are discussed. An overview of the role and function of the home care nurse relating to pediatric clients is presented, with guidelines for specific types of clients. In addition, special considerations for nurses to be aware of when making the transition from the hospital to high-tech pediatric home care are discussed. These special considerations are applicable whether the child's level of care includes skilled intermittent nursing visits or private duty block-time nursing. Children requiring the types of high-tech care discussed in this section will often require private duty nursing overseen by a clinical nurse case manager or supervisor. Generic care plans for various client situations are found in Appendix J and will assist the home care nurse in planning individualized care for children and their families.

Factors Contributing to the Need for High-Tech Pediatric Home Care

There are four major factors contributing to the need for high-tech pediatric home care. First, there are approximately *10 million* chronically ill children in the United States. The numbers of these children has increased steadily over the past two decades because of the tremendous advances in medical and surgical technologies. Premature and low-birth-weight infants, who previously would have died from severe respiratory problems, are now surviving. These infants, however, are often left with bronchopulmonary dysplasia, apnea, and tracheal stenosis.

Surgical advances have meant that children with congenital defects, such as heart disease and spina bifida, are surviving, but also may be left with ongoing deficits. Children with illnesses acquired later in childhood are also reaping the benefits of advanced technology. Children with cancer, asthma, cystic fibrosis, diabetes, muscular dystrophy, cerebral palsy, infections, and injuries are now living full and productive lives into adulthood.

The second major factor contributing to the increase in pediatric home care is *advanced equipment technology*, which allows more high-risk and chronically ill children to be cared for at home. Availability and ease in use of equipment, such as ventilators, infusion pumps, monitors, suction machines, phototherapy lights, and nebulizers, have allowed children to receive tracheostomy care, dialysis, enteral and parenteral nutrition, IV antibiotics, and respiratory therapy in the comfort of their homes.

The *cost-effectiveness* of pediatric home care, as compared with hospital care, is an important third factor contributing to the use of pediatric home care. Although the general cost-effectiveness of pediatric home care can be supported by several studies, it cannot be applied in all cases (Cabin, 1985). Macmarik and Thompson (1986) found that the average cost of caring for a ventilator-dependent child at home is 87% less than in a hospital setting. Other studies have shown that home care costs of caring for children with other high-tech needs are about 70% less than hospital costs (Goldberg, Faure, Vaughn, Sharski, & Seleny, 1984), and it appears that over time the cost of home care declines. The longer the child is home and the more the child's health improves, the overall plan becomes simplified and other family members participate in the care plan. Third-party payers are beginning to recognize these cost savings and are looking at improving benefits for home care coverage, especially to prevent rehospitalization (Hill & Thompson, 1994).

The final and most significant factor for the increase is the *benefit of home care* to the child. A child's development in the hospital tends to regress, whereas the child's development at home tends to advance, despite the presence of a chronic, debilitating illness. Normal interactions with parents and siblings have a positive effect on the physical, emotional, and social well-being of ill children. The most successful pediatric home care plans are those that combine optimal medical technology and support with the benefits of normal family relationships to promote growth and development in ill children.

Planning for High-Tech Pediatric Home Care

Initial Planning

Planning for the unique and individual home care needs of the ill child presents many challenges but also offers the satisfaction of giving the child and family the opportunity to continue living in a cohesive family unit. A commitment to normalizing the life of the child while providing adequate medical, nursing, and emotional support to the family is the primary goal in bringing the ill child home. Planning for home care services may occur during a period of hospitalization or may occur after the child has been in a community-based setting. Occasionally families may bring children home anticipating they will be able to manage the child's care without the support of home care services. In these situations, the initial assessment for services would occur in the home (Grammatica, 1989).

Planning and coordination of home care services must be a team effort. The primary physician, nurse, social worker, and home care agency must all work together to provide the best continuity and quality of care possible. Initial planning involves researching the family's health insurance coverage. If there is a lack of adequate reimbursement for home care, any type of home care plan, no matter how basic, becomes problematic.

Funding

Private insurance companies, health maintenance organizations (HMOs), and managed care organizations have greatly varying policies and procedures for pediatric home care. It is often possible to negotiate with insurance companies and other payment sources by documenting that the cost of home care would be considerably less expensive than hospital care. Each state has an individual Medicaid policy, which is specific regarding income eligibility and covered services and equipment. Other sources of funding are local community organizations and private foundations or the State Crippled Children's Program (Ahmann, 1986; Bernbaum & Hoffman-Williamson, 1991).

Hospital Discharge Assessment

The next phase of planning for pediatric home care is assessing the child's and family's needs, determining the nursing care plan, and setting up a working relationship between the family and health professionals. Family assessment includes looking at the family's understanding of the diagnosis, prognosis, and actual care required. What is the family's attitude toward the child's illness? Are parents able to demonstrate adequate responsibility? Is the physical environment of the home conducive to home care?

Regular predischarge conferences assist in communicating needs, setting goals, and determining readiness for discharge. To enhance continuity of care, the conferences should include all appropriate hospital and home care personnel. Parents should also be involved because they need to become increasingly comfortable with their role in advocating for their child, identifying their own learning needs, and with the total home care plan.

Implementing the Home Care Plan

Implementation of the home care plan involves conducting parental and professional education, ordering equipment, and making appropriate referrals for community services. Parent or caregiver teaching should stress the details of routine and potential emergency care. Discussion, written materials, and demonstration by the nurse are the usual techniques. Return demonstration of materials learned is essential and will provide evidence of confidence and competence. Caregivers should be given extended periods of time when they are totally responsible for the child's care in the hospital while having easy access to professional support.

Home care nurses and other personnel who will be providing services in the home also need to be confident and comfortable with the different aspects of the child's care. They, too, must have the opportunity to become familiar with the child's care before discharge from the hospital. Parents should *never* be responsible for training professional home care personnel.

Selection of an appropriate pharmacy and equipment vendor is imperative to providing a positive home care experience for the family of the pediatric high-tech client. According to Szulnyog (1994) and Hartsell and Ward (1985), the following are important criteria to consider for choosing a pharmacy and equipment vendor:

- 24-hour availability
- home visits to provide follow-up instruction and support
- pediatric experience and equipment
- ability to service and replace equipment
- provision of written instructions on operation/ maintenance of equipment and information on medications

Referrals to community services may include not only the local home health agency but also private duty home care nursing agencies, parent-infant education programs, and parent support groups. Referrals should be made well before the anticipated date of discharge to avoid gaps in service. Notification of the need for home care should occur as early as possible to allow the home care nurse ample time to become familiar with the care, visit the child while hospitalized, and make a predischarge home visit, if necessary. Teaching checklists and a written plan of care should be provided for the home care nurse from the institution. Other therapeutic needs the child may have might indicate physical, occupational, speech, and respiratory therapy referrals. Referrals for professional respite care may be needed as well, based on the family's need for extended hours of nursing care. Several agencies may need to be involved to provide adequate coverage.

Role of the Home Health Agency in High-Tech Pediatric Home Care

It is important that the home health agency accepting the pediatric home care referral have a formal pediatric home care program in operation, because home care nursing holds a key case management function in caring for a child in the home. Ideally, the program should have a pediatric clinical nurse specialist and trained pediatric home care nurses. The pediatric clinical nurse specialist takes responsibility for staff education, case consultation, and quality management activities. The agency should have written policies and procedures regarding care of children in the home that are separate from other agency policies.

A standard pediatric assessment form and care planning tool should be used in the home health agency to document each pediatric home visit. This pediatric assessment form includes a prenatal history and a significant health history of the child, including a review of systems and information regarding nutrition, safety, development, and social information. The nurse, as case manager, is responsible for performing accurate assessments, teaching, documentation, and an update of the care plan. The nurse is in a key position to provide ongoing communication with the physician and other health care personnel on the child's health status. The physician depends on the nurse's assessments to manage and prescribe home treatments or medications.

The needs of ill children at home may be quite complex and involve many different types of personnel. The home care nurse, physician, physical therapist, occupational therapist, speech therapist, nutritionist, social worker, home health aide, teacher, and private duty nurse must all function as a team. If the personnel involved do not all work for the same agency, there needs to be an even greater effort made at communication and coordination. The nurse may find it beneficial to call team meetings periodically to facilitate the coordination and continuity of care, and the home health agency should facilitate this function in any way possible.

Guidelines for Nurses and Families of High-Tech Pediatric Home Care Clients

Often, nurses selected to care for technology-dependent children at home have recently worked in an acute care, institutional setting. With these children the nurse may be in the home for a short visit or for hours or shifts on a continuous basis. Because these children have usually been hospitalized for an extended period of time, the child, the nurse, and the family have ad-justments to make from hospital to home-based care. In order to make this transition as smooth as possible, this section outlines some of the issues and situations that may be encountered and suggests ways the nurse can intervene.

Adjustment Period for Nurses and Families New to Home Care

Initially, when home care is started, there is a period when trust is built among the parents, the nurse, and the agency. Parents are anxious about their abilities to care for the child without the immediate support of hospital personnel. Nurses new to home care may also be nervous about their ability to function independently outside of the hospital. It can be a time of stress and tension for all. Nurses need to be understanding and accommodating with families as they learn to care for a child at home (Ray & Ritchie, 1993; Teague et al., 1993).

Clients As Authority in the Home versus Nurse As Authority in the Hospital

The home care nurse must remember that the child would not be discharged from the hospital unless the parents had demonstrated to hospital and medical staff that they could adequately care for the child. In the home, the parents are in a position to be continuously observed and possibly criticized for the care they provide, so they can be, understandably, very nervous and defensive of their expertise. Parents may need help in understanding that although they may feel that with all the training they have had they are the "experts" in the care of their child, they may not have the experience and broad knowledge base that a professional nurse does. Thus, they may need to ask questions and take direction from the nurse. Additionally, because home care nurses always need to function under physician orders, this may at times come in conflict with what the parents see as their "orders" for the nurse, catching the nurse in the middle. This means that both the nurse and the parents must constantly look for ways to communicate openly and empathize with each other's position.

Maintaining Professional Relationships versus Personal Relationships

The role of the home care nurse is not as clearly defined as that of the hospital nurse. In the home, the nurse has the opportunity to be exposed to daily family dynamics and interactions that, at times, may be distressing. In these situations, the family may try to draw the nurse into family or marital issues, wanting her to take sides. It is important that the nurse set boundaries from the onset of care and continuously reinforce those boundaries as situations arise. Even in the best situations and with the nurse always vigilant of her role, there may be a point at which the nurse cannot separate her personal feelings and value judgments from the professional objectivity needed to provide optimal care. If that happens, she may need to come off the case.

Supporting Family Relationships

Home care nurses are not in the home to replace the parent. Nurses who work with families in the home must be sensitive to not undermining the parents' authority with the child, especially in the area of discipline. With an ill child, often parents are too lax in their discipline or can be so stressed that they are very harsh with the child. Even when the discipline the parent imparts is not appropriate, communication with the child about family members needs to remain positive. There will be many opportunities to discuss developmental stages, discipline principles, and parenting skills with the parent, and this should be an integral part of the family's care plan.

The relationship of the ill child to siblings is also a component of supporting family relationships. One of the major reasons for children to be cared for at home is to promote the development of normal socialization skills with all members of the family and with friends and relatives. Nurses should allow normal interaction and play between siblings and encourage parents to spend adequate time with the siblings of the ill child so they do not feel neglected.

Reporting Abuse and Neglect

Pediatric home care nurses are in a position to observe and document concerns over the parents' ability to properly care for the child. The reporting of suspected abuse or neglect is mandated through most states' child abuse and neglect reporting acts. It may be difficult for a nurse to decide if or when to report behavior that she feels is abusive or neglectful. The nurse should discuss her concerns with a supervisor and know the agency's policy on reporting abuse and neglect.

Guidelines for Specific Types of High-Tech Pediatric Home Care Clients

The following material outlines the home nursing care needed by children with various problems. Ge-

neric care plans that can be used with these clients can be found in Appendix J and should be used by the home care nurse to become familiar with the care needed for this unique group of clients.

Respiratory Problems

Home care for the child with a respiratory problem may involve one or more of the following: apnea monitor, oxygen therapy, tracheostomy, or ventilator.

Home Apnea Monitoring. Children requiring the use of apnea monitors fall into three major categories: (1) premature infants with apnea, (2) those who have experienced or are at risk for experiencing a life-threatening event, and (3) those at high risk for sudden infant death syndrome (SIDS).

Guidelines for home infant apnea monitoring are not standardized, but there are general indications for monitoring. Documented apnea lasting more than 20 seconds and an apneic episode associated with cyanosis are the most common indicators for monitor use. Monitors are discontinued when an infant has been without apnea for six to eight weeks. If an infant is on oxygen or medications, the monitor is usually continued six to eight weeks beyond the time when all therapy has been discontinued. Home monitoring for most infants is discontinued prior to one year of age. Infants and children with chronic cardiac or respiratory conditions, for example, a tracheostomy, will require monitoring indefinitely because these children remain at high risk for fatal apnea (Bernbaum & Hoffman-Williamson, 1991; Klijanowicz, 1984).

Before hospital discharge, teaching should begin and reinforcement should be provided on the follow-up home visits after discharge. Topics to be covered are normal infant breathing patterns for sleep and awake states, definition of apnea as it affects the infant, situations likely to provoke apnea, appropriate response to apnea, infant CPR, and the operation of the monitor. The family's ability to tolerate the increased stress of home infant monitoring must be assessed, and the nurse may make a referral to a support group that could be useful to the family. Home care services for the child on an apnea monitor should include:

- home nursing visits to assess the infant's cardiopulmonary status, review teaching, and assess the parents' abilities and stresses
- home visits from the monitor supplier to review monitor operation and to check home safety

Home Oxygen Therapy. Children with chronic pulmonary and cardiac conditions, which result in chronic hypoxia, are typical candidates for the use of home oxygen therapy. These children fall into two categories. The first category consists of the children who have serious cardiopulmonary dysfunction but have the potential to recover, for example, infants with bronchopulmonary dysplasia. Goals for these children are to wean the child from oxygen, prevent respiratory infections, control cor pulmonale, and enhance growth and development. The second category of children needing oxygen therapy consists of those who have an end-stage disease (e.g., cystic fibrosis) that is stable or progressing. Nursing goals with these children are to promote comfort and quality of life for as long as possible.

The type of oxygen delivery varies with the age and diagnosis of the child and equipment availability. Infants will most likely use a nasal cannula or hood, whereas an older child may benefit more from a face mask. Home care services for the child receiving oxygen therapy should include the following:

- home care nursing visits to assess the child's cardiopulmonary and nutritional status, assess if oxygen delivery is appropriate and equipment is being used correctly, review teaching (especially safety precautions and CPR), and evaluate the infant's respiratory status
- home visits from the oxygen supplier to replace the supply on a regular basis. The oxygen company should have a backup supply available in case of equipment malfunction or oxygen depletion.

Home Tracheostomy Care. Common reasons for tracheostomies in children are airway obstruction and inability to raise secretions. The cause of airway obstruction may be central nervous system vocal cord paralysis, subglottic web, cystic hygroma, subglottic hemangioma, or subglottic stenosis. Inability to raise secretions may be caused by bronchopulmonary dysplasia, cystic fibrosis, pneumonia, or diaphragm dysfunction.

Before hospital discharge, the home care nurse should be informed about what the parents have been taught so that appropriate plans for teaching and home follow up can be made by the primary caregiver in the hospital. A predischarge home visit may be helpful if assessment of the home environment is needed. Home care services for the child with a tracheostomy include:

- home care nursing visits to assess the child's respiratory status, quality of secretions, appropriateness of equipment and supplies, and parents' competence in all aspects of tracheostomy care (which includes suctioning, changing tubes, CPR, and emergency procedures)
- home visits from equipment vendor for instruction and servicing of equipment

Home Ventilator Care. The reasons for using mechanical ventilation in children range from congenital to acquired conditions involving cardiopulmonary, neuron, skeletal, or central nervous control of breathing. Home care may not be appropriate for all children who are ventilator dependent. Factors that must be considered before beginning discharge planning for these children are stability of the disease process, motivation of the family to learn the necessary care, adaptability of the home environment, and availability of a community support system (Ahmann, 1986; Szulnyog, 1994).

As previously mentioned, the home care nurse should be informed of all teaching done in the hospital and the need for reinforcement once the child is home. Extensive education with all caregivers is essential in suctioning, tracheostomy care, operation and cleaning of equipment, identifying signs of respiratory distress, and performing CPR. Home care services for the ventilator-dependent child include:

- home care nursing visits to assess the child's clinical status, teach and reinforce skills of caregivers, implement infection control measures, and assess appropriateness of equipment and supplies
- respiratory therapy to assess the functioning and effectiveness of oxygen administration and ventilation, and to perform oxygenation studies
- home visits from the equipment vendor to teach operation and maintenance of ventilator and oxygen administration, and to assess the safety of the home environment

Gastrointestinal Problems

Tube Feedings. Home care for the child with a gastrointestinal or nutritional problem will usually involve tube feedings or colostomy care. Tube feedings become necessary when a child cannot accept adequate oral feedings. Common reasons include prematurity, cardiopulmonary conditions, and gastroesophageal reflux. Tube feedings may be all or part of the child's total nutritional requirements, depending on the child's tolerance of the procedure and physical condition.

Methods of tube feedings are nasogastric (NG), gastrostomy (G), nasojejunal, and jejunostomy. NG or G tube feedings may be done as a bolus or over a long period of time using a feeding pump. G tubes have changed dramatically over the last ten years. Most children now have skin-level devices allowing for decreased chance of removal and a more aesthetically appealing appearance (Haas-Beckert & Heyman, 1993). A feeding pump is almost always used with jejunal feedings.

Before the hospital discharge, the family must demonstrate complete responsibility for feeding over a 24-hour period. The home care nurse should be aware of all teaching done, the family's demonstrated abilities, and all equipment and supplies needed. Home care services for the child receiving tube feedings include:

- home care nursing visits to teach and assess tube feeding techniques, positioning of child, positioning of tube, aspiration precautions, skin care, and growth and development
- home visits from the equipment vendor to teach operation and maintenance of feeding pump
- when oral feedings are instituted, consulting a speech therapist to assist in developing a feeding plan (McNichol, 1989)

Colostomy Care. Colostomies are placed in infants because of an anorectal malformation (e.g., imperforate anus, rectal atresis) or Hirschsprung's disease (an absence of ganglia cells in an intestinal segment resulting in a lack of peristalsis). Older children may require colostomies for inflammatory bowel disease (ulcerative colitis or Crohn's disease). Ostomy care in infants under a year is usually done without an appliance, whereas older children will usually have an appliance. The use of a gauze square dressing placed over the ostomy and secured with a diaper is usually adequate for infants and toddlers. However, pediatric appliances are available if there are concerns regarding skin breakdown around the ostomy. Some parents will choose to alternate methods depending upon convenience and cost. As with adult ostomy care, there are many skin care creams, ointments, and powders available. Some trial and error may be necessary to determine which products are most effective for each individual child.

Before hospital discharge, the family must demonstrate total responsibility for ostomy care over a 24-hour period. The home care nurse should be aware of all teaching that was done in the hospital, the family's demonstrated abilities, and all supplies needed. Home care services for the child with an ostomy include:

- home care nursing visits to assess knowledge level and teach ostomy care, various ostomy care techniques, ostomy irrigations (if ordered), skin care, symptoms of dehydration, expectations of volume and consistency of ostomy drainage, and growth and development

- possibly consulting with an enterostomal therapist to develop a final, comprehensive care plan with long-term issues considered

Pediatric Home IV Therapy

Home IV therapy for children is a more recent development in high-tech pediatric home care, but it is often a viable and safe alternative to hospitalization. IV therapy may be peripheral or central and serves the purpose of providing hydration, administration of antibiotics, pain medications, or chemotherapy. IV therapy often is used for total parenteral nutrition. The success of home IV therapy for children is strongly dependent on client and family suitability. Not all clients who could be managed at home are able to meet eligibility criteria (Szulnyog, 1994).

A critical aspect of pediatric home IV therapy is the predischarge planning and screening for eligibility to participate in the program. Screening criteria should include:

- ability of client and family to demonstrate adequate skills
- minimal risk for abusing IV site or supplies
- backup plan for restarting peripheral IV
- family's lifestyle and environment suitability to supporting home IV
- clinical stability of child
- parents' signing of informed consent form to indicate understanding of their responsibilities for home IV

Prior to discharge, the family must demonstrate complete responsibility for care of the IV over a 24-hour period. The home care nurse should be aware of all teaching done, the family's demonstrated abilities, and all equipment and supplies needed. Home care services for the child with an IV include:

- home care nursing visits to teach and assess patency of IV site, IV complications, and the child's clinical response to the IV therapy
- home visits from equipment vendor to teach operation and maintenance of IV pumps (see generic care plan, Appendix J)

Home Phototherapy

Home phototherapy is a proven safe and effective method for treating full-term newborns with physiological jaundice. The benefits of phototherapy are cost savings by reducing lengthy hospitalizations and an uninterrupted parent-infant attachment process. Families who receive careful screening and training have done well with home phototherapy programs (Wilkerson, 1989).

There are two methods of delivering home phototherapy. The traditional method is placing the unclothed infant with eye protection under a standard type of light. The major concern here is maintaining the infant's body temperature. The new technology for phototherapy involves the use of the fiberoptic blanket that is wrapped around the infant's torso. The major advantages with this treatment is that there is no need for eye patching, it is easier to maintain the infant's body temperature, it avoids damage to sensitive genital areas and promotes parent-child bonding. (Savinetti-Rose, Kemper-Kline, & Mabry, 1990).

Regardless of which method of phototherapy is selected, families must demonstrate knowledge of necessary observations and procedures to follow while the infant is receiving treatment. With the advent of newborn discharge within 24 hours of delivery, home phototherapy may be initiated in the home rather than the hospital. Written instructions on infant care and equipment use are essential. To ensure that parents understand the care requirements, a signed teaching or consent form is used. Home care services for the child under home phototherapy include:

- daily home care nursing visits to assess the status of the newborn, to reinforce teaching with the family, and to assess the family's continued ability to carry out home phototherapy safely
- home visits by the equipment vendor to teach operation and maintenance of the fiberoptic blanket or lights
- home blood specimens drawn for laboratory testing (see generic care plan, Appendix J)

Terminally Ill Children

The high-tech home care needs for terminally ill children can include many of the aspects of care discussed previously. Home care may also include a home hospice program in which palliative care is provided to the child rather than curative care. The general considerations and overall services needed to care for the terminally ill child are discussed in this section.

Home hospice care for the terminally ill child has many advantages. In a hospice program, the main goal of care is keeping the child as pain free and comfortable as possible. Children are more tolerant of pain, discomfort, and fatigue when they are in familiar surroundings. Additionally, family members feel less loss

of control when they are allowed to participate in the child's care and may cope more realistically with the impending death while experiencing the gradual decline of the child. Parents' anxiety may sometimes increase as the child's death approaches, and they may decide to admit the child to the hospital if they become unable to deal with death at home.

A terminally ill child can be kept at home if there is a parent or other caregiver willing to take responsibility for the child's care. Discharge planning should take into consideration the family's needs, resources, and ability to cope with the stress of home care. Home care services for the terminally ill child include:

- home care nursing visits to assess and teach the family about pain management, nutrition, sleep and rest, elimination, skin care, and preparation for death
- social work visits to assist the family in coping with emotional, psychosocial, and financial concerns
- medical equipment and supply vendor visits to teach operation of equipment and service
- death pronouncement in the home by the nurse if allowed by the individual state

General Considerations for All Pediatric Home Care

Although each type of pediatric home care has its own unique aspects, there are several general considerations.

- There are no specific visit frequencies for children. Visit frequency is individualized based on the teaching needs of the family and the acuity level of the child.
- All home nursing services and equipment vendors must provide 24-hour availability.
- Nurses must refer to other professionals, such as physical and speech therapists, social workers, nutritionists, and home health aides.
- Nurses must keep open lines of communication with physicians and other personnel involved.
- Respite care always must be available to family caregivers.

Family and caregiver burnout is always a possibility in pediatric home care. The home care nurse is in the best position to evaluate continually the appropriateness and safety of the home care plan. Families may forget that there are options to home care. It may be the nurse who suggests that home care may not be the optimal plan. Alternatives available can include long-term care in a skilled nursing facility or foster care, depending on community resources.

Medical Day-Care Programs

As an extension of pediatric home care services, some home health agencies offer day care for technology-assisted, medically fragile children. In these special centers, all the child's needs are met in one location. In addition to receiving the needed care, such as tracheostomy suctioning, physical therapy, and G tube feedings, the child also experiences the usual day-care activities, such as fingerpainting, music, and gross motor play. The centers are mainly staffed with nurses with support from home health aides, therapists, and special education teachers. All health-related activities are incorporated into the child's daily routine with special consideration of the child's developmental level (Porter, 1992).

Community Resources

Sources of funding for pediatric home care can include the following:

- private insurance and HMOs
- Medicaid
- Supplemental Security Income (SSI)
- Women, Infants and Children (WIC) Program
- state crippled children's services
- state and local social service agencies
- community or disease-specific organizations
- religious organizations
- state and local public health and education programs
- private contributions

Sources of support and informational resources can be obtained from local chapters of many national organizations. Appendix K is a brief list of these organizations.

HOSPICE HOME CARE

The History of Hospice

The hospice concept was originated in medieval Europe, where places of refuge were provided for travelers as they journeyed to the many sites of pilgrimage, often with great hardship. As early as the nineteenth century, hospices in England provided palliative care to terminally ill clients in hospitals and then provided care in the client's home. Historically, dying

has been viewed as a natural process in which family and friends provided all of the care that was needed. As the health care system became more complex and impersonal, the common place for death shifted from the home to the hospital. The experience of dying in a hospital has changed the nature of dying for both the client and the family. The need to humanize the health care system has made room for the development of the hospice concept in America.

In the United States, the impetus for the development of hospice care came in 1974 in New Haven, Connecticut, where a hospice was established starting with a home care program and then subsequently adding an inpatient facility. A group of professionals (doctors, nurses, social workers, clergy, etc.) and lay volunteers modeled this first American hospice after St. Christopher's Hospice in England, where all care was provided in the home and by volunteers. As the Connecticut hospice grew in the number of clients served and the types of care provided, there was the beginning of paid professional care within the organization. The Connecticut hospice was the first free-standing hospice in the United States, providing a model for terminal care that many organizations have followed. Today there are 1,459 certified hospices in the United States (National Association for Home Care, [NAHC], 1994).

The Hospice Philosophy

Hospice refers to a concept of care that is practiced anywhere by anyone when support is offered to people who are dying whether or not it is formally recognized as hospice care (Sheehan, 1988). Most students of the hospice concept agree that it is a philosophy of care rather than a place of care. This means that hospice nursing can be provided in the home, a hospice inpatient facility, an acute care hospital, or an extended care facility. Although clients and families dealing with a terminal illness often prefer to stay at home with home care services, the place of care is much less important than the type of care that is provided.

Hospice care couples the most up-to-date principles of pain control and symptom management with the centuries' old principles of compassionate, individualized care and concern for the dignity of the dying client. It is much more than the coordination of care from a variety of caregivers. The practice of hospice care revolves around careful attention to the physiological, psychosocial, and spiritual needs of the client and his or her significant others. The care usually begins sometime in the last six months of the client's life and extends through the bereavement period with the family.

The hospice nurse must possess a firm foundation in the home care principles and skills found throughout this text. Furthermore, the nurse working with hospice clients must function as a member of an interdisciplinary team, possess the ability to address the emotional needs of the hospice client and family, and have a broad knowledge of community resources (Stanhope & Lancaster, 1992). There are specific, recognizable elements that are part of all hospice programs and go beyond just medical care for the terminally ill. The basic tenets of the hospice philosophy are described by Lack (1979) and are discussed below.

A Comprehensive Approach to Care. Attention to the physiological, psychological, sociological, and spiritual needs of the client and family constellation is the focus of all care given to hospice clients. This also implies continuity of care, whether the client is at home or in an inpatient setting. A holistic approach to the client and the family is an integral component of the hospice philosophy. The client and family benefit from the availability of skilled professionals trained to meet their physical, psychological, sociological, and spiritual needs.

Concentration on the Client and Family As the Unit of Service. Consistent with the philosophy of home care nursing, hospice care recognizes the family as the unit of care. As such, care is provided with the recognition that the family and the client must be the recipients of care. If the family is unable to cope emotionally with some aspect of the client situation, interventions should be provided to the family as well as the client. Recognition of the family's role in the provision of care is also a component of this principle. Hospice interventions may be focused on assisting the family in the development of the necessary skills to care for a dying relative.

An Interdisciplinary Team Approach to Care. The interdisciplinary team includes physicians, nurses, social workers, home health aides, specialized therapists, pastoral counselors, and clergy. One health professional cannot have all the answers, the collaboration of many health professionals is essential in meeting the complex needs of the dying client and his or her family.

The hospice home care nurse plays a major role as a member of the interdisciplinary team. Most commonly, the hospice nurse makes the initial home visit and identifies the client and family needs. As other disciplines become involved in the situation, the hospice nurse retains responsibility for the planning, implementation, evaluation, and coordination of the nursing care.

Clients may not want or need the services of all members of the hospice team. All services are available to the client and family at any point in the client's illness, but the use of all services is not a requirement of hospice care.

Utilization of Direct Service Volunteers As Part of the Interdisciplinary Team. The use of volunteers as part of the hospice interdisciplinary team originated in the early days of the hospice movement in the United States. Because hospice care was developed through the efforts of a volunteer work force, the tradition of using volunteers continues to have a strong influence and is a requirement of the federal regulations concerning hospice. Volunteers provide a variety of services, including respite care, meal preparation, and friendly visiting.

Concentration of Care on the Improvement of the Quality of Life, not the Extension of Life. Pain control and symptom control, elements of palliative care, are very important aspects of the hospice philosophy and are probably the elements with which clients are most familiar. Unlike health care that focuses on curing diseases, palliative care is described as care that focuses on the relief from symptoms and discomfort. For example, if an abdominal tumor is causing severe pain as a result of compression of organs, palliative care could involve relief of that pain through the use of analgesics rather than removal of the tumor through surgical intervention.

Palliative care is fundamentally different from the chronic care model to which many home care nurses are accustomed. In the palliative care model, nothing is done "to the client" beyond those measures that relate to symptom control. The client and family have full authority in determining the care that will be provided. For example, monitoring the diet of a diabetic in his or her final weeks of life may not be done at all by the hospice nurse. Vital signs may not be taken on a terminally ill cardiac client. This difference in approach may be difficult for nurses in agencies that serve both hospice clients and traditional home care clients. Recognition of the differences in nursing approaches will be helpful in meeting the needs of all clients and families. Symptom control is achieved through noninvasive assessment of the client's problems followed by interventions that involve an individually titrated medication administration to control pain and retain alertness (Blues & Zerwekh, 1984).

Service Availability on a 24-Hour, 7-Day-per-Week Basis. The type of care required by dying clients and their families is not restricted to an eight-hour period during the day. Many clients feel most frightened and alone at night when the visitors have left and the environment is quiet. For hospice clients and their families, around-the-clock availability of professionals and services is essential to help the family feel that they can cope with situations that arise. This constant availability often makes the difference between keeping clients at home and admitting them to the hospital (Jarvis, 1985).

Bereavement Follow Up. Bereavement care is available to the family, usually for one year following the death of the client or until services are no longer needed or wanted. Services include helping the family adjust to the emotional, social, spiritual, and economic changes that come as a result of the death of a loved one. Bereavement services can be provided in the form of individual home visits with the family, self-help groups, or therapeutic groups led by a professional. Families may determine which strategy they feel would be most comforting and beneficial.

The Medicare Hospice Benefit

In order for a home care agency to be able to bill Medicare for hospice care, the agency must be a certified hospice provider. Just as agencies must go through a certification process to be a traditional Medicare home health agency provider, agencies must meet all the Medicare Hospice Conditions of Participation to be a hospice provider for Medicare beneficiaries. This certification process details all the personnel who must be part of the interdisciplinary team and the minimum standards of care for hospice clients.

Like home care agencies, hospice providers must bill for the services provided to their clients so they can remain fiscally solvent. The regulations and restrictions that are part of the traditional Medicare program are not well suited to the terminally ill client. In order to deal with the differences between client needs and Medicare regulations, legislation was enacted in 1983 that resulted in the development of a Medicare hospice benefit for terminally ill clients.

In order for a client to be admitted to a hospice program, regardless of the payment source, certain admission criteria must be considered. For home care services, the usual admission criteria include:

- A diagnosis of a terminal illness; the client's terminal illness must be certified by the attending physician and the medical director of the hospice providing the care
- A prognosis of six months or less
- Informed consent by the client authorizing hospice services
- A referral to the hospice by the client's attending physician

When a client elects to use the Medicare hospice benefit for either inpatient or home care, he or she must waive the traditional Medicare benefit that provides for more curative interventions rather than palliative. The Medicare hospice benefit is technically structured in periods. During his or her lifetime, a client who is terminally ill may elect to receive hospice care for two 90-day periods, a subsequent period of 30 days, and a final period of unlimited duration. It is interesting to note that from 1983 to 1988 and in 1990, the final period was limited to 30 days (Commerce Clearing House, 1993). The client is now eligible to receive several services and resources that were previously unavailable. The two 90-day election periods must be used before the 30-day period, which must precede the unlimited extension period (Commerce Clearing House, 1993).

The client elects to receive hospice care from a certified hospice provider for one of the "periods" defined by the hospice program. Clients may revoke their hospice election before the period has expired, thereby reinstating their eligibility for other Medicare benefits. For example, a client who is terminally ill may first decide he or she wants only palliative care so he or she elects the Medicare hospice benefit. Sixty days into the first 90-day period, the client changes his or her mind and decides to pursue aggressive, curative therapy. The client can transfer back to the traditional Medicare benefit, which would make him or her eligible for all the traditional Medicare services.

A client must meet all Medicare criteria for home care, except be homebound, to be eligible for the Medicare hospice benefit. The Medicare hospice benefit covers:

- nursing, home health aide, and social work visits deemed necessary by the hospice care team
- services, including pastoral care, dietary counseling, and other supportive programs
- therapy services, such as physical therapy, deemed necessary by the hospice care team
- prescription drugs related to the condition requiring hospice care, which are covered at the rate of 95% of cost
- DME needed for hospice home care, which is covered at 100%

Types of Hospice Providers

There are many ways to provide hospice care. Some agencies offer only services for the client in the home, whereas other providers couple home care with inpatient hospital services. Recognizing that the hospice concept is a philosophy of care rather than a place where care is given, it seems appropriate that hospice care can be given in a variety of settings. The following are the commonly seen types of hospice care providers:

- A home care agency, certified as a hospice provider, delivers care to the terminally ill in the home. Care is provided to the hospice clients using the interdisciplinary team approach.
- An independent agency may provide care that serves hospice clients exclusively. These agencies are licensed as home care agencies and are certified as hospice providers. Some of these independent agencies have inpatient facilities, whereas others contract with local hospitals for the care of acutely ill hospice clients.
- An acute care hospital may have either hospice units or specially designated hospice beds. When the client is discharged from the hospital, home care is provided by one of the other types of hospice home care providers.

In summary, hospice care is a philosophy that is a humane alternative for terminally ill clients. Using an interdisciplinary team approach, terminal care that focuses on palliative care, specific symptom control, emotional support, and pain management is provided to the clients and their families. Recognizing the complex needs of dying clients and their families, care is focused on meeting their physiological, psychological, social, and spiritual needs. Clients receiving hospice care can waive the traditional Medicare benefit for a more comprehensive Medicare hospice benefit that is designed to meet their health care needs.

PSYCHIATRIC HOME CARE

The Health Care Financing Administration (HCFA) formally acknowledged psychiatric home care as a reimbursable service in 1979. Growth in psychiatric home care was slow in the 1980s, with home care agencies employing psychiatric nurses mainly as consultants to their staff nurses. Currently, psychiatric home care has demonstrated substantial growth. In 1992, 3.1% of all clients receiving home care had a psychiatric diagnosis listed as the primary reason for referral to the home care agency (NAHC, 1994). The recent growth in psychiatric home care has paralleled the growth in home care in general, which has resulted in many agencies developing psychiatric home care programs that care for psychiatric clients of all ages.

The primary purpose of a psychiatric home care program is to provide services that are adjunctive to outpatient treatment with a psychiatrist or as a viable alternative to hospitalization. Goals of a psychiatric home care program include:

- developing a collaborative relationship with psychiatrists and other referral sources
- providing comprehensive care to assist the client to remain in the community
- easing the transition from hospital to the home
- acting as a resource to medical providers, the client, the family, and the community in general on issues related to the mental health of populations
- providing educational opportunities for future mental health professionals through consultation with professionals and contracts with nursing schools (Pelletier, 1988)

Medicare is the primary payer for psychiatric home care services, yet many HMOs and preferred provider organizations (PPOs) are recognizing the cost savings of psychiatric care in the home and have included psychiatric home care in their benefit packages. In order for psychiatric services to be covered by Medicare, the following three criteria must be met:

1. The evaluation and psychotherapy needed by the client requires the skills of a psychiatrically trained nurse.
2. The services are provided under a plan of care established and reviewed by a physician, not necessarily a psychiatrist.
3. The client must meet the criteria for Medicare home care services, which include being homebound and needing intermittent, part-time care that is reasonable and necessary.

Medicare defines a psychiatrically trained nurse as one who has special training and/or experience beyond the standard curriculum required for an RN (see Appendix O, Transmittal 222). Many nurses demonstrate the distinction of being specially trained in psychiatric nursing by obtaining certification in psychiatric nursing by the American Nurses Association (ANA). Master's-level preparation as a clinical nurse specialist in psychiatric nursing is not required for reimbursement by Medicare.

The homebound criterion is one that often precludes psychiatric clients from receiving home care services reimbursed by Medicare. There is the perception that a psychiatric diagnosis would not render a client homebound. In many situations, secondary physiological diagnoses or exacerbation of physiological symptoms prevents the client from leaving the home without great effort. In other situations, even though clients may be physically capable of ambulation, their mental status makes it difficult, risky, or impossible to leave the home safely (Miller & Duffey, 1993).

There are many advantages and disadvantages to providing psychiatric home care. The psychiatric home care nurse will be able to view clients within the context of family and environment, allowing for the most comprehensive assessment. Complete assessments are essential to the development of appropriate treatment regimes. Exhibit 11–2 provides a description of the es-

sential components of a home psychiatric assessment that can be used as a guideline for an initial nursing visit. This information is also helpful for the home care nurse to determine if the client is in need of an evaluation by a psychiatric nurse.

Psychiatric care provided in the home is often perceived as less threatening, especially to the elderly and the chronically mentally ill. The disadvantage of psychiatric home care is that the home care nurse

Exhibit 11–2
COMPONENTS OF A HOME PSYCHIATRIC ASSESSMENT

This outline provides a format for the home care nurse to follow when making a psychiatric assessment in the home. Much of the information should be integrated into the agency's documentation system, but there are other areas the nurse needs to specifically address to ensure a comprehensive psychiatric assessment.

Reason for Referral:
Primary problem presented
Person from whom the referral was made
Client's understanding of the problem and of the nurse's involvement

General Physical Status:
Existing medical conditions (acute or chronic)
Medications
Nutrition
Elimination
Hygiene
Sleep/rest pattern
Activities of daily living
Vital signs

Psychiatric History:
Past psychiatric history (hospitalizations, outclient treatment, medications)
Psychiatric clinician currently involved in client's care (if any)
Any previous episodes similar to current problem and response to treatment

Mental Status:
General appearance (dress, posture, facial expression, motor activity, specific mannerisms)
Emotional state (mood, affect, level of anxiety, self-esteem, feelings of unreality, suicidal or homicidal thoughts)
Speech (quantity, quality, organization)
State of consciousness (alertness, responsiveness, fluctuation)

Content of thought (preoccupations, disturbances, ruminations)
Perceptual state (illusions, delusions, hallucinations)
Cognitive functioning (orientation to person, place, and time; recent and remote memory; attention and concentration; judgment)

Lifestyle:
Education
Work/job background
Socialization
Leisure activities
Religion
Limitations because of current problems
Important relationships/significant others

Home Environment:
Type of dwelling (apartment, own home)
General appearance of home (cleanliness, appropriateness)
Adequate heat, light, food

Appropriate Actions/Planning:
Immediate referral to psychiatric services (emergency room, mobile crisis unit, community mental health center)
Referral to home care agency mental health clinician
Return visit to gather further information
Discussion with primary physician
Referral to community agency (Protective Services Agency, Department of Aging, or other social services agency)
Utilization of resources already in place for client

Source: Reprinted with permission from P. Harris, "Psychiatric Assessment in the Home: Applications to Home Care," *Quality Review Bulletin,* Vol. 13:4, Mosby-Year Book, © 1987.

is isolated in the home environment without the benefit of other professionals and other services (Harris, 1987).

In summary, psychiatric home care has become an essential component of a multispecialty home health care delivery system. Bringing the specialized skills of the psychiatric nurse into the home has resulted in improved quality of life for many clients who would otherwise have to receive care in institutional settings. Psychiatric home care programs have allowed clients to remain active and functional in their own homes and environments.

EARLY NEWBORN DISCHARGE PROGRAMS

Postpartum home visiting programs are being developed throughout the country in response to the shortened hospital length of stay for healthy mothers and babies. Third-party payers, such as commercial insurance and HMOs, often require that mothers and infants be discharged from the hospital following an uncomplicated vaginal delivery within 24 hours in order to reduce the overall cost of care. Early discharge with a limited number of home care visits is less costly than an extended hospital stay. Early discharge programs require the home care nurse to have a new set of skills, ones that focus on the delivery of care to well mothers and babies.

In addition to the cost savings experienced by third-party payers, shortened hospital stays are often preferred by new mothers. In situations where there are adequate prenatal preparation and support systems, a shortened length of stay allows the mother to quickly return to her home and family. But for other mothers, early discharge can pose problems for the health of the infant and the adaptation of the family. In some cases, these mothers are considered high risk because of lack of education, inadequate prenatal care, low socioeconomic status, poor or absent support systems, or the presence of significant barriers to care. These high-risk mothers can present the home care nurse with significant challenges in the development of a comprehensive care plan.

Studies have found that, in most situations, 12- to 24-hour discharge is safe for both mother and infant (Avery, Fournier, & Jones, 1982). Yet it must be recognized that the care and teaching that would ordinarily occur in the hospital must be transferred to the home setting. In the first 24 hours following delivery, there may be little opportunity for the hospital nurses to provide the needed teaching for self-care and

infant care. In addition, the mother may be experiencing physiologic changes that prevent her from focusing on the teaching she is receiving. The third day following delivery is an optimal time for a home visit because the mother will have had an opportunity to care for her infant and subsequently formulate questions.

A comprehensive and detailed discussion of the essential interventions for both mother and infant in the postpartum period is beyond the scope of this text. Home care nurses who provide postpartum home visits are encouraged to consult current maternity nursing and pediatric nursing texts. The focus of the home visit is to provide the necessary information to ensure that the mother can meet her own self-care needs and care for the needs of the infant. In addition, the home care nurse should assess the adaptation of the family to the addition of the new family member and offer assistance in the accessing of any appropriate or necessary social support system.

To give the nurse a brief overview of what items to look for in a visit and what types of services are provided by home health agencies to newborns and their mothers, see Exhibit 11–3. Home care nurses participating in postpartum home visits to healthy mothers and babies must remember that the home visit requires focusing on two clients, the mother and the baby, in the context of the family unit. Assessment of both the physiologic and psychosocial needs is essential for identifying issues that require intervention. Issues important to address with the mother on a home visit following delivery include physical self-care, signs and symptoms of infection, infant safety and care, and integration of the infant into the family unit. The infant should be assessed for physiological functioning, bonding, and age-appropriate developmental behaviors. The outcome of these assessments provides the foundation for the development of the most appropriate care plan for the mother and child.

In summary, home care nurses may be asked to participate in an early newborn discharge program for their agency or have the need to refer families to those services. There are many similarities and differences between traditional home care and the home care that is provided to new mothers and infants. Traditional home care focuses on the care of one client who is usually ill. The early newborn discharge program has both mothers and babies who are well as the primary clients. As with traditional home care, the focus of the home visit is education for self-care. The home care nurse must provide the mother with the information she needs to care for herself and her new infant within the family unit.

Exhibit 11–3
ASSESSMENTS FOR POSTPARTUM HOME VISIT

Mother:
Assessment of:
  Vital signs
  Postpartal physiological changes
  Uterine involution
  Episiotomy/laceration repair
  Breasts
    Engorgement
    Lactation stage
    Nipple engorgement
  Parents' ability to provide routine care
    Bathing
    Feeding
    Diapering
    Cord and circumcision care
    Stimulation

Parents' ability to provide basic health care
  Rectal temperature
  Administering vitamins and medicines
  Suctioning with a bulb syringe
Psychosocial adaptation to the postpartum period
  Depression
  Anxiety

Infant:
Assessment of:
  Nutrition and hydration status/feeding patterns
  Healing of the umbilicus
  Healing of the circumcision site
  Urinary and bowel elimination patterns
  Sleep/wake patterns
  Age-appropriate development milestones

Source: Reprinted with permission from S. Cohen, C.A. Kenner, and A. Hollingsworth, *Maternal, Neonatal, and Women's Health Nursing*, Springhouse Corporation, © 1991.

TEST YOURSELF

1. What issues must be considered before sending a high-tech client home from the hospital? What are the similarities and differences to consider when the client is a child?

2. Name and describe the three "Rs" for high-tech home care.

3. When teaching a client to perform a hook-up and disconnect procedure for TPN, what concepts do you need to include in your teaching plan? What emergency interventions would you incorporate into your care plan?

4. Name four criteria you would use to determine a client's eligibility for high-tech home care.

5. Name two things you would need to do to prepare for emergencies with a client on home ventilator therapy.

6. When visiting a client who is receiving enteral feedings, you assess that the client has nausea and vomiting. What interventions, including client teaching, would you incorporate into your care plan?

7. Identify one high-tech pediatric illness you see in your agency (or have read about in this or another text). Identify the services needed to keep this pediatric client at home.

8. Explain why it may be difficult for a pediatric home care nurse to avoid overinvolvement in the family's daily life.

9. What is another type of care setting for the high-tech pediatric home care client and what could be its advantages?

10. Describe in your own words how hospice care differs from traditional care of a terminally ill client.

11. What steps would you take to refer a client to a hospice provider in your community?

12. Describe the differences between the traditional Medicare benefit and the Medicare hospice benefit.

13. Identify the agencies in your area (possibly including your own) that have (1) a psychiatric home care program, (2) an early newborn discharge program, and (3) other specialty home care programs.

REFERENCES

Ahmann, E. (1986). *Home care for the high-risk infant.* Gaithersburg, MD: Aspen Publishers.

Avery, M.D., Fournier, L.C., & Jones, P.L. (1982). An early postpartum hospital discharge program: Implementation and evaluation. *Journal of Obstetric, Gynecologic, & Neonatal Nursing, 11,* 233–235.

Bernbaum, J., & Hoffman-Williamson, M. (1991). *Primary care of the preterm infant.* St. Louis, MO: Mosby-Year Book.

Blues, A., & Zerwekh, J. (1984). *Hospice and palliative nursing care.* New York: Grune & Stratton.

Cabin, B. (1985). Cost effectiveness of pediatric home care. *Caring, 4,* 45–53.

Commerce Clearing House. (1993). *Medicare and Medicaid guide.* Hospice Services Section 1500–1590. Washington, DC: U.S. Department of Commerce.

Goldberg, A., Faure, E., Vaughn, C., Sharski, R., & Seleny, F. (1984). Home care for life-supported persons: An approach to program development. *Journal of Pediatrics, 104*(5), 785–795.

Grammatica, G. (1989). Developing a quality home care program for children. *Pediatric Nursing, 15,* 33–35.

Haas-Beckert B., & Heyman, M.B. (1993). Comparison of two skin-level gastrostomy feeding tubes for infants and children. *Pediatric Nursing, 19*(4), 351–364.

Harris, P. (1987). Psychiatric assessments in the home. *Quality Review Bulletin, 13*(4).

Hartsell, M., & Ward, J. (1985). Selecting equipment vendors for children on home care. *The American Journal of Maternal-Child Nursing, 10,* 26–28.

Hill, L., & Thompson, M. (1994). Case management of technology-dependent children: A family-centered approach. *Journal of Home Health Care Practice, 6*(2), 37–41.

Jarvis, L. (1985). *Community health nursing: Keeping the public healthy* (2nd ed.). Philadelphia: F.A. Davis.

Klijanowicz, A.S. (1984). Psychosocial aspects of home apnea monitoring. *Perinatology Neonatology, 8*(5), 28–36.

Lack, S.A. (1979). Hospice: A concept of care in the final stage of life. *Connecticut Medicine, 3,* 365–369.

Macmarik, R., & Thompson, J. (1986). Respiratory care of the ventilator-assisted infant in the home. *Respiratory Care, 31,* 605.

McNichol, J. (1989). When eating doesn't come naturally. *The American Journal of Maternal-Child Nursing, 1*(14), 23–26.

Miller, M., & Duffey, J. (1993). Planning and Program Development for Psychiatric Home Care. *Journal of Nursing Administration, 23*(11).

National Association for Home Care. (1994). *Basic statistics about home care.* Washington, DC: Author.

Pelletier, L. (1988). Psychiatric home care. *Journal of Psychosocial Nursing, 26*(3), 136–139.

Porter, S.A. (1992). Infant medical day care: A natural extension of home care. *Caring 9,* 90–94.

Ray, L., & Ritchie, J. (1993). Caring for chronically ill children at home: Factors that influence parents' coping. *Journal of Pediatric Nursing, 8*(4), 217–225.

Savinetti-Rose, R., Kemper-Kline, R., & Mabry, C. (1990). Home phototherapy with the fiberoptic blanket: The nurse's role in caring for newborns and their caregivers. *Journal of Perinatology, 10*(4), 21–25.

Sheehan, C. (1988). Hospice licensure: A philosophical and conceptual framework. *Caring, 7,* 8–11.

Stanhope, M., & Lancaster, J. (1992). *Community health nursing* (2nd ed.). St. Louis, MO: Mosby.

Szulnyog, C. (Ed.). (1994). *Home therapy standards, policies, and procedures.* Gaithersburg, MD: Aspen Publishers.

Teague, B., Fleming, J., Castle, A., Kiernan, B., Lobo, M., Riggs, S., & Wolfe, J. (1993). High-tech home care for children with chronic health conditions: A pilot study. *Journal of Pediatric Nursing, 8*(4), 226–232.

Wilkerson, M.N. (1989). Treating hyperbilirubinemia. *The American Journal of Maternal-Child Nursing, 14*(1), 32–36.

NANDA-Approved Nursing Diagnoses

appendix

A

This list represents the NANDA-approved nursing diagnoses for clinical use and testing (1994).

PATTERN 1: EXCHANGING

1.1.2.1	Altered Nutrition: More than Body Requirements
1.1.2.2	Altered Nutrition: Less than Body Requirements
1.1.2.3	Altered Nutrition: Potential for More than Body Requirements
* 1.2.1.1	Risk for Infection
* 1.2.2.1	Risk for Altered Body Temperature
1.2.2.2	Hypothermia
1.2.2.3	Hyperthermia
1.2.2.4	Ineffective Thermoregulation
1.2.3.1	Dysreflexia
1.3.1.1	Constipation
1.3.1.1.1	Perceived Constipation
1.3.1.1.2	Colonic Constipation
1.3.1.2	Diarrhea
1.3.1.3	Bowel Incontinence
1.3.2	Altered Urinary Elimination
1.3.2.1.1	Stress Incontinence
1.3.2.1.2	Reflex Incontinence
1.3.2.1.3	Urge Incontinence
1.3.2.1.4	Functional Incontinence
1.3.2.1.5	Total Incontinence
1.3.2.2	Urinary Retention
1.4.1.1	Altered (Specify Type) Tissue Perfusion (renal, cerebral, cardiopulmonary, gastrointestinal, peripheral)
1.4.1.2.1	Fluid Volume Excess
1.4.1.2.2.1	Fluid Volume Deficit
* 1.4.1.2.2.2	Risk for Fluid Volume Deficit
1.4.2.1	Decreased Cardiac Output
1.5.1.1	Impaired Gas Exchange
1.5.1.2	Ineffective Airway Clearance
1.5.1.3	Ineffective Breathing Pattern
1.5.1.3.1	Inability To Sustain Spontaneous Ventilation
1.5.1.3.2	Dysfunctional Ventilatory Weaning Response (DVWR)
* 1.6.1	Risk for Injury
1.6.1.1	Risk for Suffocation
* 1.6.1.2	Risk for Poisoning
* 1.6.1.3	Risk for Trauma
* 1.6.1.4	Risk for Aspiration
* 1.6.1.5	Risk for Disuse Syndrome
1.6.2	Altered Protection
1.6.2.1	Impaired Tissue Integrity
1.6.2.1.1	Altered Oral Mucous Membrane
1.6.2.1.2.1	Impaired Skin Integrity
* 1.6.2.1.2.2	Risk for Impaired Skin Integrity
# 1.7.1	Decreased Adaptive Capacity: Intracranial
# 1.8	Energy Field Disturbance

PATTERN 2: COMMUNICATING

2.1.1.1	Impaired Verbal Communication

PATTERN 3: RELATING

3.1.1	Impaired Social Interaction
3.1.2	Social Isolation
# 3.1.3	Risk for Loneliness
3.2.1	Altered Role Performance
3.2.1.1.1	Altered Parenting
* 3.2.1.1.2	Risk for Altered Parenting
# 3.2.1.1.2.1	Risk for Altered Parent/Infant/Child Attachment
3.2.1.2.1	Sexual Dysfunction
3.2.2	Altered Family Processes
3.2.2.1	Caregiver Role Strain
* 3.2.2.2	Risk for Caregiver Role Strain
# 3.2.2.3.1	Altered Family Process: Alcoholism
3.2.3.1	Parental Role Conflict
3.3	Altered Sexuality Patterns

PATTERN 4: VALUING

4.1.1	Spiritual Distress (Distress of the Human Spirit)

#	4.2	Potential for Enhanced Spiritual Well-Being	6.5.3	Dressing/Grooming Self Care Deficit

4.2   Potential for Enhanced Spiritual Well-Being

PATTERN 5: CHOOSING

	5.1.1.1	Ineffective Individual Coping
	5.1.1.1.1	Impaired Adjustment
	5.1.1.1.2	Defensive Coping
	5.1.1.1.3	Ineffective Denial
	5.1.2.1.1	Ineffective Family Coping: Disabling
	5.1.2.1.2	Ineffective Family Coping: Compromised
	5.1.2.2	Family Coping: Potential for Growth
#	5.1.3.1	Potential for Enhanced Community Coping
#	5.1.3.2	Ineffective Community Coping
	5.2.1	Ineffective Management of Therapeutic Regimen (Individuals)
	5.2.1.1	Noncompliance (Specify)
#	5.2.2	Ineffective Management of Therapeutic Regimen: Families
#	5.2.3	Ineffective Management of Therapeutic Regimen: Community
#	5.2.4	Ineffective Management of Therapeutic Regimen: Individual
	5.3.1.1	Decisional Conflict (Specify)
	5.4	Health Seeking Behaviors (Specify)

PATTERN 6: MOVING

	6.1.1.1	Impaired Physical Mobility
*	6.1.1.1.1	Risk for Peripheral Neurovascular Dysfunction
#	6.1.1.1.2	Risk for Perioperative Positioning Injury
	6.1.1.2	Activity Intolerance
	6.1.1.2.1	Fatigue
*	6.1.1.3	Risk for Activity Intolerance
	6.2.1	Sleep Pattern Disturbance
	6.3.1.1	Diversional Activity Deficit
	6.4.1.1	Impaired Home Maintenance Management
	6.4.2	Altered Health Maintenance
	6.5.1	Feeding Self Care Deficit
	6.5.1.1	Impaired Swallowing
	6.5.1.2	Ineffective Breastfeeding
	6.5.1.2.1	Interrupted Breastfeeding
	6.5.1.3	Effective Breastfeeding
	6.5.1.4	Ineffective Infant Feeding Pattern
	6.5.2	Bathing/Hygiene Self Care Deficit

	6.5.3	Dressing/Grooming Self Care Deficit
	6.5.4	Toileting Self Care Deficit
	6.6	Altered Growth and Development
	6.7	Relocation Stress Syndrome
#	6.8.1	Risk for Disorganized Infant Behavior
#	6.8.2	Disorganized Infant Behavior
#	6.8.3	Potential for Enhanced Organized Infant Behavior

PATTERN 7: PERCEIVING

	7.1.1	Body Image Disturbance
	7.1.2	Self Esteem Disturbance
	7.1.2.1	Chronic Low Self Esteem
	7.1.2.2	Situational Low Self Esteem
	7.1.3	Personal Identity Disturbance
	7.2	Sensory/Perceptual Alterations (Specify) (visual, auditory, kinesthetic, gustatory, tactile, olfactory)
	7.2.1.1	Unilateral Neglect
	7.3.1	Hopelessness
	7.3.2	Powerlessness

PATTERN 8: KNOWING

	8.1.1	Knowledge Deficit (Specify)
#	8.2.1	Impaired Environmental Interpretation Syndrome
#	8.2.2	Acute Confusion
#	8.2.3	Chronic Confusion
	8.3	Altered Thought Processes
#	8.3.1	Impaired Memory

PATTERN 9: FEELING

	9.1.1	Pain
	9.1.1.1	Chronic Pain
	9.2.1.1	Dysfunctional Grieving
	9.2.1.2	Anticipatory Grieving
*	9.2.2	Risk for Violence: Self-Directed or Directed at Others
*	9.2.2.1	Risk for Self-Mutilation
	9.2.3	Post-Trauma Response
	9.2.3.1	Rape-Trauma Syndrome
	9.2.3.1.1	Rape-Trauma Syndrome: Compound Reaction
	9.2.3.1.2	Rape-Trauma Syndrome: Silent Reaction
	9.3.1	Anxiety
	9.3.2	Fear

#New diagnoses added in 1994 classified at level 1.4 using new Criteria for Staging

*Diagnoses with modified label terminology in 1994 (This change was recommended by the NANDA Taxonomy Committee and adopted to remain consistent with the ICD.)

Source: Reprinted with permission from NANDA, *Nursing Diagnoses: Definitions & Classification 1995–1996*, North American Nursing Diagnosis Association, © 1994.

Standardized Care Plan

CORONARY ARTERY DISEASE: ANGINA PECTORIS/MYOCARDIAL INFARCTION

Potential Complications

1. arrhythmias
2. congestive heart failure
3. thromboembolism
4. Dressler's syndrome (post-MI syndrome)
5. cardiogenic shock
6. ventricular aneurysm or rupture
7. sudden death

Types of Clients/Clinical Conditions Seen by Home Health Agencies

1. Persistent or recurrent chest pain; instruction and evaluation of client's response to newly ordered or changing medications; reporting significant changes in cardiac status to physician.
2. Recent MI: discharged home with inclusive teaching program regarding prescribed post-MI rehabilitation and treatment regimen.
3. Post-MI client with an unstable cardiovascular status, requiring changes in prescribed medications and treatment regimen: need for instruction and assessment of response to therapy changes.
4. Discharged home after hospitalization for post-MI complications.

Long-Term Goal

To meet the metabolic demands of the body and maintain optimal cardiac function through restoration of balance between oxygen demand and supply.

Short-Term Goals

The client with coronary artery disease: angina pectoris/myocardial infarction will be able to:

1. Verbalize nature of disease process, risk factors, S&S of new or recurring complications to report to home health nurse or physician.
2. Take pulse rate/describe alterations in rate or rhythm to report to physician.
3. Verbalize importance of well-balanced diet with prescribed dietary restrictions.
4. Demonstrate compliance with prescribed medication therapy/identify complications, toxicity.
5. Verbalize importance of taking pulse before taking digitalis, when to hold medication and call physician.
6. Verbalize/demonstrate compliance with prescribed anticoagulant therapy, safety precautions with use, adverse reactions to report to physician.
7. Verbalize purpose of prescribed blood work.
8. Verbalize factors that precipitate angina/identify measures to relieve chest pain or require calling physician if pain persists.
9. Verbalize characteristics of MI and angina pectoris and actions to take with each/verbalize S&S to report to home health nurse or physician.
10. Demonstrate compliance with graded exercise program and activities/verbalize allowances and restrictions within the threshold of cardiac limitations, and of planned rest periods.
11. Demonstrate correct use of prescribed oxygen therapy/identify safety principles with use.
12. Verbalize understanding/identify measures to decrease dryness and breakdown of oral mucous membrane when on oxygen therapy.

13. Verbalize purpose/demonstrate correct use and application of antiembolic stocking.
14. Verbalize importance of not straining at stool and of prescribed measures to improve bowel functioning.
15. Verbalize importance of/wear Medic-Alert bracelet.
16. Verbalize how to summon help in an emergency situation.
17. Exhibit decreased level of anxiety and apprehension with positive adaptation to cardiac condition.

Related Nursing Diagnosis

Activity Intolerance

related to:
imbalance between oxygen supply and demand

as seen by:
fatigue; weakness; abnormal heart and respiratory rates and BP in response to activity; exertional dyspnea; chest pain

Anxiety

related to:
1. increase in anginal attacks with partial relief from nitrates and rest
2. altered body image and lifestyle changes
3. fear of recurrent "heart attack" and death
4. knowledge deficit regarding prescribed home care treatment regimen

as seen by:
increased facial tension and apprehension; expressed fearfulness regarding heart condition and effect on life; increased questioning of managing at home post-MI

Bowel Elimination, Alteration in: Constipation

related to:
1. prescribed activity restrictions
2. inadequate dietary fiber and fluid intake

as seen by:
straining at stool; frequency and amount less than usual pattern

Breathing Pattern, Ineffective

related to:
1. chest pain
2. decreased energy or fatigue

as seen by:
exertional dyspnea; shortness of breath, altered depth of respiration; verbal report of fatigue

Cardiac Output, Alterations in: Decreased

related to:
decreased myocardial contractility and altered conductivity secondary to myocardial damage

as seen by:
weakness and fatigue, irregular heart rate, dizziness, restlessness; chest pain; changes in mental status

Comfort, Alteration in: Pain

related to:
myocardial ischemia

as seen by:
c/o restlessness; chest pain; apprehension; guarding behavior; diaphoresis; BP and pulse rate changes; increased or decreased respiratory rate

Gas Exchange, Impaired

related to:
Altered oxygen supply secondary to:
1. decreased cardiac output
2. ineffective breathing patterns

as seen by:
dyspnea; irritability; restlessness; cough; rales; pink, frothy sputum

Grieving

related to:

"heart attack" and alteration in body image and lifestyle changes

as seen by:

alterations in activity level; verbalization of distress over cardiac condition and effect on life; anger

Knowledge Deficit (Specify)

related to:

1. disease process and related S&S
2. prescribed plan of treatment for management of cardiac condition
3. potential complications and S&S to report to home health nurse or physician

as seen by:

verbalization of lack of information, inadequate understanding; inability to perform skills necessary to meet health care needs at home

Injury, Potential for: Increased Risk of Falls and Injuries

related to:

1. generalized weakness posthospitalization
2. dizziness
3. changes in mental status

as seen by:

unsteady gait, weakness, and fatigue; changes in alertness

Mobility, Impaired Physical

related to:

1. activity intolerance
2. chest pain
3. prescribed activity restrictions

as seen by:

weakness and fatigue; decreased endurance; reluctance to attempt movement; medically imposed restrictions

Oral Mucous Membrane, Alteration in

related to:

dehydration of oral mucous membrane secondary to oxygen therapy

as seen by:

oral pain or discomfort; thirst; coated tongue; halitosis

Self-Care Deficit: Feeding, Bathing/Hygiene, Dressing/Grooming, Toileting (Specify)

related to:

1. activity intolerance
2. impaired physical mobility
3. prescribed activity restrictions

as seen by:

reluctance to participate in daily activities and meet self-care needs, associated with weakness and fatigue; chest pain; exertional dyspnea

Nursing Actions/Treatments

1. Assess cardiovascular status/identify complications.
2. Assess vital signs/identify trends (e.g., hypo- or hypertension, pulse deficit)/instruct how to take and record pulse and about alterations in rate and rhythm to report to physician.
3. Instruct about nature of disease process (e.g., CAD, angina pectoris, MI), risk factors (e.g., obesity, smoking, stress, diet high in saturated fat and cholesterol, inactivity), importance of compliance with prescribed treatment regimen, S&S of complications to report to physician.
4. Assess and evaluate nutritional status/instruct about prescribed diet with restrictions (e.g., sodium, saturated fats and cholesterol, calories, caffeine)/obtain dietary consultation as needed.
5. Observe/instruct about taking medications as ordered, purpose and action, side effects, toxicity/evaluate medication effectiveness.
6. Observe/instruct to take resting pulse for 1 minute before taking digitalis and to notify physician if pulse rate is below 60 or above 120 beats per minute or more irregular than usual before taking medication.
7. Assess/instruct about anticoagulant therapy, safety precautions to reduce risk of bleeding (e.g., avoid straining at stool; hard-bristled toothbrushes; aspirin or aspirin-containing products), adverse reactions to report to physician (e.g., bleeding, including bruises and petechiale, hematuria, tarry stools)/educate regarding measures to control any bleeding (e.g., apply firm manual pressure for 10 minutes).
8. Monitor/instruct about purpose of prescribed blood work (e.g., coagulation times, digitalis levels, arterial blood gas analysis, cardiac enzyme levels to screen for evidence of progression of MI and need to rehospitalize).

9. Assess and evaluate clinical manifestations associated with angina pectoris, circumstances under which it occurs, factors that may precipitate it (e.g., specific activities; temperature extremes; emotional stress; nicotine)/ instruct to modify activities, rest, and take prescribed nitrates, call physician if pain persists.

10. Assess/instruct about patterns of chest pain (e.g., angina compared to MI), actions to take with each, S&S to report to home health nurse or physician.

11. Observe and evaluate level of physical tolerance to perform self-care activities and ADL (e.g., angina, exertional dyspnea, fatigue, excess anxiety)/instruct about graded exercises and activities, allowances and restrictions within threshold of cardiac limitations/planned rest periods.

12. Observe/instruct about prescribed oxygen therapy: delivery method, flow rate, duration, care of equipment; safety principles with use (e.g., danger of smoking near oxygen system), care of equipment, obtain respiratory consultation as needed/evaluate effectiveness of oxygen therapy.

13. Assess and evaluate oral mucous membrane for dryness and breakdown when on oxygen therapy/instruct about good oral hygiene and adequate hydration.

14. Assess bowel elimination patterns/instruct about importance of not straining at stool and prescribed measures to treat or avoid constipation (e.g., stool softeners/laxatives, increased dietary fiber, adequate hydration)/evaluate effectiveness of bowel regimen.

15. Observe/instruct about importance of wearing Medic-Alert bracelet with information on medical condition and anticoagulant medication.

16. Assess and evaluate alterations in functional skills, self-care deficits/refer to rehabilitative services as ordered to instruct in prescribed graded cardiac exercise program and energy conservation techniques.

17. Assess/instruct how to summon help in an emergency situation (e.g., dialing 911).

18. Assess anxiety and apprehension associated with altered body image and changes in lifestyle/ encourage to verbalize concerns about sexual activity to condition/refer to social services to assist with adjustment to illness and provide information regarding community services for assistance with cardiac rehabilitation (e.g., American Heart Association, Smokenders, counseling services).

Source: Reprinted with permission from C.A. Bedrosian, *Home Health Nursing: Nursing Diagnoses and Care Plans,* Appleton & Lange, © 1989.

In-Home Log

Client Name _____

This record should be kept readily available in your home so that your nurses can record basic information related to your care. You may want to take this with you when you go to see your doctor **BUT PLEASE BRING IT BACK HOME WITH YOU.**

Homebound due to: _____

DATE/ INIT'S	VITAL SIGNS	WOUND MEASUREMENT/ APPEARANCE	NEW ORDERS/ MEDICATIONS	BLOOD SUGAR	STATUS CHANGES	TEACHING PLAN/ CODE*	INS CHECK

*Teaching Code

A. Initial instruction started/needs further instruction   B. Requires assistance/reinforcement   C. Independent in procedure/verbalizes understanding

Courtesy of Caretenders of Louisville, Louisville, Kentucky.

HCFA Form 485
with Instruction Sheet

HOME HEALTH CERTIFICATION AND PLAN OF CARE

1. Patient's HI Claim No.	2. Start Of Care Date	3. Certification Period From: To:	4. Medical Record No.	5. Provider No.

6. Patient's Name and Address	7. Provider's Name, Address and Telephone Number

8. Date of Birth	9. Sex ☐ᴹ ☐ᶠ	10. Medications: Dose/Frequency/Route (N)ew (C)hanged

11. ICD-9-CM	Principal Diagnosis NEW EXACERBATION *Primary reason for service*	Date	NEW or CHANGED *Are meds related to diagnosis #11 and #13?* *Are problems with meds noted in the clinical findings?* *Are orders present to instruct?* *Are problems with teaching the patient or caregiver noted in* *clinical findings?*
12. ICD-9-CM	Surgical Procedure *Related to principal diagnosis?*	Date	
13. ICD-9-CM	Other Pertinent Diagnoses *List all that support the skilled* *services being provided.*	Date	

14. DME and Supplies *Are these used and needed in the* *patient's treatment? Related to diagnosis and treatment?*	15. Safety Measures: *Relate to functional limits and barriers to care.*
16. Nutritional Req. *Are orders needed to instruct?*	17. Allergies: *Any conflicts with meds being taken?*

18.A. Functional Limitations

1 ☐ Amputation	5 ☐ Paralysis	9 ☐ Legally Blind
2 ☐ Bowel/Bladder (incontinence)	6 ☐ Endurance 7 ☐ Ambulation	A ☐ Dyspnea With Minimal Exertion
3 ☐ Contracture	8 ☐ Speech	B ☐ Other (Specify)
4 ☐ Hearing		

Are these items described in clinical findings?

18.B. Activities Permitted

1 ☐ Complete Bedrest	6 ☐ Partial Weight Bearing	A ☐ Wheelchair
2 ☐ Bedrest BRP	7 ☐ Independent At Home	B ☐ Walker
3 ☐ Up As Tolerated*		C ☐ No Restrictions
4 ☐ Transfer Bed/Chair	8 ☐ Crutches	
5 ☐ Exercises Prescribed	9 ☐ Cane	D ☐ Other (Specify)

*If used, is patient homebound?

19. Mental Status:
Any impact on treatment?

1 ☐ Oriented	3 ☐ Forgetful	5 ☐ Disoriented	7 ☐ Agitated	*Does this conflict with*
2 ☐ Comatose	4 ☐ Depressed	6 ☐ Lethargic	8 ☐ Other	*goals?*

20. Prognosis:
1 ☐ Poor	2 ☐ Guarded	3 ☐ Fair	4 ☐ Good	5 ☐ Excellent

21. Orders for Discipline and Treatments (Specify Amount/Frequency/Duration)

Are orders related to diagnosis, clinical findings, problems, and assessments?
Have you described any problems with implementing these orders in the clinical findings section?
Do these orders justify the frequency and duration stated?
Are any other disciplines needed? Are any disciplines duplicating treatments?
This section is the professional's intervention phase of process (nursing process, therapy process, social work process).
Describe special orders or procedures that complicate the treatment plan implementation due to patient or family situations.

22. Goals/Rehabilitation Potential/Discharge Plans

This is the outcome phase of providing care. Are goals related to the services and treatment? Can the goals be achieved in view of
  functional limitations? Are goals realistic and does the plan relate to the goals? Rehabilitation potential: if poor, why therapy now?

23. Nurse's Signature and Date of Verbal SOC Where Applicable:	25. Date HHA Received Signed POT
24. Physician's Name and Address	26. I certify/recertify that this patient is confined to his/her home and needs intermittent skilled nursing care, physical therapy and/or speech therapy or continues to need occupational therapy. The patient is under my care, and I have authorized the services on this plan of care and will periodically review the plan.
27. Attending Physician's Signature and Date Signed	28. Anyone who misrepresents, falsifies, or conceals essential information required for payment of Federal funds may be subject to fine, imprisonment, or civil penalty under applicable Federal laws.

HOME HEALTH CERTIFICATION AND PLAN OF CARE

1. Patient's HI Claim No.	2. Start Of Care Date	3. Certification Period	4. Medical Record No.	5. Provider No.
000 00 0000A	031795	From: 031795 To: 051695	07632	72-0000

6. Patient's Name and Address	7. Provider's Name, Address and Telephone Number
Jones, David P. 2635 Tree View Lane Oak City, MI 43725	Home Health Care Services 107 True Care Lane Oak City, MI 43725

8. Date of Birth 07/21/23	9. Sex ☒M ☐F	10. Medications: Dose/Frequency/Route (N)ew (C)hanged

11. ICD-9-CM 890.1	Principal Diagnosis open wound, R hip	Date 03 15 95
12. ICD-9-CM 79.35	Surgical Procedure open reduction, R femur	Date 03 10 95
13. ICD-9-CM 820.9 491.2	Other Pertinent Diagnoses fracture, R femur Chronic obstructive bronchitis	Date 03 09 95 10 06 75

10. Medications: Dose/Frequency/Route (N)ew (C)hanged

Vitamin–Mineral Supplement 1 cap qd (N)
Ibuprofen tab q4° for pain (N)
Theophylline tab qd (C)
Prednisone   5 mg qd × 3 weeks
              2.5 mg qd × 2 weeks (N)
              1.5 mg qd 1 week then D/C

14. DME and Supplies walker, nasal cannula	15. Safety Measures: clear walkways to facilitate ambulation, remove throw rugs, proper footwear, O₂ precautions
16. Nutritional Req. 2000 caloric ADA	17. Allergies: none known

18.A. Functional Limitations

1	☐ Amputation	5	☐ Paralysis	9	☐ Legally Blind
2	☐ Bowel/Bladder (incontinence)	6	☒ Endurance	A	☒ Dyspnea With Minimal Exertion
		7	☒ Ambulation		
3	☐ Contracture	8	☐ Speech	B	☐ Other (Specify)
4	☐ Hearing				

18.B. Activities Permitted

1	☐ Complete Bedrest	6	☒ Partial Weight Bearing	A	☐ Wheelchair
2	☐ Bedrest BRP	7	☐ Independent At Home	B	☒ Walker
3	☐ Up As Tolerated			C	☐ No Restrictions
4	☒ Transfer Bed/Chair	8	☐ Crutches		
5	☒ Exercises Prescribed	9	☐ Cane	D	☐ Other (Specify)

19. Mental Status:

1	☒ Oriented	3	☐ Forgetful	5	☐ Disoriented	7	☐ Agitated
2	☐ Comatose	4	☐ Depressed	6	☐ Lethargic	8	☐ Other

20. Prognosis:

1	☐ Poor	2	☐ Guarded	3	☐ Fair	4	☒ Good	5	☐ Excellent

21. Orders for Discipline and Treatments (Specify Amount/Frequency/Duration)

Wound care to R hip daily. Irrigate wound with NS and pack with Clorpactin-soaked gauze. Dress with bulky dressing.
Skilled nursing 7 wk 4, 3 wk 3, 2 wk 1, for assessment of wound healing, performance of wound care and teaching high-protein, high-vitamin diet to facilitate wound healing.
Teaching re: effective coughing technique, effective breathing patterns, and pulmonary exercises to improve respiratory efficiency.
Assess for side effects of medications.
Physical therapy 3 wk 4, 2 wk 4, for evaluation of functional ability, gait training, transfer techniques, and teaching use of walker.
Home care aide: daily for 2 wk and 3x/wk for 6 wk.
Personal care: assist with therapeutic exercises and assist with transfers.

22. Goals/Rehabilitation Potential/Discharge Plans

Rehabilitation potential good to achieve full healing of the open wound on R hip by 5/16/95. Walking independently with walker by 4/30/95. Compliant with diet, medications, and therapy regimen by discharge. Plan to discharge to self-care with daughter's assistance when goals met.

23. Nurse's Signature and Date of Verbal SOC Where Applicable:	25. Date HHA Received Signed POT

24. Physician's Name and Address James Pinker, MD 2364 Dixwell Avenue Oak City, MI 43725	26. I certify/recertify that this patient is confined to his/her home and needs intermittent skilled nursing care, physical therapy and/or speech therapy or continues to need occupational therapy. The patient is under my care, and I have authorized the services on this plan of care and will periodically review the plan.
27. Attending Physician's Signature and Date Signed	28. Anyone who misrepresents, falsifies, or conceals essential information required for payment of Federal funds may be subject to fine, imprisonment, or civil penalty under applicable Federal laws.

Source: Blank forms from the Health Care Financing Administration, 1994.

HCFA Form 486 with Instruction Sheet

MEDICAL UPDATE AND PATIENT INFORMATION

1. Patient's HI Claim No.	2. SOC Date	3. Certification Period From: To:		4. Medical Record No.	5. Provider No.

6. Patient's Name and Address		7. Provider's Name

8. Medicare Covered: ☐ Y ☐ N	9. Date Physician Last Saw Patient:	10. Date Last Contacted Physician:

11. Is the Patient Receiving Care in an 1861 (J)(1) Skilled Nursing Facility or Equivalent? ☐ Y ☐ N ☐ Do Not Know	12. ☐ Certification ☐ Recertification ☐ Modified

13. Dates of Last Inpatient Stay: Admission Discharge	14. Type of Facility:

15. Updated information: New Orders/Treatments/Clinical Facts/Summary from Each Discipline

OVERALL—In order with dates

CLINICAL FACTS: Describe SOC <u>assessments</u> (assessment phase of process). Describe current <u>assessments</u> in measurable terms. Do these support the diagnosis? Relate to orders and treatments? Relate to the functional limitations? Any conflicts with diagnosis, treatment, and goals?

<u>HAVE YOU CREATED A CLINICAL PICTURE? BE GRAPHIC AND SPECIFIC.</u>

State any problems in teaching, learning, and implementing the treatment plan.

NEW ORDERS: Put information in chronological order; note date and details of changes, was there hospitalization?

SUMMARY: What has happened? What have you tried? What works? What doesn't work? What is the current status of the patient? How much more service is needed? Check HCFA Form 485 for conflicting information in orders, limitations, meds, and goals. Any change in patient condition will support continued service and should show the continued need for skilled care. This area should demonstrate that the assessment process or any other skill has occurred.

16. Functional Limitations (Expand From 485 and Level of ADL) Reason Homebound/Prior Functional Status

Prior level of function: In detail with <u>dates</u>. Were there multiple hospitalizations?

Current functional level: Why is this patient homebound? Are there any conflicts with #15 above? If diagnosis is over 2 months old, describe why home health care is necessary now. Was there prior therapy? For how long?

17. Supplementary Plan of Care on File from Physician Other than Referring Physician: ☐ Y ☐ N
    (If Yes, Please Specify Giving Goals/Rehab. Potential/Discharge Plan)

18. Unusual Home/Social Environment

Describe barriers to treatment, teaching, or goals.

19. Indicate Any Time When the Home Health Agency Made a Visit and Patient was Not Home and Reason Why if Ascertainable	20. Specify Any Known Medical and/or Non-Medical Reasons the Patient Regularly Leaves Home and Frequency of Occurrences

21. Nurse or Therapist Completing or Reviewing Form	Date (Mo., Day, Yr.)

MEDICAL UPDATE AND PATIENT INFORMATION

1. Patient's HI Claim No. 000 00 0000 A	2. SOC Date 031795	3. Certification Period From: 031795 To: 051695	4. Medical Record No. 07632	5. Provider No. 72-0000

6. Patient's Name and Address Jones, David P. 2635 Tree View Lane Oak City, MI 43725	7. Provider's Name Home Health Care Services

8. Medicare Covered: ☒ Y ☐ N	9. Date Physician Last Saw Patient: 031695	10. Date Last Contacted Physician: 031995

11. Is the Patient Receiving Care in an 1861 (J)(1) Skilled Nursing Facility or Equivalent? ☐ Y ☒ N ☐ Do Not Know	12. ☒ Certification ☐ Recertification ☐ Modified

13. Dates of Last Inpatient Stay: Admission 030995 Discharge 031695	14. Type of Facility: A

15. Updated information: New Orders/Treatments/Clinical Facts/Summary from Each Discipline

SN: On admission, patient had an open wound measuring 8x4x2 cm with purulent drainage.
Uses O_2 when ambulating. SN performed wound care daily, taught medications and side effects, diet and O_2 precautions. Wound measures 4x2x1 cm. with serosanguineous drainage. Compliant with therapeutic regime.

PT: On admission, patient was unstable using walker. Could only walk 3–4 steps with maximal assistance due to poor endurance. PT instructed in use of walker and therapeutic exercises to improve endurance. Can ambulate with walker 15 feet.

AIDE: Aide assists with personal care and therapeutic exercise program. Patient able to assist with self-care on 3/31/95. On 04/01/95, decreased to 3x week.

16. Functional Limitations (Expand From 485 and Level of ADL) Reason Homebound/Prior Functional Status

Limited weight bearing on R leg. Can ambulate only 10 feet with assistance. Needs assistance with ADLs due to difficulty with ambulation.

17. Supplementary Plan of Care on File from Physician Other than Referring Physician: (If Yes, Please Specify Giving Goals/Rehab. Potential/Discharge Plan)   ☐ Y ☒ N

18. Unusual Home/Social Environment

Lives alone in a two-story walk-up

19. Indicate Any Time When the Home Health Agency Made a Visit and Patient was Not Home and Reason Why if Ascertainable None	20. Specify Any Known Medical and/or Non-Medical Reasons the Patient Regularly Leaves Home and Frequency of Occurrences None

21. Nurse or Therapist Completing or Reviewing Form	Date (Mo., Day, Yr.) 04/10/95

Source: Blank forms from the Health Care Financing Administration, 1994.

Critical Path
Agency Forms

HomeCare-Path Assessment Visit

Hospital Name
City, State
Home Health Agency

Patient Name _____ MR# _____

Date _____ Time In _____ Time Out _____   WM=Written Material   NA=Not Applicable

NURSING INTERVENTIONS	COMPLETED	NOT COMPLETED	COMMENTS
1. Assess patient for appropriateness for home care and level of learning.			
2. Complete admission packet (process)—Bill of Rights, Advance Directive, Consent Form—obtain appropriate signatures.			
3. Assess environmental and psychosocial needs.			
4. Do physical assessment.			
5. Instruction: a. Call system—WM			
b. Emergency numbers—WM			
c. Home safety—WM			
d. Medication schedule—WM			
6. Evaluate need for referrals: MOW _____ PT _____ MSW _____ ST _____ HHA _____ Other _____			
7. Discuss general plan of care and tentative plan of discharge.			
8. Other			

PATIENT OUTCOME	MET	NOT MET	EXPLAIN VARIANCE
1. Verbalizes home health call system.			
2. States two measures to promote home safety.			
a.			
b.			
3. Other			
SIGNATURE		PATIENT INITIAL	

Source: Copyright © 1994, Clinton Memorial Hospital, Wilmington, Ohio.

HomeCare-Path Visit

Hospital Name
City, State
Home Health Agency

Patient Name _____ MR# _____

Nursing Assessment of Signs & Symptoms: Problem (+) No Problem (–)   WM=Written Material NA=Not Applicable

☐ NEUROLOGICAL	☐ RESPIRATORY	☐ G.I.	☐ G.U.	☐ MUSCULOSKELETAL
☐ Alert	☐ Crackles	☐ Nausea/vomiting	☐ Burning/pain	☐ Weakness
☐ Anxious	☐ Rhonchi	☐ Anorexia	☐ Frequency/urgency	☐ Bed/chair bound
☐ Confused	☐ Cough/SOB	☐ Diarrhea	☐ Hesitancy	☐ Balance/gait unsteady
☐ Disoriented	☐ Wheezes	☐ Constipation	☐ Distention/retention	☐ Functional status
☐ Lethargic	☐ O₂	☐ Bowel sounds	☐ Incontinent	☐ Independent
☐ Vertigo	☐ Other	☐ Last BM _____	☐ Catheter	☐ Assist
☐ Sensory			Size _____	☐ Dependent
			Urine _____	☐ Assistive device
☐ VITAL SIGNS	☐ CARDIOVASCULAR	☐ DIET/HYDRATION	Color _____	☐ Cane
			Odor _____	☐ Walker
☐ Temp. _____	☐ Arrhythmia	☐ Regular	Clear _____	☐ Wheelchair
☐ Pulse _____	☐ Chest pain	☐ ADA _____	Cloudy _____	☐ Other:
☐ Resp. _____	☐ Peripheral pulses	☐ Blood sugar ____		
☐ B/P _____	☐ Edema:	☐ Appetite		☐ PAIN
	RUE __ LUE __	☐ Weight _____		
	RLE __ LLE __			☐ Location
				☐ Intensity
☐ HOME SAFETY	☐ PSYCHOSOCIAL	☐ SKIN	☐ MED COMPLIANCE	0–10 _____
				☐ Pain med. effectiveness
	Strengths:	☐ Color	☐ New	
	☐ Family support	☐ Turgor	☐ Changes	☐ HHA SERVICE
☐ OTHER	☐ Willing	☐ Dry	☐ Other:	
	☐ Available	☐ Wound		☐ Patient satisfaction
	☐ Able	☐ Other:		☐ HHA to continue
				☐ HHA plan of care revised
	☐ LAST MD APPT.			☐ HHA following assignment

NURSING INTERVENTION/EDUCATION	COMPLETED	NOT COMPLETED	COMMENTS

PATIENT OUTCOME	MET	NOT MET	EXPLAIN VARIANCE
PLAN			

TIME IN	TIME OUT	DATE	RN SIGNATURE		PATIENT INITIAL

Source: Copyright © 1994, Clinton Memorial Hospital, Wilmington, Ohio.

CHF—HomeCare-Path—Visit #1

Hospital Name
City, State
Home Health Agency

Patient Name _____ MR# _____

Nursing Assessment of Signs & Symptoms: Problem (+) No Problem (–)   WM=Written Material   NA=Not Applicable

☐ **NEUROLOGICAL**

☐ Alert
☐ Anxious
☐ Confused
☐ Disoriented
☐ Lethargic
☐ Vertigo
☐ Sensory

☐ **VITAL SIGNS**

☐ Temp. _____
☐ Pulse _____
☐ Resp. _____
☐ B/P _____

☐ **HOME SAFETY**

☐ **OTHER**

☐ **RESPIRATORY**

☐ Crackles
☐ Rhonchi
☐ Cough/SOB
☐ Wheezes
☐ O₂
☐ Other

☐ **CARDIOVASCULAR**

☐ Arrhythmia
☐ Chest pain
☐ Peripheral pulses
☐ Edema:
   RUE __ LUE __
   RLE __ LLE __

☐ **PSYCHOSOCIAL**

Strengths:
☐ Family support
   ☐ Willing
   ☐ Available
   ☐ Able

☐ **LAST MD APPT.**

☐ **G.I.**

☐ Nausea/vomiting
☐ Anorexia
☐ Diarrhea
☐ Constipation
☐ Bowel sounds
☐ Last BM _____

☐ **DIET/HYDRATION**

☐ Regular
☐ ADA _____
☐ Blood sugar _____
☐ Appetite
☐ Weight _____

☐ **SKIN**

☐ Color
☐ Turgor
☐ Dry
☐ Wound
☐ Other:

☐ **G.U.**

☐ Burning/pain
☐ Frequency/urgency
☐ Hesitancy
☐ Distention/retention
☐ Incontinent
☐ Catheter
   Size _____
   Urine _____
   Color _____
   Odor _____
   Clear _____
   Cloudy _____

☐ **MED COMPLIANCE**

☐ New
☐ Changes
☐ Other:

☐ **MUSCULOSKELETAL**

☐ Weakness
☐ Bed/chair bound
☐ Balance/gait unsteady
☐ Functional status
   ☐ Independent
   ☐ Assist
   ☐ Dependent
☐ Assistive device
   ☐ Cane
   ☐ Walker
   ☐ Wheelchair
☐ Other:

☐ **PAIN**

☐ Location
☐ Intensity
   0–10 _____
☐ Pain med. effectiveness

☐ **HHA SERVICE**

☐ Patient satisfaction
☐ HHA to continue
☐ HHA plan of care revised
☐ HHA following assignment

NURSING INTERVENTION/EDUCATION	COMPLETED	NOT COMPLETED	COMMENTS
1. Instruct patient/caregiver on home O₂ if applicable—WM.			
2. Instruct patient/caregiver on medication #1–3—WM.			
3. Begin instruction to patient/caregiver on pathophysiology/disease process CHF—WM.			
4. Instruct patient/caregiver on low/no salt diet—WM.			
5. Instruct patient/caregiver on importance of weighing every day or as ordered by MD, and record—WM.			
6. Other			

PATIENT OUTCOME	MET	NOT MET	EXPLAIN VARIANCE
1. States 3 O₂ safety measures, if applicable.			
2. Verbally returns medication administration and major side effects for each medication taught today.			
3. Verbally defines CHF.			
4. States 3 foods high in sodium to avoid.			
5. Verbally understands when to weigh and record.			
6. Other			
PLAN			

TIME IN	TIME OUT	DATE	RN SIGNATURE	PATIENT INITIAL

Source: Copyright © 1994, Clinton Memorial Hospital, Wilmington, Ohio.

Example of Advance Directive

Connecticut Health Care Document

These are my health care instructions. My appointment of a health care agent, my appointment of an attorney-in-fact for health care decisions, the designation of my conservator of the person for my future incapacity and my document of anatomical gift.

To any physician who is treating me: These are my health care instructions including those concerning the withholding or withdrawal of life support systems, together with the appointment of my health care agent and my attorney-in-fact for health care decisions, the designation of my conservator of the person for future incapacity and my document of anatomical gift. As my physician, you may rely on any decision made by my health care agent, attorney-in-fact for health care decisions, or conservator of my person if I am unable to make a decision for myself.

PART I. HEALTH CARE INSTRUCTIONS

I _____, the author of this document, request that, if my condition is deemed terminal or if I am determined to be permanently unconscious, I be allowed to die and not be kept alive through life support systems. By terminal condition, I mean that I have an incurable or irreversible medical condition which, without the administration of life support systems, will, in the opinion of my attending physician, result in death within a relatively short time. By permanently unconscious I mean that I am in a permanent coma or persistent vegetative state, which is an irreversible condition in which I am at no time aware of myself or the environment and show no behavioral response to the environment. The life support systems that I do not want include, but are not limited to: artificial respiration, cardiopulmonary resuscitation, and artificial means of providing nutrition and hydration. I do want sufficient pain medication to maintain my physical comfort. I do not intend any direct taking of my life, but only that my dying not be unreasonably prolonged.

Other Instructions

(If you wish to give additional instructions, you may do so. If none, write "None" on the lines below.)

_____

_____

_____

_____

Courtesy of Promed Resources, Inc., St. Louis, Missouri, 1995.

continues

PART II. APPOINTMENT OF HEALTH CARE AGENT AND ATTORNEY-IN-FACT

I appoint _____,

(name, address, city, state, and telephone number)

to be my health care agent and attorney-in-fact for health care decisions. If my attending physician determines that I am unable to understand and appreciate the nature and consequences of health care decisions and unable to reach and communicate an informed decision regarding treatment, my health care agent and attorney-in-fact for health care decisions is authorized to:

1. Convey to my physician my wishes concerning the withholding or removal of life support systems
2. Take whatever actions are necessary to ensure that any wishes are given effect
3. Consent, refuse, or withdraw consent to any medical treatment as long as such action is consistent with my wishes concerning the withholding or removal of life support systems
4. Consent to any medical treatment designed solely for the purpose of maintaining physical comfort

Designation of Alternate Agent and Attorney-in-Fact (Optional)

(You are not required to designate one or more alternates, but you may do so. An alternate agent and attorney-in-fact may make the same health care decisions as your designated agent and attorney-in-fact if the designated agent and attorney-in-fact is unable or unwilling to act.)

If my agent and attorney-in-fact named by me shall die, become legally disabled, incapacitated or incompetent, or resign, refuse to act, or be unavailable, I name the following (each to act successively in the order named) as my alternate agent and attorney-in-fact.

First Alternate Agent

Name: _____

Address: _____

Second Alternate Agent

Name: _____

Address: _____

Special Instructions (Optional)

(You may give your agent(s) any special instructions in this section. If you do not wish to do so, put "None" on the lines provided.)

_____

_____

_____

_____

continues

Limitations (Optional)

(You may wish to put additional limitations on your agents in this section. If you do not wish to do so, put "None" on the lines provided.)

_____

_____

_____

_____

PART III. APPOINTMENT OF CONSERVATOR

If a conservator of my person should need to be appointed, I designate _____ be appointed my conservator. If _____ is unwilling or unable to serve as my conservator, I designate _____.

No bond shall be required of either of them in any jurisdiction.

PART IV. ANATOMICAL GIFT DONATION

(Initial one of the following statements.)

___ I do not wish to make any anatomical gift.
___ I hereby make this anatomical gift, if medically acceptable, to take effect upon my death.

I give: (check one)
    ___ 1. any needed organ or parts
    ___ 2. only the following organs or parts

_____

to be donated for: (check one)
    ___ 1. any of the purposes stated in subsection (a) of section 19A-279(f) of the general statutes
    ___ 2. these limited purposes _____

_____

_____

AUTHOR'S SIGNATURE

These requests, appointments, and designations are made after careful reflection, while I am of sound mind. Any party receiving a duly executed copy or facsimile of this document may rely upon it unless such party has received actual notice of my revocation of it.

_____   _____
(signature)   (date)

_____   _____
(print or type name)   (Social Security number)

_____
(address)

_____
(city, state, ZIP code)

continues

WITNESS SIGNATURES

We, the subscribing witnesses, being duly sworn, say that we witnessed the execution of these health care instructions, the appointment of a health care agent and an attorney-in-fact, the designation of a conservator for future incapacity, and a document of anatomical gift by the author of this document; that the author subscribed, published, and declared the same to be the author's instructions, appointments, and designation in our presence; that we thereafter subscribed the document as witnesses in the author's presence, at the author's request, and in the presence of each other; that at the time of the execution of said document the author appeared to us to be eighteen years of age or older, of sound mind, able to understand the nature and consequences of said document, and under no improper influence, and we make this affidavit at the author's request this _____ day of _____ 19 ___.

_____   _____
(witness)   (witness)

_____   _____
(print or type name)   (print or type name)

_____   _____
(address)   (address)

_____   _____
(city, state, ZIP code)   (city, state, ZIP code)

NOTARY

STATE OF CONNECTICUT   )
) ss.
COUNTY OF _____   )

We, the undersigned, being duly sworn, depose and say:
That on this date, the within named _____
                               (author of document)

signed the foregoing Health Care Document in our presence as witnesses; that we

_____ and _____
(witness)   (witness)

thereupon subscribed our names thereto as witnesses in (his/her) presence and at (his/her) request and in the presence of each other; that at the time of the execution of said Health Care Document the said

_____
(author of document)

appeared to be more than eighteen years of age and of sound mind and memory, and to the best of our judgment not under any improper restraint or influence or in any respect incompetent to make said Health Care Document; and that we make this affidavit at (his/her) request this   day of _____, 19____.

Subscribed and sworn to before me, on this _____ day of _____, 19__.

_____
Notary Public
Commissioner of Superior Court

Standard High-Tech Care Plans

PLAN OF CARE: HOME IV THERAPY

GOALS:

NAME: _____   **TYPE OF SERVICE:** _____

DIAGNOSIS(es): 1. Home IV therapy _____   2. _____

Date	Patient and/or Family Needs and Problems	Unusual Problems	Planned Steps To Meet Needs and Solve Problems	By Whom	Date	Review and Signature
	Hookup and disconnect procedure		Client will be instructed, per procedure, on: • aseptic technique • spiking IV bag and priming tubing • how to access IV line • regulation of fluid rate • heparinization of line • proper securing with tape The client/caregiver must demonstrate proficiency (to the satisfaction of the nurse) in performing and maintaining therapy to initially enroll and to continue in the home care program.			

	Teaching needs: indications for and concept of home IV therapy		The client will be taught:
			
			• the concept of home IV therapy
			• indications for home IV therapy (e.g., hydration, antibiotics)
			• benefits of home IV therapy
			  –decreased cost
			  –early return to work and activities of daily living
			  –shorter length of hospitalization
			  –decreased incidence of contracting nosocomial infections			

	IV site observation and care		Patient will be instructed to keep site dry (no shower, only sponge baths). Patient will be taught to observe site for redness, streaking, swelling, pain and/or leaking at site, and to notify RN. Patient will be taught the side effects of the specific medication that is being administered.			

PLAN OF CARE: HICKMAN CARE

GOALS:

NAME: _____   TYPE OF SERVICE: _____

DIAGNOSIS(es): 1. __Hickman Care_____   2. _____

Date	Patient and/or Family Needs and Problems	Unusual Problems	Planned Steps To Meet Needs and Solve Problems	By Whom	Date	Review and Signature
	Performance of *daily* site care		1. Caregiver will have successfully completed training in Hickman care. 2. Caregiver will be able to demonstrate knowledge of what a Hickman catheter is and of general safety precautions. Hickman catheter care: a. Clean work area with alcohol. b. Wash hands with liquid soap for 3 minutes. c. Gather supplies and open packages. d. Remove old dressing and inspect the site for: • leaking of fluids • blood or pus • redness, swelling, or tenderness *Any of the above should be reported immediately to the client's MD or home care nurse. e. Using peroxide-soaked sterile cotton tip applicator, clean exit site following Hickman catheter care instructions, and apply bandage.			
	Performance of *daily* heparin flush		1. Immediately following daily site care, wash hands. 2. Prepare supplies for flush procedure. 3. Flush Hickman catheter with 2.5 cc of heparin following flush procedure instructions.			
	Performance of *weekly* cap change		1. Once weekly (or more often if indicated) immediately following site care procedure, and preceding heparin flush, change injection cap following cap change instructions. 2. Remove old tape from clamping site and apply new tape. Place tape on a rotating basis, moving from a position close to the skin, outward. Write date on tape.			
	Hickman catheter complications		1. Report immediately any signs and symptoms indicated on signs and symptoms checklist to MD or home care nurse.			

PLAN OF CARE: PORT-A-CATH MAINTENANCE

GOALS:

NAME: _____   **TYPE OF SERVICE:** _____

DIAGNOSIS(es): 1. __Port-A-Cath Maintenance__   **2.** _____

Date	Patient and/or Family Needs and Problems	Unusual Problems	Planned Steps To Meet Needs and Solve Problems	By Whom	Date	Review and Signature
	Patient responsibility immediately post-op		Indication for, and explanation of Port-A-Cath will be done by MD and/or nurse. A. Initially, gauze will be applied post-op (with or without Huber needle inserted in Port-A-Cath, per MD discretion). Dressing will be changed after 24 hours and then every 3 days until incision is healed. B. Patient will be instructed to avoid showering for first 10 days, and that when showering to direct spray on his/her back. Dressing must be changed if it becomes wet or loose. C. Patient will be aware of possibility of swelling around site for up to 2 weeks post-op.			
	Long term		A. Patient will be taught to inspect site for leakage of fluid/infiltration/hematoma, redness, streaking, or tenderness along catheter track. B. If patient is to access Port-A-Cath he/she will be taught per agency procedure specifically hookup, disconnection, and heparinization of Port-A-Cath.			
	Accessing line		Using aseptic technique: A. Set up sterile field, per procedure. B. Using #18g Huber needle and extension tubing, prime with NS, and clamp. C. Clean site, per procedure, with Betadine. D. Palpate Port-A-Cath with one hand, locating center. E. With other hand, push needle perpendicularly through skin into center of device until needle stops. F. Open clamp on extension tubing and infuse solution.			
	Long-term therapy		For continuous or long-term therapy: A. An air occlusive window dressing will be applied. B. The needle and occlusive dressing will be changed by an RN weekly. C. Line will be primed, per procedure. D. Dressing will be applied, per procedure. E. Dressing will be secured with tape to form a window frame, and extension tubing will be secured on top.			

continues

PLAN OF CARE: PORT-A-CATH MAINTENANCE

GOALS:

NAME: _____   TYPE OF SERVICE: _____

DIAGNOSIS(es): 1. Port-A-Cath Maintenance   2. _____

Date	Patient and/or Family Needs and Problems	Unusual Problems	Planned Steps To Meet Needs and Solve Problems	By Whom	Date	Review and Signature
	Disconnecting line		Using aseptic technique: A. Draw up NS and heparin, per procedure. B. Clean connection with three alcohol wipes between extension tubing and cap, or pump tubing. C. Inject NS and heparin, per procedure. Close clamp. D. Remove dressing. E. With Betadine, cleanse site, per procedure. F. Place thumb and forefinger of one hand on either side of needle, grip hub and pull upward. With other hand, apply pressure to decrease incidence of hematoma.			
	Troubleshooting		A. For spontaneous blood backflow, patient should check connections and tighten, and check pump function. B. Leaking: Check connections and tighten; retape. C. Catheter occlusion: Clamp extension tubing and notify MD/nurse. Instruct patient not to flush. D. For extravasation: Instruct patient to notify MD/nurse. Note needle placement, backflow of blood, catheter disconnection, attempt to aspirate bid. Consider: cracked or separated catheter from Port-A-Cath. E. Withdrawal occlusion: Check needle placement, have patient change position. Consider: thrombosis, cracked or separated catheter. Instruct patient to notify MD/nurse with the following signs and symptoms A. fever greater than 101° B. swelling, redness, tenderness or discharge at site, or blood backup in tubing C. swelling and/or pain in area of collarbone, neck, face, or upper arm D. prominent veins in neck, face, arm, or chest E. difficulty swallowing F. sores in mouth, diarrhea, nausea, or vomiting			

PLAN OF CARE: TPN

GOALS:

NAME: _____   **TYPE OF SERVICE:** _____

DIAGNOSIS(es): 1. __TPN_____   **2.** _____

Date	Patient and/or Family Needs and Problems	Unusual Problems	Planned Steps To Meet Needs and Solve Problems	By Whom	Date	Review and Signature
	Observation/recording and precautions		Need to monitor: • serum electrolytes—P_{12} weekly • urine dipsticks for greater than 1+ glycosuria • weight/nutritional status • vital signs • Hickman catheter site (see care plan) • distended veins in neck, arms, hands secondary to central venous thrombosis • swelling/edema in face, neck, head secondary to infiltration of solution into surrounding tissues			
	Teaching needs: patient and significant others		• Check temperature (M-W-F), notify nurse of elevation. Check temperature more frequently if patient feels ill. • Weight/urine dipstick (M-W-F) and document. Check more frequently if patient feels ill. • Importance of balanced diet and adequate elimination. • Notify nurse of weight gain or loss more than 2 lbs. • Notify nurse of any of the following symptoms: Excessive cramping, gas accumulation, diarrhea, nausea, vomiting, constipation, large urine output, decrease in appetite, if applicable • Teaching and reinforcement of aseptic handwashing technique and maintaining sterility of IV solution delivery system.			

Clinical Flowsheet

	DATE	DATE	DATE	DATE
Vital Signs				
Intake: Oral Intravenous Enteral				
Output: Urine Stool Other				
Neurological: (confusion, orientation)				
Respiratory (SOB, rales, rhonchi)				
Gastrointestinal (N/V/D, constipation)				
Genitourinary (color, characteristics)				
Hematological (bleeding, bruising)				
Cardiac (palpitations, edema, syncope, heart sounds)				
Musculoskeletal (pain, decreased ROM)				
Medication reactions (describe relative to prescribed medications)				
Intravenous: Catheter site: (appearance, dressing change) Restart/re-access Flow/troubleshooting				
Enteral: (describe flow and tolerance) Placement checked				
Lab tests drawn				
Teaching topics (describe topic and patient reaction)				
See care plan (yes/no)				
See physician orders (yes/no)				
See narrative note (yes/no)				
Signature				

Generic Pediatric Home Care Plan for Families with an Ill Child

GENERAL PSYCHOSOCIAL ISSUES FOR FAMILIES

Assessment

Overall, ongoing observation of home environment and family interaction:

- Is the family nurturing and supportive to the ill child?
- Is parental anxiety interfering with parent-child bonding?
- Are interactions between parents positive and supportive?
- Are parents able to communicate appropriately with health professionals?
- How are siblings reacting and adjusting?
- Are parents feeling isolated and exhausted from the ongoing responsibilities of home care?

Nursing Interventions

1. Promote parents' self-esteem and confidence by commending their accomplishments with the child.
2. Act as a role model in meeting the ill child's and siblings' physical, developmental, and emotional needs.
3. Allow parents the time and opportunity to discuss their lives and feelings.
4. Offer emotional support without encouraging dependency.
5. Identify a case manager (usually the primary home care nurse) and clearly define what needs to be communicated.
6. Suggest appropriate support groups, organizations, or agencies to assist with financial, social, or mental health needs.
7. Assist parents in problem solving by identifying respite programs, arranging for private duty nursing, or identifying friends/family who could offer assistance.

see specific care plans, next four pages

GENERIC HOME CARE PLANS

Generic Home Care Plan for the Child Receiving IV Therapy

Assessment

Physical

1. State the child's diagnosis and its associated high-tech management (e.g., osteomyelitis of right tibia requiring 6 weeks IV antibiotic treatment)
2. Describe pertinent health history
3. Record baseline vital signs cardiopulmonary, HEENT, GI, GU, neuro, musculoskeletal, and integumentary status
4. Describe functional disabilities relating to play or ADLs
5. Describe location of IV site and if peripheral or central
6. State how often peripheral IV site dressing or central IV dressing to be changed

Psychosocial

1. Describe child's and family's reaction to venipuncture and IV procedures
2. Observe general parenting skills and parental support

Developmental

1. Describe the child's behavior reactions to IV therapy and if appropriate for developmental stage
2. Note if child is able to participate in regular school program or requires home tutoring

Nursing Interventions

Equipment

1. List all types of equipment necessary. The following is a comprehensive list:
   • IV solution(s)
   • IV pump
   • IV needles (angiocath or butterfly)
   • Syringes and needles
   • Medications
   • Arm board
   • Tubex
   • Transparent dressing (e.g., Tegarderm, Opsite, DuoDERM)
   • Heparin solution
   • Saline
   • Heparin lock adaptor
   • Alcohol and Betadine swabs
   • Injection cap
   • Padded clamp
   • Needle disposal container
   • Hydrogen peroxide
   • Central line catheter repair kit

Teaching

1. Review's child's diagnosis and reasons for IV and medications
2. Signs of IV complications: infiltration, infection
3. Demonstrate and redemonstrate IV setup procedure using appropriate sterile technique
4. Demonstrate and redemonstrate use of equipment
5. Who and when to call in event of complications or equipment malfunction

Safety Checklist

1. Are there adequate trained caregivers?
2. Are equipment and supplies child proofed or in a safe location?
3. Is there a backup plan if peripheral IV cannot be started at home?

Generic Home Care Plan for the Child with a Respiratory Problem
(Apnea Monitor, Oxygen, Tracheostomy, Ventilator)

Assessment

Physical

1. State the child's diagnosis and its associated high-tech management (e.g., tracheal stenosis requiring tracheostomy, oxygen, and apnea monitor)
2. Describe pertinent health history
3. Record baseline weight, height, head circumference, vital signs, breath sounds, retractions, color, nasal flaring
4. Describe type, amount of feedings, position for feedings, special bottles, nipples, spoons
5. Describe functional disabilities relating to play or ADLs
6. Describe sleep/wake patterns

Psychosocial

Observe and record:
1. Parenting skills
2. Parent-child bonding
3. Siblings' response to ill child
4. Parent sharing and support

Developmental

1. Observe child's developmental stage in relation to actual age (e.g., no verbal skills for 3-year-old)
2. Describe child's limitations and potential (e.g., tires quickly with motor activity but has good muscle tone)
3. Note infant stimulation programs or school programs child may be involved in or referred to

Nursing Interventions

Equipment

1. List all types of equipment necessary. The following is a comprehensive list:
   - Ventilator
   - Oxygen source
   - Oxygen tent
   - Nasal cannula
   - Trach mask
   - Extra tubing
   - Humidity source
   - Ambu bag
   - Sterile water or saline
   - Suction machine and catheters
   - Monitor leads and electrode pads
   - Monitor belt
   - Battery pack

Teaching

1. Signs of respiratory distress specific to this child
2. How to respond to alarms
3. Infant/child CPR
4. Review plan in event of emergency
5. Suctioning and chest physiotherapy
6. Review child's diagnosis and reasons for equipment
7. Demonstration with redemon-stration on use and cleaning of equipment
8. Review oxygen monitor ventilator settings
9. Medications: actions, side effects, and contraindications

Safety Checklist

1. Are there adequately trained caregivers?
2. Can alarms be heard from all locations?
3. Are emergency numbers posted?
4. Are equipment and medications child proofed or in a safe location?
5. Are equipment manuals available?
6. Are no sources of combustion present?
7. Is a fire extinguisher available?
8. Is there a source of power in event of blackout?

Generic Home Care Plan for the Child with a Gastrointestinal/Nutritional Problem
(Feeding Tubes, Colostomies, Feeding Pumps)

Assessment

Physical

1. State the child's diagnosis and its associated high-tech management (e.g., gastroesophageal reflux requiring duodenal tube feedings and gastrostomy tube placement)
2. Describe pertinent health history
3. Record baseline weight, height, head circumference, growth percentiles, bowel function/sounds, vomiting, oral feedings, skin around stoma
4. Describe type, amount, rate of feedings
5. Describe functional disabilities relating to play or ADLs
6. Describe sleep/wake pattern in relation to feedings

Psychosocial

Observe and record:
1. Parenting skills
2. Parent-child bonding
3. Siblings' response to altered feeding procedure
4. Parent sharing and support

Developmental

1. Observe child's developmental stage in relation to actual age
2. Describe child's limitations and potential (e.g., child will suck on pacifier but refuses to swallow)
3. Note infant stimulation or school programs child may be involved in or referred to

Nursing Interventions

Equipment

1. List all types necessary. The following is a comprehensive list:
   - Nasogastric tubes
   - Gastrostomy tube
   - Stethoscope
   - Syringes
   - Feeding pump and bags
   - Liquid food
   - Colostomy bags
   - Stoma protectant
   - Catheter adapters

Teaching

1. Review child's diagnosis and reasons for equipment
2. Signs of feeding intolerance
3. Demonstration with redemonstration on use and cleaning of equipment
4. Skin care and/or dressing changes for stoma
5. Medications: actions, side effects, administration

Safety Checklist

1. Are there adequately trained caregivers?
2. Are equipment and medications child proofed and in a safe location?
3. Are equipment manuals available?
4. Is there a backup method of feeding in the event of pump malfunction?

Generic Home Care Plan for the Infant Receiving Home Phototherapy

Assessment

Physical

1. State the infant's diagnosis and its associated high-tech management (e.g., hyperbilirubinemia requiring phototherapy)
2. Describe pertinent health history
3. Record baseline vital signs, weight, general appearance, skin, hydration status, elimination patterns
4. Sleep/wake patterns in relation to feedings

Psychosocial

1. Parenting skills
2. Parent-child bonding
3. Siblings' response
4. Parent sharing and support

Developmental

1. Infant's behavioral response to phototherapy (lethargy, irritability, quiet, alert, etc.)
2. Is infant held and touched when away from lights for feedings?

Nursing Interventions

Equipment

1. List all types of equipment necessary. The following is a comprehensive list:
   - Eye patches
   - Thermometers

Teaching

1. Review diagnosis and reasons for equipment
2. Demonstration and redemonstration of axillary temperature procedure and frequency
3. Turn infant every 2–3 hours
4. Demonstration and redemonstration of application and positioning of eye patches
5. Documentation procedure for feedings, elimination, temperature, and position changes
6. Guidelines for when to call health professionals
7. Necessity for regular heel-stick bilirubin levels

Safety Checklist

1. Are caregivers available to observe the infant at all times?
2. Are equipment and supplies out of reach of siblings?

Pediatric Home Care Resource List

appendix
K

American Cancer Society
1599 Clifton Road, NE
Atlanta, GA 30329
800-4-CANCER

American Lung Association
1740 Broadway
New York, NY 10019
212-315-8700 or 800-586-4872

**Association for the Care of Children's Health
(ACCH)**
7910 Woodmont Avenue
Suite 300
Bethesda, MD 20814
301-654-6549

Candlelighters Childhood Cancer Foundation
7910 Woodmont Avenue
Suite 460
Bethesda, MD 20814
301-657-8401 or 800-366-2223

Children's Hospice International
700 Princess Street
Lower Level
Alexandria, VA 22314

Cystic Fibrosis Foundation
6931 Arlington Road
Bethesda, MD 20814
800-344-4823

Leukemia Society of America
600 Third Avenue
4th Floor
New York, NY 10017
212-573-8484 or 800-654-1247

Muscular Dystrophy Association of America
10 East 40th Street
Room 4110
New York, NY 10016
212-689-9040

National Easter Seal Society
230 West Monroe Street
Suite 1800
Chicago, IL 60606-4802
312-726-6200 or 800-221-6827

**National Information Center for Children and
Youth with Disabilities**
P.O. Box 1492
Washington, DC 20013
202-844-8200 or 800-695-0285

Parents Helping Parents, Inc.
3041 Olcott Street
Santa Clara, CA 95054
408-727-5775

United Cerebral Palsy Association, Inc.
105 Madison Avenue
New York, NY 10016
212-683-6700

Glossary of General Home Health Terms and Abbreviations

The following terms and abbreviations are defined in order to aid the reader in using this text. Commonly used diagnosis abbreviations are not defined.

Audit. A review of a random selection of an agency's medical records to determine whether payment of services was justified. The reviewers look at the clinical record documentation to determine if the beneficiary was entitled to the service and if the service provided complied with coverage criteria. Audits can be performed quarterly, postpayment, or at random.

Beneficiary. A person (patient) eligible to receive Medicare or Medicaid benefits or benefits of other health insurance programs.

Branch office. A location or site from which a home health agency provides services within a portion of the total geographic area served by the parent agency. The branch office is part of the home health agency and is located sufficiently close to share administration, supervision, and services in a manner that renders it unnecessary for the branch independently to meet the conditions of participation as a home health agency.

Case conference. A meeting or phone conversation to coordinate, solve problems, and plan for effective home health care services. Case conferences are frequently multidisciplinary.

Case management. A collaborative process in which participants assess, plan, implement, coordinate, monitor, and evaluate the options and services required to meet an individual's health needs, using communication and available resources, to promote quality, cost-effective outcomes.

Case manager. (1) In the context of a person working for an insurance company, health maintenance organization (HMO), or other payer of services, a case manager is someone who helps identify appropriate providers and facilities throughout the continuum of services, while ensuring that available resources are being used in a timely and cost-effective manner in order to obtain optimal value for both the patient and the reimbursement source. (2) In terms of a provider of care, such as a home health agency, a case manager is someone who assesses the patient's needs, coordinates the other providers within the agency, and delivers some or all of the direct care to the patient. This person does not usually have total responsibility for coordinating the payment for the patient's services (other than those directly being provided by the agency).

Claim. The billing form known as the UB-92, which is submitted (usually electronically) to the fiscal intermediary or any third-party payer following the rendering of services and after the physician's plan of care (HCFA Form 485) is on file at the agency. This form is usually submitted once a month.

Clinical note. A written notation of a contact with a patient by a member of the health care team, dated and signed (with title). Clinical notes describe signs and symptoms, treatments, care rendered, drugs given, patient reactions, information or teaching provided, patient comprehension, and changes in physical or emotional condition.

Community Health Accreditation Program (CHAP). An arm of the National League for Nursing, accredits home care agencies based on established standards.

Copayment. This is the payment made by the patient to his or her hospital or physician. Copayments are usually referred to in terms of dollars, such as $10 per prescription or $20 per physician visit. The health

271

benefits company picks up the balance owed to the hospital or physician.

Covered services. These are the services performed by health care provider for which the insurance company agrees to pay—either in full or in part. Some health care services are not "covered services" because they are not essential to treatment.

Database. All the information (including referral information, laboratory reports, the initial assessment, and evaluations) collected by the agency about a client.

Discharge summary. A documented report that summarizes the home health care services, treatments, and goals achieved for the entire period of time that the patient received home health care.

Durable medical equipment (DME). Also referred to as home medical equipment.

Health maintenance organization (HMO). An HMO is a prepaid insurance plan that provides for comprehensive health care for enrollees within the plan's specific policy requirements.

Home care record. The compilation of a patient's total home health agency and related documentation, including history, service agreements, assessments, clinical notes, physician's plan of care, discharge summaries, laboratory notes, notifications of noncoverage, and any other documentation unique to the agency.

Home medical equipment (HME). Such equipment, often referred to as DME, includes items that are purchased or rented for the care of in-dividuals in the home (e.g., wheelchairs, hospital beds, etc.).

Joint Commission on Accreditation of Healthcare Organizations. The Joint Commission conducts home health agency surveys for accreditation based on its established standards.

Licensed practical nurse (LPN). A person who is licensed as a practical nurse by the state in which he or she is practicing.

Licensed vocational nurse (LVN). A person who is licensed as a vocational nurse by the state in which he or she is practicing.

Managed care. Managed care has five parts: (1) preadmission certification of any proposed hospitalization; (2) concurrent review, meaning a reviewer continues to monitor hospitalization; (3) case management or individual benefits management, meaning the managers will strongly suggest cheaper alternatives to long hospital stays and other high-cost services; (4) second opinions; and (5) bonuses or penalties for the physician depending upon the cost of care.

Medical social worker. An individual who has a master's degree from a school of social work accredited by the Council on Social Work Education and has one year of social work experience in a health care setting.

Nonprofit agency. An agency exempt from federal income taxation under section 501 of the Internal Revenue Code of 1954.

Parent home health agency. The agency that develops and maintains administrative control of subunits or branch offices.

Patient. Any individual receiving home health care.

Peer review organization (PRO). A utilization and quality control review organization mandated by the Omnibus Budget Reconciliation Act of 1986 to review beneficiary complaints about the quality of home health services and to review samples of early hospital readmission cases.

Plan of care (POC) or plan of treatment (POT). Medical treatment plan established by the treating physician with the assistance of the home health care nurse.

Preferred provider organization (PPO). A PPO is an insurance plan that provides comprehensive care only through contracted providers.

Primary care physician (PCP). This is the physician who is turned to first for any medical care. This physician will either treat patients or refer them to a specialist whose practice is limited to specific areas of expertise. The PCP is responsible for coordinating all aspects of care.

Primary diagnosis. The illness or injury that is responsible for the patient's greatest need for treatment and most intensive skilled services.

Primary home health agency. The agency that is responsible for the services furnished to patients and for implementation of the plans of care.

Private payer. An individual who pays for home health services directly.

Progress note. A written notation by a member of the health care team, dated and signed (with title) that summarizes the facts about care and the patient's response during a given period of time.

Proprietary agency. A private, profit-making home health agency.

Provider. This can be any physician or hospital—or any company with the appropriate medical licensing—that provides health care services or medical equipment. A participating provider is one that has agreed with a health benefits company to accept its payment as payment in full for covered services and has agreed not to bill the patient for any balance. A nonparticipating provider has no such agreement and may bill the patient for any balance.

Public agency. An agency operated by a state or local government.

Regulation. Medicare program regulations are the general and permanent rules formally approved and issued by the Secretary of Health and Human Services and implemented by the Health Care Financing Administration (HCFA). Regulations have the force and effect of law and are binding on all parties until amended or revoked.

Subdivision. A component of a multifunction health care agency (e.g., the home care department of a hospital or the nursing division of a health department) that independently meets the Medicare Conditions of Participation for home health agencies. A subdivision that has subunits or branch offices is considered a parent agency.

Subunit. A semiautonomous organization that services patients in a geographic area different from that of the parent agency and must independently meet the conditions of participation for home health agencies because it is too far from the parent agency to share administration, supervision, and services on a daily basis.

Summary report. A compilation of pertinent facts from a patient's clinical and progress notes. Summary reports are submitted to the patient's physician.

Surveyor. A professional, usually a registered nurse, employed by a state agency, HCFA, or an accrediting body (e.g., the Joint Commission and CHAP) to review and evaluate home health agencies' initial or ongoing compliance with Medicare Conditions of Participation and state regulations for the purpose of Medicare/Medicaid certification, accrediting body certification, or state licensure.

Third-party payer. A government or commercial entity that reimburses for health care services on behalf of the insured person.

UB-92. A universal billing form used as a claim (bill) for reimbursement by the third-party payers. It is usually electronically submitted monthly for payment of services rendered and items supplied.

Visit. Personal contact in the patient's place of residence made for the purpose of providing home health care services by a member of the home health team.

Glossary of Medicare and Medicaid Home Health Terms

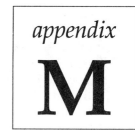

appendix

M

Administrative law judge (ALJ). The judge who hears the appeal of a denied claim in a court of law. This is the last stage of the appeal process.

Advisories. A written notification from the fiscal intermediary regarding important changes or interpretations in the regulations or new material from the Health Care Financing Administration (HCFA). Some fiscal intermediaries call them admissions newsletters or bulletins.

Certification. The *original* plan of care (HCFA Form 485) completed upon the patient's admission to the home health agency.

Certification of a home health agency. The process by which a home health agency is granted approval to participate in the Medicare program by complying with the Conditions of Participation.

Conditions of Participation (COPs). Federal regulations that govern the Medicare home health program and provide guidelines for agency management, personnel, and patient care. There is a manual in each home care agency that outlines the COPs. When state licensure surveyors perform annual visits, they look for compliance with the COPs.

Coverage. The criteria outlined by the payer source that determine if an agency will be reimbursed for the services delivered to the client.

Denial. Refusal by a fiscal intermediary or third-party payer to pay for a claim because it did not meet Medicare or third-party payer guidelines. A medical necessity denial is a denial by Medicare based on the grounds that the care provided was not skilled, not reasonable and necessary, not intermittent, or was excessive or unsafe. A technical denial is a denial by

Medicare based on the grounds that the patient was not homebound, did not require intermittent skilled care, or lacked appropriate physician's orders.

Fiscal intermediary (FI) (sometimes called home health regional imtermediary [HHRI]). One of the nine insurance companies that have been designated by HCFA to oversee the financial and clinical management of the Medicare home health benefit program, including the processing of claims.

Guidelines. The instructions in the HIM-11 for implementation of the Medicare home health benefit. These guidelines are HCFA's interpretation of the regulations.

Health Care Financing Administration (HCFA). HCFA, which is in the Department of Health and Human Services, is responsible for the administration of the Medicare program.

The HCFA Form 485 series. Includes HCFA Forms 485, 486, 487. A HCFA Form 488 is used by some states as a request for further information. HCFA Form 485 (Home Health Certification and Plan of Care) includes data elements required by federal regulation and meets the physician's plan of care requirements. It is used for both certification and recertification (see Appendix D). A HCFA Form 485 covers physician orders for no longer than 62 days at a time.

HCFA Form 486 (Medical Update and Patient Information). An update on a Medicare patient that is required only if the fiscal intermediary requests additional information (see Appendix E).

HCFA Form 487 (Addendum to the Plan of Care/Medical Update). This form is used for additional information and data carried over from HCFA Form 485 or 486.

HCFA Form 488 (Home Health Agency Intermediary Medical Information Request or other form used by the fiscal intermediary). This form is used by the fiscal intermediaries to request additional information required to make a coverage determination on a submitted claim. Some fiscal intermediaries have developed other forms that substitute for the HCFA Form 488.

Health insurance claim number (HICN). HICNs contain numeric and alpha indicators (e.g., 344-24-6890A) and are issued by the Social Security Administration. The HICN is the patient identification number that appears on a Medicare card.

HIM-11. The Medicare Home Health Agency Manual Publication 11, of HCFA, which contains the guidelines for the Medicare program, coverage issues, services, and billing procedures.

Home Health Agency (HHA). A HHA provides home health care.

Medicaid. A medical assistance program that is jointly administered by the federal government (HCFA) and the states. It is established to assist families with dependent children, the aged, blind, and disabled persons who cannot pay for health care because of limited financial resources. Each state has different guidelines for the Medicaid program.

Medical claim reviewer. A person, generally a nurse, employed by the fiscal intermediary to review the documentation submitted by an agency on HCFA Forms 485 and 487. The reviewer's objective is to determine whether the supporting documentation meets Medicare regulations and how the information relates to the UB-92 for the purpose of approving or denying payment.

Medicare. A federal health care coverage program for those over 65, some disabled persons, and those with end-stage renal disease under Title XVIII of the 1965 Amendments of the Social Security Act. Part A covers hospitalizations, related inpatient services, and home care. Part B covers outpatient services, including physician visits, lab work, covered home medical equipment (at 80%) and certain supplies.

Recertification. The *subsequent* plan of care (HCFA Form 485) that is required if the patient stays on service beyond the length of the original HCFA Form 485. A recertification is necessary for every 62 days the patient is on service by the home health agency.

Reconsideration of a claim (Recon). When a denial is received by the agency from the fiscal intermediary there is a process for appeal. This process is called a reconsideration.

Regulations (Regs). Rules and guidelines set up by various bodies that regulate home health care. For example, HCFA sets regulations to implement the Medicare home health benefit as legislation outlines.

Transmittals. Periodic updates to the HIM-11. These indicate new coverage guidelines or clarify interpretations of coverage of criteria so agencies can better understand and comply with coverage. These are mailed by the fiscal intermediary to agencies participating in the Medicare program.

Glossary of Legal Terms

Abandonment. The unilateral severance of the professional relationship between a health care provider, without reasonable notice, at a time when there is still a need for continuing health care.

Affidavit. A written statement that is taken under oath.

Appeal. A petition to a higher court to review and retry the legal issues and correct or reverse a judgment or decision by a lower court.

Appellant. A party who appeals the decision of a lower court to a court of higher jurisdiction.

Appellee. The party against whom an appeal to a higher court is taken.

Civil law. The division of American law that does not deal with crimes.

Comparative negligence. A defense theory in negligence cases where the degree of negligence by the plaintiff is compared to that of the defendant and apportioned accordingly for the purpose of monetary damages. Used by a majority of states instead of contributory negligence.

Complaint. The first pleading on the part of the plaintiff in a civil action.

Consent. Voluntary agreement by a competent person to make a choice to allow someone else to do something.

Contract. An agreement between two or more persons to do or to refrain from doing something. May be an express contract based on declarations, either oral or in writing, or an implied contract implied by law from the circumstances surrounding a transaction.

Contributory negligence. A defense theory in negligence cases based on the idea that the injured party contributed to his or her own negligence and thus should be barred from recovering any monetary damages.

Corporate negligence. Liability of an institution for its failure to use reasonable care in conducting its business.

Damages. A monetary sum or compensation awarded by the court or jury for the loss or harm suffered by the plaintiff.

Defamation. Injury to a person's reputation or character by willful and malicious statements to a third person. Libel is by use of written words; slander by use of spoken words.

Defendant. The person against whom a lawsuit is initiated. The defendant defends himself or herself against allegations by the plaintiff, who seeks legal redress.

Deposition. Testimony of a witness taken in writing under oath in answer to oral or written questions. Usually used in pretrial phase to prepare for litigation. A person who is being deposed is called a *deponent.*

Due process. A legal concept requiring that legal proceedings or those of a legal nature be conducted with rules and principles that protect an individual's rights.

Evidence. Anything offered to prove or disprove a claim or fact in a legal proceeding. May include documents, objects, testimony of witnesses, or other records.

Indemnify. The process of repaying a party for losses brought on when the obligation to repay exists under a contractual provision.

Inference. A conclusion reached by the jury from the facts proved.

Interrogatories. Written questions about the case submitted to a party by another party that are answered under oath. Part of the pretrial discovery process, but may be used later as evidence.

Issue. A single and material point resulting from the allegations of the parties in the lawsuit.

Judgment. The decision of the law as given by the court after the legal proceedings.

Liability. A legally recognized responsibility one is bound to perform. In negligence law, it is the legal responsibility for the loss of another person for one's failure to act or failure to act appropriately.

Liability insurance. A contract to have someone else (the insurer) pay for any loss or liability on the part of the insured in exchange for the payment of premiums. Occurrence basis policy covers incidents occurring at the time when premiums were paid. Claims-made basis policy covers only if in effect when the claim is made (i.e., it is not retroactive to the time of an earlier incident).

Litigation. A trial in a court for the purpose of establishing rights and duties between parties in a lawsuit.

Negligence. The failure to use that degree of care equal to a reasonably prudent or careful person acting under the same or similar circumstances. This could involve commission of an act or failure to carry out an act by omission.

Plaintiff. The person who initiates the lawsuit against the defendant and seeks legal redress, usually in the form of monetary damages.

Precedent. A ruled case or court decision used as an example of authority for a similar case or one that raises similar issues.

Release. A written contract for which some claim or interest in something is surrendered to another person. An example is a release by a client to disclose information to an insurer.

Respondent superior. Means "let the master answer." The employer (master) answers for the wrongful acts or negligence of the employee (servant) when acting within the scope of his or her employment.

Risk management. A system of identifying potential liability exposure to prevent financial loss. A business concept that identifies and evaluates the probability of financial loss in order to prevent its occurrence.

Standard of care. In negligence law, that degree of care and skill that a reasonably prudent person should exercise. In malpractice cases or professional negligence, that degree of skill, care, and knowledge exercised by members of the same discipline.

Statute. An act of the legislature declaring, prohibiting, or commanding something. For example, a state nurse practice act is a statute regulating the practice of nurses in a particular state.

Statute of limitations. The statutory time limit that a plaintiff has to file a lawsuit. Exceptions include an extension for the time it would reasonably take to "discover" a wrong, or a longer time extension if the plaintiff is a minor.

Subpoena. An order by the court for a person to appear at a certain time and place to testify on a matter. A *subpoena duces tecum* commands a witness to produce certain documents in his or her possession.

Summons. A legal document called a writ that directs the sheriff or other officer to notify a person that an action (lawsuit) has been started against him or her. Requires the named party or parties (defendants) to appear on a certain day to answer the complaint against them.

Tort. A legal wrong committed against a person or the property of another for which the law gives a civil remedy. Exists independent of a contract.

Vicarious liability. Liability of a corporation or organization for the negligence of its employees. Based on the idea that the employer receives the benefits of the employees' acts and, therefore, should also be responsible for the burdens of the employees' acts. The employer is in a position to control or supervise the acts of the employees.

Medicare Coverage of Services (Transmittal Revision 222)

COVERAGE OF SERVICES

Covered and Noncovered Home Health Services

203. CONDITIONS TO BE MET FOR COVERAGE OF HOME HEALTH SERVICES

Home health agency services are covered by Medicare when the following criteria are met:

° The person to whom the services are provided is an eligible Medicare beneficiary.

° The home health agency which is providing the services to the beneficiary has in effect a valid agreement to participate in the Medicare program.

° The beneficiary qualifies for coverage of home health services as described in §204.

° The services for which payment is claimed are covered as described in §§205 and 206.

° Medicare is the appropriate payer.

° The services for which payment is claimed are not otherwise excluded from payment.

203.1 Reasonable and Necessary Services

A. <u>Background.</u>—In enacting the Medicare program, Congress recognized that the physician would play an important role in determining utilization of services. The law requires that payment can be made only if a physician certifies the need for services and establishes a plan of care. The Secretary is responsible for ensuring that the claimed services are covered by Medicare, including determining whether they are "reasonable and necessary."

B. <u>Determination of Coverage.</u>—The beneficiary's health status and medical need as reflected in the home health plan of care and medical record provide the basis for determinations as to whether services provided are reasonable and necessary. A finding that services are reasonable and necessary must be based on information available in these documents, although clear inferences may be drawn from information provided in the plan of care (form HCFA 485) or in supplementary forms (forms HCFA 486, 487, 488).

A finding that care is not reasonable and necessary must be based on information provided on the forms and in the medical record with respect to the unique medical condition of the individual beneficiary. <u>That is, a coverage denial may not be made based solely on the reviewer's general inferences about patients with similar diagnoses or on data related to utilization generally, but must be based upon objective clinical evidence regarding the patient's individual need for care.</u>

> Intermediaries will assume the type and frequency of services ordered are reasonable and necessary unless objective clinical evidence clearly indicates otherwise, or there is a lack of clinical evidence to support coverage.

> A coverage determination may be made based on a review of the HCFA 485/486/487. Provide clear documentation regarding the patient's progress or lack of progress, medical condition, functional losses, and goals.

Both payment and denial decisions may be based on summary information contained in the relevant HCFA data forms; however, additional information from the medical records (either via Form 488 or a copy of the medical record) must be requested when medical information needed to support a decision is not clearly present. The following examples illustrate this statement.

Examples of cases in which development of the case is needed:

EXAMPLE 1: A plan of care provides for daily skilled nursing visits for care of a pressure sore, but the description of the pressure sore and the dressing which is contained on the form causes the reviewer to question why daily skilled care is needed. The intermediary would not reduce the number of visits but would either request additional information to support the need for daily care or would request the nursing notes to determine if the beneficiary required daily skilled care.

EXAMPLE 2: A beneficiary with a diagnosis of congestive heart failure (CHF) has been hospitalized for 5 days. Posthospital skilled nursing care is ordered 3 × wk × 60 days for skilled observation, teaching of diet medication compliance, and signs and symptoms of the disease. The documentation on the HCFA 485–486 shows that the patient has had CHF for 10 years with an exacerbation requiring recent hospitalization. The medications are not shown as changed or new. The clinical findings are contradictory. There is a possibility that this beneficiary requires skilled observation and teaching although the documentation does not give a clear picture of the beneficiary's needs. Therefore, the case would be developed further to determine if the criteria for coverage were met.

Examples of cases which would be denied without further development:

EXAMPLE 3: A plan of care calls for vitamin B12 injections 1 × mo × 60 days for a beneficiary who has been discharged from the hospital following a recent hip fracture. The beneficiary has generalized weakness but there is no diagnosis or clinical symptoms shown which support that the Medicare requirements governing coverage of skilled nursing care for B12 injections are met. The claim would be denied without development for further information since there is no support for coverage of the skilled nursing care for the B12 injections.

EXAMPLE 4: A beneficiary has a primary diagnosis of back sprain for which he was hospitalized for 7 days. The beneficiary also has a secondary diagnosis of emphysema with an onset 2 years prior to the start of care. Following the hospitalization, the physician ordered skilled nursing 2 × wk × 4 weeks for skilled observation of vital signs and response to medication and aide services 2 × wk × 4 weeks for personal care. The documentation on the HCFA 485–486 shows that the beneficiary is up as tolerated, is able to walk 10 feet without resting, and is alert. Clinical facts show normal vital signs, and no reference to emphysema. The beneficiary is on phenobarbital PO 30 mg TID. The documentation clearly does not support the medical necessity for skilled nursing care and the claim for the services would be denied without development.

Examples of cases in which payment may be made without further development:

> The length of time services will be covered is determined by the needs of each patient.

EXAMPLE 5: A beneficiary with a diagnosis of CHF has been hospitalized for five days. Post-hospital skilled nursing care is ordered 3 × wk × 60 days for skilled observation, teaching of a new diet regimen, compliance with multiple new medications, and signs and symptoms of the disease state. The documentation on the HCFA 485–486 shows the beneficiary had had an acute exacerbation of a pre-existing CHF condition which required the recent acute hospitalization. The beneficiary is discharged from the hospital with a medication regimen changed from previous medications. The HCFA forms documenting the clinical evidence of the recent acute exacerbation of the beneficiary's cardiac condition combined with changed medications support the physician's order for care. Payment may be made without further development.

> In this example the patient's need for skilled nursing is evidenced by the need for skilled observation, teaching, and monitoring the effectiveness and safety of multiple new medications. There is a reasonable potential for complicating factors occurring based on the medical history presented.

EXAMPLE 6: A plan of care provides for physical therapy treatments 3 × wk × 45 days for a beneficiary who has been discharged from the hospital following a recent hip fracture. The beneficiary was discharged using a walker 7 days before the start of home care. The HCFA form 485 and supplementary form HCFA 486 show that the beneficiary was discharged from the hospital with restricted mobility in ambulation, transfers, and climbing of stairs. The beneficiary had an unsafe gait which indicated a need for gait training and the beneficiary had not been instructed in stair climbing and a home exercise program. The goal of the physical therapy was to increase strength, range of motion and to progress from walker to cane with safe gait. Information on the relevant HCFA forms also indicates that the beneficiary had a previous functional capacity of full ambulation, mobility, and self-care. The claim may be paid without further development, since there are no objective clinical factors in the medical evidence to contradict the order of the beneficiary's treating physician.

> A patient's need for skilled physical therapy services is based primarily on documentation of functional limitations in self-care, mobility, and safety as well as ROM and strength losses which require skilled treatment and/or to establish a safe and effective maintenance program.

203.2 Impact of Other Available Caregivers and Other Available Coverage on Medicare Coverage of Home Health Services.—Where the Medicare criteria for coverage of home health services are met, beneficiaries are entitled by law to coverage of reasonable and necessary home health services.

Therefore, a beneficiary is entitled to have the costs of reasonable and necessary services reimbursed by Medicare without regard to whether there is someone available in the home to furnish them. However, where a family member or other caring person is or will be providing services that adequately meet the patient's needs, it would not be reasonable and necessary for home health agency personnel to furnish such services. Ordinarily it can be presumed that there is no able and willing person in the home to provide the services being rendered by the home health agency unless the beneficiary or family indicates otherwise, and objects to the provision of the services by the home health agency, or unless the home health agency has firsthand knowledge to the contrary.

EXAMPLE: A beneficiary, who lives with an adult daughter and who otherwise qualifies for Medicare coverage of home health services, requires the assistance of a home health aide for bathing and assistance with an exercise program to improve endurance. The daughter is unwilling to bathe her elderly father and assist him with the exercise program. Home health aide services to provide these services would be reasonable and necessary.

> Home health services are available without regard to the availability of a caregiver. (Exception: insulin injections §205.14a(2).)

Similarly, a beneficiary is entitled to have the costs of reasonable and necessary home health services reimbursed by Medicare even if the beneficiary would qualify for institutional care (e.g., hospital care or skilled nursing facility care).

EXAMPLE: A beneficiary who is being discharged from a hospital with a diagnosis of osteomyelitis and who requires continuation of the IV antibiotic therapy that was begun in the hospital was found to meet the criteria for Medicare coverage of skilled nursing facility services. If the beneficiary also meets the qualifying criteria for coverage of home health services, payment may be made for the reasonable and necessary home health services the beneficiary needs, notwithstanding the availability of coverage in a skilled nursing facility.

Medicare payment should be made for reasonable and necessary home health services where the beneficiary is also receiving supplemental services that do not meet Medicare's definition of skilled nursing care or home health aide services.

EXAMPLE: A patient who needs skilled nursing care on an intermittent basis also hires a licensed practical nurse (LPN) to provide nighttime assistance while family members sleep. The care provided by the LPN, as respite to the family members, does not require the skills of a licensed nurse (as defined in §205.1) and therefore has no impact on the beneficiary's eligibility for Medicare payment of home health services even though another third party insurer may pay for that nursing care.

Services which do not meet Medicare's definition of skilled nursing and/or aide services can also be provided without affecting home health benefits as long as these services are not furnished under the physician's plan of care to the HHA.

203.3 Use of Utilization Screens and "Rules of Thumb."—Medicare recognizes that determinations of whether home health services are reasonable and necessary must be based on an assessment of each beneficiary's individual care needs. Therefore, denial of services based on numerical utilization screens, diagnostic screens, diagnosis, or specific treatment norms is not appropriate.

Use of screens or norms may be used only to identify cases to be referred to medical review. Once in medical review, coverage determinations are based on review of the medical information on each case.

---

204. CONDITIONS THE BENEFICIARY MUST MEET TO QUALIFY FOR COVERAGE OF HOME HEALTH SERVICES

To qualify for Medicare coverage of any home health services, the beneficiary must meet each of the criteria specified in this section. Beneficiaries who meet each of these criteria are eligible to have payment made on their behalf for services which are discussed in §205 and §206.

204.1 Confined to the Home.—

A. Patient Confined to His Home.—In order for a beneficiary to be eligible to receive covered home health services under both Part A and Part B, the law requires that a physician certify in all cases that the beneficiary is confined to his home. (See §240.1.) An individual does not have to be bedridden to be considered as confined to his home. However, the condition of these patients should be such that there exists a normal inability to leave home and, consequently, leaving their homes would require a considerable and taxing effort. If the patient does in fact leave the home, the patient may nevertheless be considered homebound if the absences from the home are infrequent or for periods of relatively short duration, or are attributable to the need to receive medical treatment. Absences attributable to the need to receive medical treatment include attendance at adult day centers to receive medical care, ongoing receipt of outpatient kidney dialysis, and the receipt of outpatient chemotherapy or radiation therapy. It is expected that in most instances absences from the home which occur will be for the purpose of receiving medical treatment. However, occasional absences from the home for nonmedical purposes, e.g., an occasional trip to the barber, a walk around the block, or a drive, would not necessitate a finding that the individual is not homebound so long as the absences are undertaken on an infrequent basis or are of relatively short duration and do not indicate that the patient has the capacity to obtain the health care provided outside rather than in the home.

The patient is homebound if he/she experiences:
° A normal inability to leave home;
° A considerable and taxing effort to leave; and
° Absences from home are infrequent, of short duration, or to receive medical care.

Homebound eligibility is not affected by frequent absences from the home when the reason to leave is to receive medical care.

Homebound criteria may be met when the beneficiary attends adult day care when the purpose is attributable to the patient receiving medical care.

The aged person who does not often travel from his home because of feebleness and insecurity brought on by advanced age would not be considered confined to his home for purposes of receiving home health services unless he meets one of the above conditions. A patient who requires speech therapy but does not require physical therapy or nursing services must also meet one of the above conditions in order to be considered as confined to his home.

Although a patient must be confined to his home to be eligible for covered home health services, some services cannot be provided at the patient's residence because equipment is required which cannot be made available there. If the services required by an individual involve the use of such equipment, the home health agency may make arrangements with a hospital, SNF, or a rehabilitation center to provide these services on an outpatient basis. (See §§200.2 and 206.5.) However, even in these situations, for the services to be covered as home health services the patient must be considered as confined to his home; and to receive such outpatient services it may be expected that a homebound patient will generally require the use of supportive devices, special transportation, or the assistance of another person to travel to the appropriate facility.

If for any reason a question is raised as to whether an individual is confined to his home, the agency will be requested to furnish the intermediary with the information necessary to establish that the beneficiary is homebound as defined above.

B. Patient's Place of Residence.—A patient's residence is wherever he makes his home. This may be his own dwelling, an apartment, a relative's home, a home for the aged, or some other type of institution. However, an institution may not be considered a patient's residence if it:

1. Meets at least the basic requirement in the definition of a hospital, i.e., it is primarily engaged in providing by or under the supervision of physicians, to inpatients, diagnostic and therapeutic services for medical diagnosis, treatment, and care of disabled, or

sick persons, or rehabilitation services for the rehabilitation of injured, disabled, or sick persons, or

2. Meets at least the basic requirement in the definition of an SNF, i.e., it is primarily engaged in providing to inpatients skilled nursing care and related services for patients who require medical or nursing care, or rehabilitation services for the rehabilitation of injured, disabled, or sick persons. All nursing homes that participate in Medicare and/or Medicaid as skilled nursing facilities and most facilities that participate in Medicaid as intermediate care facilities meet this basic requirement. In addition, many nursing homes which do not choose to participate in Medicare or Medicaid meet this test. Check with your fiscal intermediary or Medicare regional office before serving nursing home patients.

Thus, if an individual is a patient in an institution or distinct part of an institution which provides the services described in (A) or (B) above, he is not entitled to have payment made for home health services under either Part A or Part B since such an institution may not be considered his residence.

When a patient remains in a participating SNF following his discharge from active care, the facility may not be considered his residence for purposes of home health coverage.

Check with your intermediary if you are not sure whether a facility can be a beneficiary's home.

204.2 Services Are Provided Under a Plan of Care Established and Approved by a Physician.—

A. Content of the Plan of Care.—The plan of care must contain all pertinent diagnoses, including the beneficiary's mental status, the types of services, supplies, and equipment ordered, the frequency of the visits to be made, prognosis, rehabilitation potential, functional limitations, activities permitted, nutritional requirements, medications and treatments, safety measures to protect against injury, discharge plans, and any additional items the home health agency or physician chooses to include.

The plan of care refers to the HCFA 485. All information stated above must be completed on the form when it is sent to the physician for signature.

NOTE: This manual uses the term "plan of care" to refer to the medical treatment plan established by the treating physician with the assistance of the home health care nurse. The term we used in the past was "plan of treatment." However, the term we used in the past was changed to "plan of care" in the Omnibus Budget Reconciliation Act of 1987 (OBRA '87) without a change in definition. It is anticipated that a discipline-oriented plan of care will be established, where appropriate, by a home health agency nurse regarding nursing and home health aide services and by skilled therapists regarding specific therapy treatment. These plans of care may be incorporated within the physician's plan of care or separately prepared.

B. Specificity of Orders.—The orders on the plan of care must indicate the type of services to be provided to the beneficiary, both with respect to the professional who will provide them and with respect to the nature of the individual services, as well as the frequency of the services.

EXAMPLE: SN × 7/wk × 1 wk; 3/wk × 4 wk; 2/wk × 3 wk (skilled nursing visits 7 times per week for 1 week; three times per week for 4 weeks; and two times per week for 3 weeks) for skilled observation and evaluation of the surgical site, for teaching sterile dressing changes and to perform sterile dressing changes. The sterile change consists of . . . (detail of procedure).

Orders for care can indicate a specific range in the frequency of visits to ensure that the most appropriate level of services is provided to home health beneficiaries. When a range of visits is ordered the upper limit of the range is to be considered the specific frequency.

EXAMPLE: SN × 2–4/wk × 4 wk; 1–2/wk × 4 wk for skilled observation and evaluation of the surgical site. . . .

Example of inappropriate specificity: Skilled nursing visits 3 times per week and PRN as needed. (This order is not specific because: 1) the number of weeks is not specified; 2) "PRN" is open-ended; and 3) the nature of the service is not specified.)

A HCFA 488 will be sent to you when orders are missing or incomplete. When a range is used for frequency of visits, the upper limit is considered the physician's order. The upper limit of the range is also considered for medical review of intermittent. Orders for PRN should indicate a projected number of visits and reason for the visits.

NOTE: If care is being ordered for 2 months (and you are using weeks in the duration), then you may need to use 9 weeks instead of 8 weeks.

C. Who Signs the Plan of Care.—The physician who signs the plan of care must be qualified to sign the physician certification as described in 42 CFR 424 subpart B.

The qualified physician must sign the plan. A stamped signature is not acceptable.

D. Timeliness of Signature.—The plan of care must be signed before the bill is submitted to the intermediary for payment.

E. Use of Verbal Orders.—

(1) Services which are provided from the beginning of the certification period and before the physician signs the plan of care are considered to be provided under a plan of care established and approved by the physician where there is a verbal order for the care prior to rendering the services which is documented in the medical record and where the services are included in a signed plan of care.

Acceptable Verbal Order Documentation and Confirmation:

° Receipt of verbal order is identified by the nurse's signature and date on item 23 of the HCFA 485 and the form is signed by the physician.
° The HCFA 485 is signed by the physician and contains the verbal order(s) written, signed, and dated in the clinical record.
° The form on which the verbal order is written, signed, and dated by agency staff is countersigned by the physician.
° A document signed by the physician contains the written signed and dated verbal order in the clinical record.
° There are no required forms or formats for documentation or confirmation of verbal orders.

EXAMPLE: The HHA acquires a verbal order for venipuncture for a beneficiary to be performed on August 1. The HHA provides the venipuncture on August 1 and evaluates the beneficiary's need for continued care. The physician signs the plan of care for the venipuncture on August 15. Since the HHA has acquired a verbal order prior to the delivery of services, the visit is considered to be provided under a plan of care established and approved by the physician.

(2) Services which are provided in the subsequent certification period are considered to be provided under the subsequent plan of care where there is a verbal order before the services provided in the subsequent period are furnished and the order is reflected in the medical record. However, services which are provided after the expiration of a plan of care, but before the acquisition of a verbal order or a signed plan of care, cannot be considered to be provided under a plan of care.

If the recertification is not signed before the previous certification expires, there must be a verbal order.

EXAMPLE 1: The beneficiary is under a plan of care in which the physician orders venipuncture every 2 weeks. The last day covered by the initial plan of care is July 31. The beneficiary's next venipuncture is scheduled for August 5, and the physician signs the plan of treatment for the new period on August 1. The venipuncture on August 5 was provided under a plan of care established and approved by the physician.

EXAMPLE 2: The beneficiary is under a plan of care in which the physician orders venipuncture every 2 weeks. The last day covered by the plan of care is July 31. The beneficiary's next venipuncture is scheduled for August 5th, and the physician does not sign the plan of treatment until August 6th. The HHA acquires a verbal order for the venipuncture before the August 5th visit, and therefore the visit is considered to be provided under a plan of care established and approved by the physician.

EXAMPLE 3: The beneficiary is under a plan of care in which the physician orders venipuncture every 2 weeks. The last day covered by the plan of care is July 31. The beneficiary's next venipuncture is scheduled for August 5th, and the physician

does not sign the plan of treatment until August 6th. The HHA <u>does not</u> acquire a verbal order for the venipuncture before the August 5 visit, and therefore the visit cannot be considered to be provided under a plan of care established and approved by the physician. The prior plan of care expired and neither a verbal order nor a signed plan of care was in effect on the date of the service. The visit is not covered.

(3) Any increase in the frequency of services or addition of new services during a certification period must be authorized by a physician by way of a verbal order or written order prior to the provision of the increased or additional services.

F. <u>Periodic Review of the Plan of Care.</u>—The plan of care must be reviewed and signed by a physician no less frequently than every 2 months. The physician who reviews and signs the plan of care must be qualified under 42 CFR 424 subpart B to sign the physician certification and plan of care.

204.3 <u>Under the Care of a Physician.</u>—The patient must be under the care of a physician who is qualified to sign the physician certification and plan of care in accord with 42 CFR 424 subpart B.

A beneficiary is expected to be under the care of the physician who signs the plan of care and the physician certification. It is expected, but not required for coverage, that the physician who signs the plan of care will see the patient, but there is no specified interval of time within which the patient must be seen.

204.4 <u>Needs Skilled Nursing Care on an Intermittent Basis, or Physical Therapy or Speech Therapy or Has a Continued Need for Occupational Therapy.</u>—The patient must need one of the following types of services:

° Skilled nursing care which:
  – Is reasonable and necessary as defined in §205.1 A and B, and
  – Is needed on an "intermittent" basis as defined in §205.1C, or
° Physical therapy as defined in §205.2A and B, or
° Speech therapy as defined in §205.2A and C, or
° Have a continuing need for occupational therapy as defined in §205.2A and D.

The beneficiary has a continued need for occupational therapy when:
° The services which the beneficiary requires meet the definition of "occupational therapy" services of §205.2A and D, and
° The beneficiary's eligibility for home health services has been established by virtue of a prior need for skilled nursing care, speech therapy, or physical therapy in the current or prior certification period.

EXAMPLE: A beneficiary who is recovering from a cerebral vascular accident has an initial plan of care that called for physical therapy, speech therapy, and home health aide services. In the next certification period, the physician orders only occupational therapy and home health aide services because the beneficiary no longer needs the skills of a physical therapist or a speech therapist, but needs the services provided by the occupational therapist. The beneficiary's need for occupational therapy qualifies him or her for home health services, including home health aide services (presuming that all other qualifying criteria are met).

In this example, the patient was not discharged from home health services, although the need for PT and ST is ending or ended. A qualifying service established the benefit and OT is needed in the <u>next certification period</u>. The OT service may qualify the beneficiary's need for continuing home health benefits.

204.5 <u>Physician Certification.</u>—The home health agency must be acting upon a physician certification which is part of the plan of care (HCFA form 485) and which meets the requirements of this section for home health agency services to be covered.

A. <u>Content of the Physician Certification.</u>—The physician must certify that:

1. The home health services are or were needed because the beneficiary is or was confined to his home as defined in §204.1;

2. The beneficiary needs or needed skilled nursing services on an intermittent basis or physical therapy or speech therapy, or continues or continued to need occupational therapy after the need for skilled nursing care or physical therapy or speech therapy ceased;

3. A plan of care has been established and is periodically reviewed by a physician; and

4. The services are or were furnished while the individual is or was under the care of a physician.

B. <u>Periodic Recertification.</u>—The physician certification may cover a period less than but not greater than 62 days (2 months).

C. <u>Who May Sign the Certification.</u>—The physician who signs the certification must be permitted to do so by 42 CFR 424 subpart B.

205. COVERAGE OF SERVICES WHICH ESTABLISH HOME HEALTH ELIGIBILITY

For any home health services to be covered by Medicare, the beneficiary must meet the qualifying criteria as specified in §204, including having a need for skilled nursing care on an intermittent basis, physical therapy, speech therapy, or a continuing need for occupational therapy as defined in this section.

205.1 <u>Skilled Nursing Care.</u>—To be covered as skilled nursing services, the services must require the skills of a registered nurse or a licensed practical nurse under the supervision of a registered nurse, must be reasonable and necessary to the treatment of the beneficiary's illness or injury as discussed in §205.1A and B, and must be intermittent as discussed in §205.1C.

A. <u>General Principles Governing Reasonable and Necessary Skilled Nursing Care.</u>—

1. A skilled nursing service is a service which must be provided by a registered nurse, or a licensed practical nurse or a licensed vocational nurse under the supervision of a registered nurse to be safe and effective. In determining whether a service requires the skills of a nurse, consider both the inherent complexity of the service, the condition of the patient, and accepted standards of medical and nursing practice.

Document that the skills of a nurse are required based on:

° inherent complexity of the service;
° condition of the patient; and
° accepted standards of practice.

Key Documentation Questions:

1. Can the services be furnished safely and effectively without the skills of a nurse?
2. Is the care consistent with the patient's medical condition and accepted standards of practice?

Some services may be classified as a skilled nursing service on the basis of complexity alone, e.g., intravenous and intramuscular injections or insertion of catheters, and if reasonable and necessary to the treatment of the beneficiary's illness or injury, would be covered on that basis. However, in some cases the condition of the beneficiary may cause a service which would ordinarily be considered unskilled to be considered a skilled nursing service. This would occur when the beneficiary's condition is such that the service can be safely and effectively provided only by a skilled nurse.

EXAMPLE 1: The presence of a plaster cast on an extremity generally does not indicate a need for skilled care. However, the patient with a pre-existing peripheral vascular or circulatory condition might need skilled nursing and skilled rehabilitation personnel to observe for complications, to monitor medication administration for pain control, and to teach proper ambulation techniques to ensure proper bone alignment and healing.

EXAMPLE 2: The condition of a beneficiary who has irritable bowel syndrome, or who is recovering from rectal surgery, may be such that he can be given an enema safely and effectively only by a skilled nurse. If the enema is necessary to treat the illness or injury, then the visit would be covered as a skilled nursing visit.

2. A service is not considered a skilled nursing service merely because it is performed by or under the direct supervision of a licensed nurse. Where a service can be safely and effectively performed (or self-administered) by the average nonmedical person without the direct supervision of a licensed nurse, the service cannot be regarded as a skilled nursing service although a skilled nurse actually provides the service. Similarly, the unavailability of a competent person to provide a nonskilled service, notwithstanding the importance of the service to the beneficiary, does not make it a skilled service when the skilled nurse provides it.

EXAMPLE 1: Giving a bath does not ordinarily require the skills of a licensed nurse and therefore would not be considered as a skilled nursing service unless the beneficiary's condition is such that the bath could be given safely and effectively only by a licensed nurse (as discussed in §205.1A.1. above).

EXAMPLE 2: A beneficiary with a well-established colostomy absent complications may require assistance changing the colostomy bag because he cannot do it himself and there is no one else to change it. Notwithstanding the need for the routine colostomy care, the care does not become a skilled nursing service when it is provided by the licensed nurse.

3. A service which, by its nature, requires the skills of a licensed nurse to be provided safely and effectively continues to be a skilled service even if it is taught to the patient, the patient's family, or other caregivers. Where the beneficiary needs the skilled nursing care and there is no one trained, able, and willing to provide it, the services of a skilled nurse would be reasonable and necessary to the treatment of the illness or injury.

A skilled service remains a skilled service even if taught to the patient, family, or caregivers.

EXAMPLE: A beneficiary was discharged from the hospital with an open draining wound which requires irrigation, packing, and dressing twice each day. The home health agency has taught the family to perform the dressing changes. The home health agency continues to see the patient for the wound care that is needed during the time that the family is not available and willing to provide it. The wound care continues to be skilled nursing care, notwithstanding that the family provides it part of the time, and may be covered as long as it is required by the patient.

4. The skilled nursing service must be reasonable and necessary to the diagnosis and treatment of the beneficiary's illness or injury within the context of the beneficiary's unique medical condition. To be considered reasonable and necessary for the diagnosis or treatment of the beneficiary's illness or injury, the services must be consistent with the nature and severity of the illness or injury, his or her particular medical needs, and accepted standards of medical and nursing practice. A beneficiary's overall medical condition is a valid factor in deciding whether skilled services are needed. A beneficiary's diagnosis should never be the sole factor in deciding that a service the beneficiary needs is either skilled or not skilled.

Skilled service need is based on the beneficiary's overall medical condition and not solely on the diagnosis.

The determination of whether the services are reasonable and necessary should be made in consideration that a physician has determined that the services ordered are reasonable and necessary. The services must, therefore, be viewed from the perspective of the condition of the patient when the services were ordered and what was, at that time, reasonably expected to be appropriate treatment for the illness or injury throughout the certification period.

EXAMPLE 1: A physician has ordered skilled nursing visits for a patient with a hairline fracture of the hip. In the absence of any underlying medical condition or illness, nursing visits would not be reasonable and necessary for treatment of the patient's hip injury.

EXAMPLE 2: A physician has ordered skilled nursing visits for injections of insulin and teaching of self-administration and self-management of the medication regimen for a beneficiary with diabetes mellitus. Insulin has been shown to be a safe and effective treatment for diabetes mellitus, and therefore, the skilled nursing visits for the injections and the teaching of self-administration and self-management of the treatment regimen would be reasonable and necessary.

The determination of whether a beneficiary needs skilled nursing care should be based solely upon the beneficiary's unique condition and individual needs, without regard to whether the illness or injury is acute, chronic, terminal, or expected to extend over a long period of time. In addition, skilled care may, dependent upon the unique condition of the beneficiary, continue to be necessary for beneficiaries whose condition is stable.

Determination of skilled nursing need is based on:

° unique condition;
° individual need; and
° regardless of whether the condition is acute, chronic, terminal, or expected to continue over a long period of time and in <u>some cases</u> if the condition is stable.

EXAMPLE 1: Following a cerebral vascular accident (CVA), a beneficiary has an in-dwelling Foley catheter because of urinary incontinence, and is expected to require the catheter for a long and indefinite period. Periodic visits to change the catheter as needed, to treat the symptoms of catheter malfunction, and to teach proper patient care would be covered as long as they are reasonable and necessary, although the beneficiary is stable and there is an expectation that the care will be needed for a long and indefinite period.

EXAMPLE 2: A beneficiary with advanced multiple sclerosis undergoing an exacerbation of the illness needs skilled teaching of medications, measures to overcome urinary retention, and the establishment of a program designed to minimize the adverse impact of the exacerbation. The skilled nursing care the beneficiary needs for a short period would be covered despite the chronic nature of the illness.

EXAMPLE 3: A beneficiary with malignant melanoma is terminally ill, and requires skilled observation, assessment, teaching, and treatment. The beneficiary has not elected coverage under Medicare's hospice benefit. The skilled nursing care that the beneficiary requires would be covered, notwithstanding that his condition is terminal, because the services he needs require the skills of a licensed nurse.

B. <u>Application of the Principles to Skilled Nursing Services.</u>— The following discussion of skilled nursing services applies the foregoing principles to specific skilled nursing services about which questions are most frequently raised.

° Document the reasons that the beneficiary's condition is likely to change to a further acute episode or medical complication.
° Document why skilled observation and assessment is needed to determine if treatment should be changed.

° Coverage for a minimum of 3 weeks will be made when your documentation indicates a reasonable potential for medical complications, or development of a further acute episode.
° Always document any modifications made to the treatment or any additional medical procedures initiated as a result of your assessments.

1. Observation and Assessment of Patient's Condition When Only the Specialized Skills of a Medical Professional Can Determine a Patient's Status.—Observation and assessment of the beneficiary's condition by a licensed nurse are reasonable and necessary skilled services when the likelihood of change in a patient's condition requires skilled nursing personnel to identify and evaluate the patient's need for possible modification of treatment or initiation of additional medical procedures until the beneficiary's treatment regimen is essentially stabilized. Where a beneficiary was admitted to home health care for skilled observation because there was a reasonable potential of a complication or further acute episode, but did not develop a further acute episode or complication, the skilled observation services are still covered for 3 weeks or as long as there remains a reasonable potential for such a complication or further acute episode.

Information from the beneficiary's medical history may support the likelihood of a future complication or acute episode and, therefore, may justify the need for continued skilled observation and assessment beyond 3-week period. Moreover, such indications as abnormal/fluctuating vital signs, weight changes, edema, symptoms of drug toxicity, abnormal/fluctuating lab values, and respiratory changes on auscultation may justify skilled observation and assessment. Where these indications are such that it is likely that skilled observation and assessment by a licensed nurse will result in changes to the treatment of the patient, then the services would be covered. There are cases where beneficiaries who are stable continue to require skilled observation and assessment (see example in §205.1 B. 13. d.). However, observation and assessment by a skilled nurse are not reasonable and necessary to the treatment of the illness or injury where these indications are part of a long-standing pattern of the beneficiary's condition, and there is no attempt to change the treatment to resolve them.

EXAMPLE 1: A beneficiary with arteriosclerotic heart disease with congestive heart failure requires close observation by skilled nursing personnel for signs of decompensation, or adverse effects resulting from prescribed medication. Skilled observation is needed to determine whether the drug regimen should be modified or whether other therapeutic measures should be considered until the patient's treatment regimen is essentially stabilized.

EXAMPLE 2: A beneficiary has undergone peripheral vascular disease treatment including a revascularization procedure (bypass). The incision area is showing signs of potential infection (e.g., heat, redness, swelling, drainage); patient has elevated body temperature. Skilled observation and monitoring of the vascular supply of the legs and the incision site are required until the signs of potential infection have abated and there is no longer a reasonable potential of infection.

EXAMPLE 3: A patient was hospitalized following a heart attack and, following treatment but before mobilization, is discharged home. Because it is not known whether exertion will exacerbate the heart disease, skilled observation is reasonable and necessary as mobilization is initiated until the patient's treatment regimen is essentially stabilized.

EXAMPLE 4: A frail 85-year-old man was hospitalized for pneumonia. The infection was resolved, but the patient, who had previously maintained adequate nutrition, will not eat or eats poorly. The patient is discharged to the home health agency for monitoring of fluid and nutrient intake, and assessment of the need for tube feeding. Observation and monitoring by skilled nurses of the patient's oral intake, output, and hydration status are required to determine what further treatment or other intervention is needed.

EXAMPLE 5: A patient with glaucoma and a cardiac condition has a cataract extraction. Because of the interaction between the eye drops for the glaucoma and cataracts and the beta blocker for the cardiac condition, the patient is at risk for serious cardiac arrhythmias. Skilled observation and monitoring of the drug actions are reasonable and necessary until the patient's condition is stabilized.

EXAMPLE 6: A patient with hypertension suffered dizziness and weakness. The physician found that the blood pressure was too low and discontinued the hypertension medication. Skilled observation and monitoring of the patient's blood pressure is required until the blood pressure remains stable and in a safe range.

2. Management and Evaluation of a Patient Care Plan.—Skilled nursing visits for management and evaluation of the patient's care plan are also reasonable and necessary where underlying conditions or complications require that only a registered nurse can ensure that essential nonskilled care is achieving its purpose. For skilled nursing care to be reasonable and necessary for management and evaluation of the beneficiary's plan of care, the complexity of the necessary unskilled services which are a necessary part of the medical treatment must require the involvement of skilled nursing personnel to promote the patient's recovery and medical safety in view of the beneficiary's overall condition.

° Briefly document the complicating factors resulting in a high potential for complication or for ensuring that essential nonskilled services are achieving their purpose to promote the beneficiary's recovery and safety.
° Skilled management and evaluation involve a finding that recovery and safety cannot be assured unless the total care, skilled or not, is planned and managed by a registered nurse.
° Skilled management and evaluation require a specific order when they are the only skilled service rendered. They may be provided at the same time as other skilled interventions.

EXAMPLE 1: An aged beneficiary with a history of diabetes mellitus and angina pectoris is recovering from an open reduction of the neck of the femur. He requires among other services, careful skin care, appropriate oral medications, a diabetic diet, a therapeutic exercise program to preserve muscle tone and body condition, and observation to notice signs of deterioration in his condition or complications resulting from his restricted, but increasing mobility. Although any of the required services could be performed by a properly instructed person, that person would not have the capability to understand the relationship among the services and their effect on each other. Since the nature of the patient's condition, his age and his immobility create a high potential for serious complications, such an understanding is essential to ensure the patient's recovery and safety. The management of this plan of care requires skilled nursing personnel until the patient's treatment regimen is essentially stabilized.

EXAMPLE 2: An aged patient is recovering from pneumonia, is lethargic, is disoriented, has residual chest congestion, is confined to the bed as a result of this debilitated condition and requires restraints at times. To decrease the chest congestion, the physician has prescribed frequent changes in position, coughing, and deep breathing. While the residual chest congestion alone would not represent a high risk factor, the patient's immobility and confusion represent complicating factors which, when coupled with the chest congestion, could create a high probability of a relapse. In this situation, skilled oversight of the nonskilled services would be reasonable and necessary pending the elimination of the chest congestion to ensure the patient's medical safety.

Where visits by a licensed nurse are not needed to observe and assess the effects of the nonskilled services being provided to treat the illness or injury, skilled nursing care would not be considered reasonable and necessary to treat the illness or injury.

EXAMPLE: A physician orders one skilled nursing visit every 2 weeks and three home health aide visits each week for bathing and washing hair for a beneficiary whose recovery from a cerebral vascular accident has left him with residual weakness on the left side. The beneficiary's cardiovascular condition is stable, and the beneficiary has reached the maximum restoration potential. There are no underlying conditions which would necessitate the skilled supervision of a licensed nurse in assisting with bathing or hair washing. The skilled nursing visits are not necessary to manage and supervise the home health aide services and would not be covered.

3. Teaching and Training Activities.—Teaching and training activities which require skilled nursing personnel to teach a beneficiary, the beneficiary's family or caregivers how to manage his treatment regimen would constitute skilled nursing services. Where the teaching or training is reasonable and necessary to the treatment of the illness or injury, skilled nursing visits for teaching would be covered. The test of whether a nursing service is skilled relates to the skill required to teach and not to the nature of what is being taught. Therefore, where skilled nursing services are necessary to teach an unskilled service, the teaching may be covered. Skilled nursing visits for teaching and training activities are reasonable and necessary where the teaching or training is appropriate to the beneficiary's functional loss, or his illness or injury.

Where it becomes apparent after a reasonable period of time that the patient, family or caregiver will not or is not able to learn or be trained, then further teaching and training would cease to be reasonable and necessary. The reason that the patient, family, or caregiver will not or is not able to learn or be trained should be documented in the record. Notwithstanding that the teaching or training was unsuccessful, the services for teaching and training would be considered to be reasonable and necessary prior to the point that it became apparent that the teaching or training was unsuccessful, as long as such services were appropriate to the beneficiary's illness, functional loss, or injury.

The beneficiary's medical condition, medications, orders, and goals must be interrelated to support the need for teaching.

Nonskilled services may be taught as long as the teaching requires the skills of a nurse (e.g., glucometer).

EXAMPLE 1: A physician has ordered skilled nursing care for teaching a diabetic who has recently become insulin dependent. The physician has ordered teaching of self-injection and management of insulin, signs and symptoms of insulin shock, and actions to take in emergencies. The teaching services are reasonable and necessary to the treatment of the illness or injury.

EXAMPLE 2: A physician has ordered skilled nursing care to teach a beneficiary to follow a new medication regimen (in which there is a significant probability of adverse drug reactions due to the nature of the drug and the beneficiary's condition), signs and symptoms of adverse reactions to new medications, and necessary dietary restrictions. After it becomes apparent that the beneficiary remains unable to take the medications properly, cannot demonstrate awareness of potential adverse reactions, and is not following the necessary dietary restrictions, skilled nursing care for further teaching would not be reasonable and necessary, since the beneficiary has demonstrated an inability to be taught.

EXAMPLE 3: A physician has ordered skilled nursing visits to teach self-administration of insulin to a beneficiary who has been self-injecting insulin for 10 years and there is no change in the beneficiary's physical or mental status that would require reteaching. The skilled nursing visits would not be considered reasonable and necessary since the beneficiary has a long-standing history of being able to perform the service.

EXAMPLE 4: A physician has ordered skilled nursing visits to teach self-administration of insulin to a beneficiary who has been self-injecting insulin for 10 years because the beneficiary has recently lost the use of the dominant hand and must be retrained to use the other hand. Skilled nursing visits to reteach self-administration of the insulin would be reasonable and necessary.

In determining the reasonable and necessary number of teaching and training visits, consideration must be given to whether the teaching and training provided constitute a reinforcement of teaching provided previously in an institutional setting or in the home or whether it represents the initial instruction. Where the teaching represents initial instruction, the complexity of the activity to be taught and the unique abilities of the beneficiary are to be considered. Where the teaching constitutes a reinforcement, an analysis of the patient's retained knowledge and anticipated learning progress is necessary to determine the appropriate number of visits. Skills taught in a controlled institutional setting often need to be reinforced when the beneficiary returns to his or her home and does not have the advantage of the controlled environment. Where the patient needs reinforcement of the institutional teaching, additional teaching visits in the home are covered.

When the teaching constitutes reinforcement, your documentation should indicate any modifications or reinforcement needed in the home environment, for safety and/or effectiveness.

EXAMPLE 5: A patient recovering from pneumonia is being sent home requiring IV infusion of antibiotics 4 times per day. The patient's spouse has been shown how to administer the drug during the last few days of hospitalization and has been told the signs and symptoms of infection. The physician has also ordered home health services for a skilled nurse to teach the administration of the drug and the signs and symptoms requiring immediate medical attention. Teaching by the skilled nurse in the home would be reasonable and necessary to continue that begun in the hospital, since the home environment, and the nature of the supplies used in the home, differ from that in the hospital.

Reteaching or retraining for an appropriate period may be considered reasonable and necessary where there is a change in the procedure or the beneficiary's condition that requires reteaching, or where the patient, family, or caregiver is not properly carrying out the task. The medical record should document the reason that the reteaching or retraining is required.

EXAMPLE 6: A well-established diabetic who loses the use of his or her dominant hand would need to be retrained in self-administration of insulin.

EXAMPLE 7: A spouse who has been taught to perform a dressing change for a postsurgical beneficiary may need to be re-taught wound care if the spouse demonstrates improper performance of wound care.

NOTE: There is no requirement that the beneficiary, family, or other caregiver be taught to provide a service if they cannot or choose not to provide the care.

Teaching and training activities which require the skills of a licensed nurse include, but are not limited to the following:

° Teaching the self-administration of injectable medications, or a complex range of medications;

° Teaching a newly diagnosed diabetic or caregiver all aspects of diabetes management, including how to prepare and to administer insulin injections, to prepare and follow a diabetic diet, to observe foot-care precautions, and to observe for and understand signs of hyperglycemia and hypoglycemia;

° Teaching self-administration of medical gases;

° Teaching wound care where the complexity of the wound, the overall condition of the beneficiary, or the ability of the caregiver makes teaching necessary;

° Teaching care for a recent ostomy or where reinforcement of ostomy care is needed;

° Teaching self-catheterization;

° Teaching self-administration of gastrostomy or enteral feedings;

° Teaching care for and maintenance of peripheral and central venous lines and administration of intravenous medications through such lines;

° Teaching bowel or bladder training when bowel or bladder dysfunction exists;

° Teaching how to perform the activities of daily living when the beneficiary or caregiver must use special techniques and adaptive devices due to a loss of function;

° Teaching transfer techniques, e.g., from bed to chair, which are needed for safe transfers;

° Teaching proper body alignment and positioning, and timing techniques of a bed-bound beneficiary;

° Teaching ambulation with prescribed assistive devices (such as crutches, walker, cane, etc.) that are needed due to a recent functional loss;

° Teaching prosthesis care and gait training;

° Teaching the use and care of braces, splints and orthotics, and associated skin care;

° Teaching the proper care and application of any specialized dressings or skin treatments (for example, dressings or treatments needed by beneficiaries with severe or widespread fungal infections, active and severe psoriasis or eczema, or due to skin deterioration from radiation treatments);

° Teaching the preparation and maintenance of a therapeutic diet; and

° Teaching proper administration of oral medication, including signs of side effects and avoidance of interaction with other medications and food.

4. Administration of Medications.—Although drugs and biologicals are specifically excluded from coverage by the statute (§1816(m)(5) of the Social Security Act), the services of a licensed nurse which are required to administer the medications safely and effectively may be covered if they are reasonable and necessary to the treatment of the illness or injury.

a. Intravenous, intramuscular, or subcutaneous injections and infusions, and hypodermoclysis or intravenous feedings require the skills of a licensed nurse to be performed (or taught) safely and effectively. Where these services are reasonable and necessary to treat the illness or injury, they may be covered. For these services to be reasonable and necessary, the medication being administered must be accepted as safe and effective treatment of the beneficiary's illness or injury, and there must be a medical reason that the medication cannot be taken orally. Moreover, the frequency and duration of the administration of the medication must be within accepted standards of medical practice, or there must be a valid explanation regarding the extenuating circumstances which justify the need for the additional injections.

(1) Vitamin B12 injections are considered specific therapy only for the following conditions:

–Specified anemias: pernicious anemia, megaloblastic anemias, macrocytic anemias, fish tapeworm anemia,

–Specified gastrointestinal disorders: gastrectomy, malabsorption syndromes such as sprue and idiopathic steatorrhea, surgical and mechanical disorders such as resection of the small intestine, strictures, anastomosis, and blind loop syndrome,

–Certain neuropathies: posterolateral sclerosis, other neuropathies associated with pernicious anemia, during the acute phase or acute exacerbation of a neuropathy due to malnutrition and alcoholism.

For an individual with pernicious anemia caused by a B12 deficiency, intramuscular or subcutaneous injection of vitamin B12 at a dose of from 100 to 1000 micrograms no more frequently than once monthly is the accepted reasonable and necessary dosage schedule for maintenance treatment. More frequent injections would be appropriate in the initial or acute phase of the disease until it has been determined through laboratory tests that the patient can be sustained on a maintenance dose.

(2) Insulin Injections.—Insulin is customarily self-injected by patients or is injected by their families. However, where a beneficiary is either physically or mentally unable to self-inject insulin and there is no other person who is able and willing to inject the beneficiary, the injections would be considered a reasonable and necessary skilled nursing service.

Documentation must support the beneficiary's inability to administer the insulin and the nonavailability of an able or willing caregiver. Where there is a caregiver in the home the documentation must indicate that the caregiver is unable or unwilling.

EXAMPLE: A beneficiary who requires an injection of insulin once per day for treatment of diabetes mellitus, also has multiple sclerosis with loss of muscle control in the arms and hands, occasional tremors, and vision loss which cause her not to be able to fill syringes or to self-inject the insulin, skilled nursing care would be reasonable and necessary for the injection of the insulin.

The prefilling of syringes with insulin (or other medication which is self-injected) does not require the skills of a licensed nurse, and therefore is not considered to be a skilled nursing service. If the beneficiary needs someone only to prefill syringes (and therefore needs no skilled nursing care on an intermittent basis, or physical therapy or speech therapy), the beneficiary, therefore, does not qualify for any Medicare coverage or home health care. Prefilling of syringes for self-administration of insulin or other medications is considered to be assistance with medications which are ordinarily self-administrered and is an appropriate home health aide service. (See §206.1.) However, where State law requires that a licensed nurse prefill syringes, a skilled nursing visit to prefill syringes is paid as a skilled nursing visit (if the beneficiary otherwise needs skilled nursing care or physical therapy or speech therapy), but is not considered to be a skilled nursing service.

b. Oral Medications.—The administration of oral medications by a licensed nurse is not a reasonable and necessary skilled nursing care except in the specific situation in which the complexity of the beneficiary's condition, the nature of the drugs prescribed, and the number of drugs prescribed require the skills of a licensed nurse to detect and evaluate side effects or reactions. The medical record must document the specific circumstances that cause administration of an oral medication to require skilled observation and assessment.

c. Eye Drops and Topical Ointments.—The administration of eye drops and topical ointments does not require the skills of a licensed nurse. Therefore, even if the administration of eye drops or ointments is necessary to the treatment of an illness or injury and the patient cannot self-administer them, and there is no one available to administer them, the visits cannot be covered as a skilled nursing service. This section does not eliminate coverage for skilled nursing visits for observation and assessment of the beneficiary's condition. (See §205.1.B.1.)

EXAMPLE 1: A physician has ordered skilled nursing visits to administer eye drops and ointments for a beneficiary with glaucoma. The administration of eye drops and ointments does not require the skills of a licensed nurse. Therefore, the skilled nursing visits cannot be covered as skilled nursing care, notwithstanding the importance of the administration of the drops as ordered.

EXAMPLE 2: A physician has ordered skilled nursing visits for a patient with a reddened area under the breast. The physician instructs the beneficiary to wash, rinse, and dry the area daily and apply A and D ointment. Skilled nursing care is not needed to provide this treatment safely and effectively.

5. Tube Feedings.—Nasogastric tube, and percutaneous tube feedings (including gastrostomy and jejunostomy tubes), and replacement, adjustment, stabilization, and suctioning of the tubes are skilled nursing services, and if the feedings are required to treat the beneficiary's illness or injury, the feedings and replacement or adjustment of the tubes would be covered as skilled nursing services.

Daily tube feedings may be covered if all other criteria are met.

6. Nasopharyngeal and Tracheostomy Aspiration.—Nasopharyngeal and tracheostomy aspiration are skilled nursing services and, if required to treat the beneficiary's illness or injury, would be covered as skilled nursing services.

7. Catheters.—Insertion and sterile irrigation and replacement of catheters, care of a suprapubic catheter, and in selected patients, urethral catheters, are considered to be skilled nursing services. Where the catheter is necessitated by a permanent or temporary loss of bladder control, skilled nursing services which are provided at a frequency appropriate to the type of catheter in use would be considered reasonable and necessary. Absent complications, Foley catheters generally require skilled care once approximately every 30 days and silicone catheters generally require skilled care once every 60–90 days and this frequency of service would be considered reasonable and necessary. However, where there are complications which require more frequent skilled care related to the catheter, such care would, with adequate documentation, be covered.

EXAMPLE: A beneficiary who has a Foley catheter due to loss of bladder control because of multiple sclerosis has a history of frequent plugging of the catheter and urinary tract infections. The physician has ordered skilled nursing visits once per month to change the catheter, and has left a "PRN" order for up to 3 additional visits per month for skilled observation and evaluation and/or catheter changes if the beneficiary or her family reports signs and symptoms of a urinary tract infection or a plugged catheter. During the certification period, the beneficiary's family contacts the HHA because the beneficiary has an elevated temperature, abdominal pain, and scant urine output. The skilled nurse visits the beneficiary and determines that the catheter is plugged and that there are symptoms of a urinary tract infection. The skilled nurse changes the catheter, and contacts the physician to advise him of her findings and to discuss treatment. The skilled nursing visit to change the catheter and to evaluate the beneficiary would be reasonable and necessary to the treatment of the illness or injury.

8. Wound Care.—Care of wounds (including, but not limited to ulcers, burns, pressure sores, open surgical sites, fistulas, tube sites and tumor erosion sites), when the skills of a licensed nurse are needed to provide safely and effectively the services necessary to treat the illness or injury, is considered to be a skilled nursing service. For skilled nursing care to be reasonable and necessary to treat a wound, the size, depth, nature of drainage (color, odor, consistency, and quantity), condition, and appearance of surrounding skin of wound must be documented in the clinical findings so that an assessment of the need for skilled nursing care can be made. Coverage or denial of skilled nursing visits for wound care may not

be based solely on the stage classification of the wound, but rather must be based on all of the documented clinical findings. Moreover, the plan of care must contain the specific instructions for the treatment of the wound. Where the physician has ordered appropriate active treatment (e.g., sterile or complex dressings, administration of prescription medications, etc.) of wounds with the following characteristics, the skills of a licensed nurse are usually reasonable and necessary:

Three basic skills are related to coverage of wound care. They may be provided separately or in conjunction:

° Direct hands-on wound care treatment;
° Teaching of the care; and
° Skilled observation and assessment of the wound.

Document size, depth, nature of drainage, and condition of surrounding skin and any special techniques required to care for the wound. Although healing may not be a realistic goal, continued wound care may be covered as long as skilled-level care is needed.

---

a. Open wounds which are draining purulent or colored exudate or which have a foul odor present and/or for which the beneficiary is receiving antibiotic therapy;

b. Wounds with a drain or T-tube which requires shortening or movement of such drains;

c. Wounds which require irrigation or instillation of a sterile cleansing or medicated solution into several layers of tissue and skin and/or packing with sterile gauze;

d. Recently debrided ulcers;

e. Pressure sores (decubitus ulcers) which present the following characteristics:

° There is partial tissue loss with signs of infection such as foul odor or purulent drainage, or

° There is full thickness tissue loss that involves exposure of fat or invasion of other tissue such as muscle or bone;

NOTE: Wounds or ulcers that show redness, edema, and induration, at times with epidermal blistering or desquamation do not ordinarily require skilled nursing care.

f. Wounds with exposed internal vessels or a mass which may have a proclivity for hemorrhage when a dressing is changed (e.g., post–radical neck surgery, cancer of the vulva);

g. Open wounds or widespread skin complications following radiation therapy, or which result from immune deficiencies or vascular insufficiencies;

h. Post-operative wounds where there are complications such as infection or allergic reaction or where there is an underlying disease which has a reasonable potential to adversely affect healing (e.g., diabetes);

Documentation should support the reasonable potential for complications or ineffective healing.

---

i. Third-degree burns, and second-degree burns where the size of the burn or presence of complications causes skilled nursing care to be needed;

j. Skin conditions which require application of nitrogen mustard or other chemotherapeutic medication which present a significant risk to the beneficiary; or

k. Other open or complex wounds which require treatment that can only be safely and effectively provided by a licensed nurse.

EXAMPLE 1: A beneficiary has a second-degree burn with full thickness skin damage on his back. The wound is cleansed, followed by an application of Sulfamylon. While the wound requires skilled monitoring for signs and symptoms of infection or complications, the dressing change requires skilled nursing services.

EXAMPLE 2: A beneficiary experiences a decubitus ulcer where the full thickness tissue loss extends through the dermis to involve subcutaneous tissue. The wound involves necrotic tissue with a physician's order to apply a covering of a debriding ointment following vigorous irrigation. The wound is then packed loosely with wet to dry dressings or continuous moist dressing and covered with dry sterile gauze. Skilled nursing care is necessary for a proper treatment and understanding of cellular adherence and/or exudate or tissue healing or necrosis.

NOTE: This section relates to the direct, hands-on skilled nursing care provided to beneficiaries with wounds, including any necessary dressing changes on those wounds. While a wound might not require this skilled nursing care, the wound may still require skilled monitoring for signs and symptoms of infection or complication (see §205.1.B.1) or skilled teaching of wound care to the beneficiary or the beneficiary's family (see §205.1.B.3).

9. Ostomy Care.—Ostomy care during the post-operative period and in the presence of associated complications where the need for skilled nursing care is clearly documented is a skilled nursing service. Teaching ostomy care remains skilled nursing care regardless of the presence of complications.

10. Heat Treatments.—Heat treatments which have been specifically ordered by a physician as part of active treatment of an illness or injury and which require observation of a licensed nurse to adequately evaluate the patient's progress would be considered as skilled nursing services.

11. Medical Gases.—Initial phases of a regimen involving the administration of medical gases which are necessary to the treatment of the beneficiary's illness or injury, would require skilled nursing care for skilled observation and evaluation of the beneficiary's reaction to the gases, and to teach the patient and family when and how to properly manage the administration of the gases.

12. Rehabilitation Nursing.—Rehabilitation nursing procedures, including the related teaching and adaptive aspects of nursing that are part of active treatment (e.g., the institution and supervision of bowel and bladder training programs) would constitute skilled nursing services.

13. Venipuncture.—Venipuncture when the collection of the specimen is necessary to the diagnosis and treatment of the beneficiary's illness or injury and when the venipuncture cannot be performed in the course of regularly scheduled absences from the

home to acquire medical treatment is a skilled nursing service. The frequency of visits for venipuncture must be reasonable within accepted standards of medical practice for treatment of the illness or injury.

For venipuncture to be reasonable and necessary:

–The physician order for the venipuncture for a laboratory test should be associated with a specific symptom or diagnosis, or the documentation should clarify the need for the test when it is not diagnosis/illness specific. In addition, the treatment must be recognized (in the Physician's Desk Reference, or other authoritative source) as being reasonable and necessary to the treatment of the illness or injury for venipunctures for monitoring the treatment to be reasonable and necessary.

–The frequency of testing should be consistent with accepted standards of medical practice for continued monitoring of a diagnosis, medical problem, or treatment regimen. Even where the laboratory results are consistently stable, periodic venipuncture may be reasonable and necessary because of the nature of the treatment.

Examples of reasonable and necessary venipuncture for stabilized beneficiaries include, but are not limited to those described below. While these guidelines do not preclude a physician from ordering more frequent venipunctures for these laboratory tests, the HHA must present justifying documentation to support the reasonableness and necessity of more frequent testing.

a. Captopril may cause side effects such as leukopenia and agranulocytosis and it is standard medical practice to monitor the white blood cell count and differential count on a routine basis (every 3 months) when the results are stable and the patient is asymptomatic.

b. In monitoring phenytoin (e.g., Dilantin) administration, the difference between a therapeutic and a toxic level of phenytoin in the blood is very slight. It is therefore appropriate to monitor the level on a routine basis (every 3 months) when the results are stable and the beneficiary is asymptomatic.

c. Venipuncture for fasting blood sugar (FBS):

–An unstable insulin- dependent or non–insulin-dependent diabetic would require FBS more frequently than once per month if ordered by the physician.

–Where there is a new diagnosis or where there has been a recent exacerbation, but the beneficiary is not unstable, monitoring once per month would be reasonable and necessary.

–A stable insulin or non-insulin dependent diabetic would require monitoring every 2–3 months.

d. Venipuncture for prothrombin

–Where the documentation shows that the dosage is being adjusted, monitoring would be reasonable and necessary as ordered by the physician.

–Where the results are stable within the therapeutic ranges, monthly monitoring would be reasonable and necessary.

–Where the results are stable within non-therapeutic ranges, there must be documentation of other factors which would indicate why continued monitoring is reasonable and necessary.

EXAMPLE: A beneficiary with coronary artery disease (CAD) was hospitalized with atrial fibrillation and was subsequently discharged to the home health agency with orders for anticoagulation therapy. Monthly venipunctures as indicated are necessary to report prothrombin (protime) levels to the physician, notwithstanding that the beneficiary's prothrombin time tests indicate essential stability.

Coverage of Venipuncture

Based on 3 conditions

° The physician orders the service;

° The frequency of the blood work is:

1. consistent with accepted standards of medical practice;

2. the nature of the treatment; and/or

3. if different from #1 above document the need or condition of the individual patient.

° The services are considered reasonable and necessary to the treatment of an illness or injury (which includes maintenance).

EXAMPLES:

1. Periodic blood work in conjunction with, e.g., gold therapy.
2. Periodic bloodwork to monitor individual levels in conjunction with medication monitoring, e.g., phenytoin therapy.
3. Periodic bloodwork to monitor patient condition and/or maintenance or changes in treatment plan.

---

14. <u>Student Nurse Visits.</u>—Visits made by a student nurse may be covered as skilled nursing care when a home health agency participates in training programs in which it utilizes student nurses enrolled in a school of nursing to perform skilled nursing services in a home setting. To be covered, the services must be reasonable and necessary skilled nursing care, and must be performed under the general supervision of a registered or licensed nurse. The supervising nurse need not accompany the student nurse on each visit.

15. <u>Psychiatric Evaluation and Therapy.</u>—The evaluation and psychotherapy needed by a patient suffering from a diagnosed psychiatric disorder that necessitated active treatment in an institution require the skills of a psychiatrically trained nurse and the costs of the psychiatric nurse's services may be covered as a skilled nursing care. Psychiatrically trained nurses are nurses who have special training and/or experience beyond the standard curriculum required for an R.N. The services of the psychiatric nurse are to be provided under a plan of care established and reviewed by a psychiatrist. A psychiatrist may also prescribe services of nonpsychiatric nursing such as intramuscular injections of behavior-modifying medications.

It is not necessary for the patient to require active treatment in an institution to be eligible.

A psychiatric nurse must furnish care under a plan established, reviewed, and signed by a psychiatrist.

Because the law precludes agencies that primarily provide care and treatment of mental diseases from participating as home health agencies, psychiatric nursing must be furnished by an agency that does not primarily provide care and treatment of mental diseases.

C. Intermittent Skilled Nursing Care.—To meet the requirement for "intermittent" skilled nursing care, an individual must have a medically predictable recurring need for skilled nursing services. In most instances, this definition will be met if a patient requires a skilled nursing service at least once every 60 days.

> This section applies if the beneficiary must qualify on the basis of a need for intermittent SN alone (e.g., no need for PT, ST, or continued OT.)

205.2 Skilled Therapy Services.—

A. General Principles Governing Reasonable and Necessary Physical Therapy, Speech Therapy, and Occupational Therapy.—

> Note that the content of the plan of care (204.2A) requires identification of functional limitations and safety measures to protect against injury. As with skilled nursing care, these measures are pertinent to justify need for skilled rehabilitation. Document functional limitations in ADL and mobility, or speech-language-voice communication, as well as safety factors requiring skilled intervention.

1. The service of a physical, speech or occupational therapist is a skilled therapy service if the inherent complexity of the service is such that it can be performed safely and/or effectively only by or under the general supervision of a skilled therapist. To be covered, the skilled services must also be reasonable and necessary to the treatment of the beneficiary's illness or injury or to the restoration or maintenance of function affected by the beneficiary's illness or injury. It is necessary to determine whether individual therapy services are skilled and whether, in view of the beneficiary's overall condition, skilled management of the services provided is needed although many or all of the specific services needed to treat the illness or injury do not require the skills of a therapist.

> Skilled management involves a finding that the patient's recovery and safety cannot be assured unless the total care, skilled or not, is planned and managed by skilled rehabilitation personnel. Document the precautions needed as well as the medical complications and safety factors present which warrant skilled management.

2. The development, implementation, management and evaluation of a patient care plan based on the physician's orders constitute skilled therapy services when, because of the beneficiary's condition, those activities require the involvement of a skilled therapist to meet the beneficiary's needs, promote recovery, and ensure medical safety. Where the skills of a therapist are needed to manage and periodically reevaluate the appropriateness of a maintenance program because of an identified danger to the patient, such services would be covered, even if the skills of a therapist are not needed to carry out the activities performed as part of the maintenance program.

> The skills of a therapist are needed to establish a reasonable and necessary maintenance program until it can be safely and effectively carried out by nonskilled individuals. However, if you identify a danger to the patient's safety which warrants the skills of the therapist to manage, and periodically reevaluate the appropriateness of the maintenance furnished, the services may be covered because the program is not yet fully established for safety and effectiveness.

3. While a beneficiary's particular medical condition is a valid factor in deciding if skilled therapy services are needed, a beneficiary's diagnosis or prognosis should never be the sole factor in deciding that a service is or is not skilled. The key issue is whether the skills of a therapist are needed to treat the illness or injury, or whether the services can be carried out by nonskilled personnel.

> The coverage decision must be based on the need for the skills of a therapist and not only on the diagnosis. For example, a patient diagnosed as "old stroke" may, in fact, need skilled rehabilitation. Document the reasons.

Since the need for "intermittent" skilled nursing care makes the individual eligible for other covered home health services, the intermediary should evaluate each claim involving skilled nursing services furnished less frequently than once every 60 days. In such cases, payment should be made only if documentation justifies a recurring need for reasonable, necessary, and medically predictable skilled nursing services. The following are examples of the need for infrequent, yet intermittent, skilled nursing services:

1. The patient with an indwelling silicone catheter who generally needs a catheter change only at 90-day intervals;

2. The person who experiences a fecal impaction due to the normal aging process (i.e., loss of bowel tone, restrictive mobility, and breakdown in good health habits) and must be manually disimpacted. Although these impactions are likely to recur, it is not possible to pinpoint a specific timeframe; or

3. The blind diabetic who self-injects insulin may have a medically predictable recurring need for a skilled nursing visit at least every 90 days. These visits, for example, would be to observe and determine the need for changes in the level and type of care which have been prescribed, thus supplementing the physician's contacts with the patient. (See Coverage Issues Appendix, §HHA-1.)

Where the need for "intermittent" skilled nursing visits is medically predictable but a situation arises after the first visit making additional visits unnecessary, e.g., the patient is institutionalized or dies, the one visit would be reimbursable. However, a one-time order; e.g., to give gamma globulin following exposure to hepatitis, would not be considered a need for "intermittent" skilled nursing care since a recurrence of the problem which would require this service is not medically predictable.

Although most patients require services no more frequently than several times a week, Medicare will pay for part-time (as defined in §206.7) medically reasonable and necessary skilled nursing care 7 days a week for a short period of time (2–3 weeks). There may also be a few cases involving unusual circumstances where the patient's prognosis indicates the medical need for daily skilled services will extend beyond 3 weeks. As soon as the patient's physician makes this judgment, which usually should be made before the end of the 3-week period, the home health agency must forward medical documentation justifying the need for such additional services and include an estimate of how much longer daily skilled services will be required.

A person expected to need more or less <u>full-time skilled nursing care over an extended period of time</u>; i.e., a patient who requires institutionalization, would usually not qualify for home health benefits.

> A beneficiary may qualify for home health benefits, if, at the onset of care, daily SN care is documented and needed for a finite and predictable period of time.
>
> Daily is defined as 5, 6, or 7 days per week. SN care (private pay or otherwise) that is not included on the POC or billed to Medicare does not impact the intermittent determination.

4. A service that is ordinarily considered nonskilled could be considered a skilled therapy service in cases in which there is clear documentation that, because of special medical complications, skilled rehabilitation personnel are required to perform or supervise the service or to observe the beneficiary. However, the importance of a particular service to a beneficiary or the frequency with which it must be performed does not, by itself, make a nonskilled service into a skilled service.

5. The skilled therapy services must be reasonable and necessary to the treatment of the beneficiary's illness or injury within the context of the beneficiary's unique medical condition. To be considered reasonable and necessary for the treatment of the illness or injury:

a. The services must be consistent with the nature and severity of the illness or injury, the beneficiary's particular medical needs, including the requirement that the amount, frequency, and duration of the services must be reasonable, and

b. The services must be considered, under accepted standards of medical practice, to be specific and effective treatment for the patient's condition, and

c. The services must be provided with the expectation, based on the assessment made by the physician of the beneficiary's rehabilitation potential, that:

+The condition of the beneficiary will improve materially in a reasonable and generally predictable period of time, or

+The services are necessary to the establishment of a safe and effective maintenance program.

> If there is not a reasonable expectation of improvement in a patient's condition, there may still be a need for skilled services to establish a maintenance program. A special <u>medical complication</u> might also necessitate skilled services to perform exercises or treatments that are normally considered nonskilled, even when no rehabilitation potential is present, e.g., for a terminally ill patient.
>
> Document the reasons.

Services involving activities for the general welfare of any beneficiary, e.g., general exercises to promote overall fitness or flexibility and activities to provide diversion or general motivation, do not constitute skilled therapy. Those services can be performed by nonskilled individuals without the supervision of a therapist.

d. Services of skilled therapists which are for the purpose of teaching the patient or the patient's family or caregivers necessary techniques, exercises, or precautions are covered to the extent that they are reasonable and necessary to treat illness or injury. However, visits made by skilled therapists to a beneficiary's home solely to train other home health agency staff (e.g., home health aides) are not billable as visits since the home health agency is responsible for ensuring that its staff is properly trained to perform any service it furnishes. The cost of a skilled therapist's visit for the purpose of training home health agency staff is an administrative cost to the home health agency.

EXAMPLE: A beneficiary with a diagnosis of multiple sclerosis has recently been discharged from the hospital following an exacerbation of her condition which has left her wheelchair bound and, for the first time, without any expectation of achieving ambulation again. The physician has ordered physical therapy to select the proper wheelchair for her long-term use, to teach safe use of the wheelchair and safe transfer techniques to the beneficiary and the family. Physical therapy would be reasonable and necessary to evaluate the beneficiary's overall needs, to make the selection of the proper wheelchair, and to teach the beneficiary and/or family safe use of the wheelchair and proper transfer techniques.

B. <u>Application of the Principles to Physical Therapy Services.</u>— The following discussion of skilled physical therapy services applies the principles in §205.2A to specific physical therapy services about which questions are most frequently raised.

1. <u>Assessment.</u>—The skills of a physical therapist to assess a beneficiary's rehabilitation needs and potential or to develop and/or implement a physical therapy program are covered when they are reasonable and necessary because of the beneficiary's condition. Skilled rehabilitation services concurrent with the management of a patient's care plan include objective tests and measurements such as, but not limited to, range of motion, strength, balance, coordination, endurance, or functional ability.

2. <u>Therapeutic Exercises.</u>—Therapeutic exercises which must be performed by or under the supervision of the qualified physical therapist to ensure the safety of the beneficiary and the effectiveness of the treatment, due either to the type of exercise employed or to the condition of the beneficiary, constitute skilled physical therapy.

3. <u>Gait Training.</u>—Gait evaluation and training furnished a beneficiary whose ability to walk has been impaired by neurological, muscular, or skeletal abnormality require the skills of a qualified physical therapist and constitute skilled physical therapy and are considered reasonable and necessary if they can be expected to improve materially the beneficiary's ability to walk.

Gait evaluation and training which is furnished to a beneficiary whose ability to walk has been impaired by a condition other than a neurological, muscular, or skeletal abnormality would nevertheless be covered where physical therapy is reasonable and necessary to restore the lost function.

The patient's ability to walk with an assistive device for a specific number of feet is never the sole basis for deciding coverage. Coverage decisions are based on all relevant factors described in the guidelines. Document the functional gait deviance or loss needing restoration and safety factors as well as the type of gait training furnished.

EXAMPLE 1: A physician has ordered gait evaluation and training for a beneficiary whose gait has been materially impaired by scar tissue resulting from burns. Physical therapy services to evaluate the beneficiary's gait, to establish a gait training program and to provide the skilled services necessary to implement the program would be covered.

EXAMPLE 2: A beneficiary who has had a total hip replacement is ambulatory but demonstrates weakness, and is unable to climb stairs safely. Physical therapy would be reasonable and necessary to teach the beneficiary to safely climb and descend stairs.

Repetitive exercises to improve gait, or to maintain strength and endurance and assistive walking are appropriately provided by nonskilled persons and ordinarily do not require the skills of a physical therapist. Where such services are performed by a physical therapist as part of the initial design and establishment of a safe and effective maintenance program, the services would, to the extent that they are reasonable and necessary, be covered.

EXAMPLE: A beneficiary who has received gait training has reached his maximum restoration potential, and the physical therapist is teaching the beneficiary and family how to safely perform the activities which are a part of the maintenance program being established. The visits by the physical therapist to demonstrate and teach the activities (which by themselves do not require the skills of a therapist) would be covered since they are needed to establish the program.

4. Range of Motion.—Only a qualified physical therapist may perform range of motion tests and therefore such tests are skilled physical therapy.

Range of motion exercises constitute skilled physical therapy only if they are part of an active treatment for a specific disease state, illness, or injury, which has resulted in a loss or restriction of mobility (as evidenced by physical therapy notes showing the degree of motion lost and the degree to be restored). Range of motion exercises which are not related to the restoration of a specific loss of function often may be provided safely and effectively by nonskilled individuals. Passive exercises to maintain range of motion in paralyzed extremities that can be carried out by nonskilled persons do not constitute skilled physical therapy.

However, as indicated in section 205.2A4, where there is clear documentation that, because of special medical complications (e.g., susceptible to pathological bone fractures), the skills of a therapist are needed to provide services which ordinarily do not need the skills of a therapist, then the services would be covered.

The documentation should clearly identify the medical complications which present a high probability that serious complications could occur without skilled supervision. The example here is not meant to include the mere possibility that a pathological FX could occur.

5. Maintenance Therapy.—Where repetitive services which are required to maintain function involve the use of complex and sophisticated procedures, the judgment and skill of a physical therapist might be required for the safe and effective rendition of such services. If the judgment and skill of a physical therapist is required to safely and effectively treat the illness or injury, the services would be covered as physical therapy services.

Repetitive maintenance exercises are noncovered if the skills of a therapist are not needed. However, therapeutic exercises can be skilled due either to the type or complexity of exercise or to the patient's condition. Repetitive maintenance exercises, on an exception basis, might require the skills of a therapist because of the level of the procedures or because of complications. Normally nonskilled heat treatments might require the skills of a therapist, due to the complications in the patient's condition.

EXAMPLE: Where there is an unhealed, unstable fracture which requires regular exercise to maintain function until the fracture heals, the skills of a physical therapist would be needed to ensure that the fractured extremity is maintained in proper position and alignment during maintenance range of motion exercises.

Establishment of a maintenance program is a skilled physical therapy service where the specialized knowledge and judgment of a qualified physical therapist are required for the program to be safely carried out and the treatment aims of the physician achieved.

EXAMPLE: A Parkinson's patient or a patient with rheumatoid arthritis who has not been under a restorative physical therapy program may require the services of a physical therapist to determine what type of exercises are required for the maintenance of his present level of function. The initial evaluation of the patient's needs, the designing of a maintenance program which is appropriate to the capacity and tolerance of the patient and the treatment objectives of the physician, the instruction of the beneficiary, family or caregivers to safely and effectively carry out the program and such re-evaluations as may be required by the beneficiary's condition, would constitute skilled physical therapy.

While a patient is under a restorative physical therapy program, the physical therapist should regularly reevaluate his condition and adjust any exercise program the patient is expected to carry out himself or with the aid of supportive personnel to maintain the function being restored. Consequently, by the time it is determined that no further restoration is possible (i.e., by the end of the last restorative session) the physical therapist will already have designed the maintenance program required and instructed the beneficiary or caregivers in carrying out the program.

6. Ultrasound, Shortwave, and Microwave Diathermy Treatments.—These treatments must always be performed by or under the supervision of a qualified physical therapist and are skilled therapy.

7. Hot Packs, Infra-Red Treatments, Paraffin Baths, and Whirlpool Baths.—Heat treatments and baths of this type ordinarily do not require the skills of a qualified physical therapist. However, the skills, knowledge and judgment of a qualified physical therapist might be required in the giving of such treatments or baths in a particular case, e.g., where the patient's condition is complicated

by circulatory deficiency, areas of desensitization, open wounds, fractures, or other complications.

> Document the complications requiring the skills of a physical therapist when these treatments are rendered alone.

C. Application of the General Principles to Speech Language Pathology Services.—The following discussion of skilled speech language pathology services applies the principles to specific speech language pathology services about which questions are most frequently raised.

1. The skills of a speech language pathologist are required for the assessment of a beneficiary's rehabilitation needs (including the causal factors and the severity of the speech and language disorders), and rehabilitation potential. Reevaluation would only be considered reasonable and necessary if the beneficiary exhibited a change in functional speech or motivation, clearing of confusion or the remission of some other medical condition that previously contraindicated speech language pathology services. Where a beneficiary is undergoing restorative speech language pathology services, routine reevaluations are considered to be a part of the therapy and could not be billed as a separate visit.

2. The services of a speech language pathologist would be covered if they are needed as a result of an illness, or injury and are directed toward specific speech/voice production.

3. Speech language pathology would be covered where the service can only be provided by a speech language pathologist and where it is reasonably expected that the service will materially improve the beneficiary's ability to independently carry out any one or combination of communicative activities of daily living in a manner that is measurably at a higher level of attainment than that prior to the initiation of the services.

4. The services of a speech language pathologist to establish a hierarchy of speech-voice-language communication tasks and cueing that directs a beneficiary toward speech-language communication goals in the plan of care would be covered speech language pathology.

5. The services of a speech language pathologist to train the beneficiary, family, or other caregivers to augment the speech-language communication, treatment or to establish an effective maintenance program would be covered speech therapy.

6. The services of a speech language pathologist to assist beneficiaries with aphasia in rehabilitation of speech and language skills are covered when needed by a beneficiary.

7. The services of a speech therapist to assist individuals with voice disorders to develop proper control of the vocal and respiratory systems for correct voice production are covered when needed by a beneficiary.

D. Application of the General Principles to Occupational Therapy.—The following discussion of skilled occupational therapy services applies the principles to specific occupational therapy services about which questions are most frequently raised.

1. Assessment.—The skills of an occupational therapist to assess and reassess a beneficiary's rehabilitation needs and potential or to develop and/or implement an occupational therapist program are covered when they are reasonable and necessary because of the beneficiary's condition.

2. Planning, Implementing, and Supervision of Therapeutic Programs.—The planning, implementing, and supervision of therapeutic programs including, but not limited to those listed below are skilled occupational therapy services, and if reasonable and necessary to the treatment of the beneficiary's illness or injury would be covered.

a. Selecting and teaching task-oriented therapeutic activities designed to restore physical function.

EXAMPLE: Use of woodworking activities on an inclined table to restore shoulder, elbow, and wrist range of motion lost as a result of burns.

b. Planning, implementing, and supervising therapeutic tasks and activities designed to restore sensory-integrative function.

EXAMPLE: Providing motor and tactile activities to increase sensory output and improve response for a stroke patient with functional loss resulting in a distorted body image.

c. Planning, implementing, and supervising of individualized therapeutic activity programs as part of an overall "active treatment" program for a patient with a diagnosed psychiatric illness.

> The treatment must relate directly to the therapeutic treatment goals in the patient's "active treatment" program. Where an individual's motivational needs are not related to a specific diagnosed psychiatric illness or are of a diversional type, the services would not generally require the specialized skills of an occupational therapist. Document how the "active treatment plan" is established, e.g., psychiatrist.

EXAMPLE: Use of sewing activities which require following a pattern to reduce confusion and restore reality orientation in a schizophrenic patient.

d. Teaching compensatory techniques to improve the level of independence in the activities of daily living.

EXAMPLE: Teaching a beneficiary who has lost use of an arm how to pare potatoes and chop vegetables with one hand.

EXAMPLE: Teaching a stroke patient new techniques to enable him to perform feeding, dressing, and other activities of daily living as independently as possible.

e. The designing, fabricating, and fitting of orthotic and self-help devices.

EXAMPLE: Construction of a device which would enable an individual to hold a utensil and feed himself independently.

EXAMPLE: Construction of a hand splint for a patient with rheumatoid arthritis to maintain the hand in a functional position.

f. Vocational and prevocational assessment and training which is directed toward the restoration of function in the activities of daily living lost due to illness or injury would be covered. Where vocational or prevocational assessment and training are related solely to specific employment opportunities, work skills, or work settings, such services would not be covered because they would not be directed toward the treatment of an illness or injury.

Documentation should indicate that the occupational therapy services are directed to functional losses in ADL rather than solely work related. For example, teaching a disabled individual a method to pick up, hold, and dial a telephone may relate to normal ADL as well as being work related and could be covered.

3. Illustration of Covered Services.—

EXAMPLE 1: A physician orders occupational therapy for a patient who is recovering from a fractured hip and who needs to be taught compensatory and safety techniques with regard to lower extremity dressing, hygiene, toileting, and bathing. The occupational therapist will establish goals for the beneficiary's rehabilitation (to be approved by the physician), and will undertake the teaching of the techniques necessary for the patient to reach the goals. Occupational therapy services would be covered at a duration and intensity appropriate to the severity of the impairment and the beneficiary's response to treatment.

EXAMPLE 2: A physician has ordered occupational therapy for a beneficiary who is recovering from a CVA. The beneficiary has decreased range of motion, strength, and sensation in both the upper and lower extremities on the right side. In addition, the beneficiary has perceptual and cognitive deficits resulting from the CVA. The beneficiary's condition has resulted in decreased function in activities of daily living (specifically bathing, dressing, grooming, hygiene, and toileting). The loss of function requires assistive devices to enable the beneficiary to compensate for the loss of function and to maximize safety and independence. The beneficiary also needs equipment such as himi-slings to prevent shoulder subluxation and a hand splint to prevent joint contracture and deformity in the right hand.

The services of an occupational therapist would be necessary to assess the beneficiary's needs, develop goals (to be approved by the physician), to manufacture or adapt the needed equipment to the beneficiary's use, to teach compensatory techniques, to strengthen the beneficiary as necessary to permit use of compensatory techniques, to provide activities which are directed towards meeting the goals governing increased perceptual and cognitive function. Occupational therapy services would be covered at a duration and intensity appropriate to the severity of the impairment and the beneficiary's response to treatment.

EXAMPLE 2:   A patient's recovery and safety can be affected by perceptual and cognitive deficits. Document how these deficits impact the functional ADL, mobility, and/or safety of the beneficiary necessitating skilled intervention.

206. COVERAGE OF OTHER HOME HEALTH SERVICES

206.1 Skilled Nursing Care, Physical Therapy, Speech Therapy, and Occupational Therapy.—Where the beneficiary meets the qualifying criteria in 204, Medicare covers skilled nursing services that meet the requirements of 205.1 A and B and 206.7, physical therapy which meets the requirements of 205.2 A and B, speech therapy which meets the requirements of 205.2 A and C, and occupational therapy which meets the requirements of 205.2 A and D.

206.2 Home Health Aide Services.—For home health aide services to be covered, the beneficiary must meet the qualifying criteria as specified in §204; the services which are provided by the home health aide must be part-time or intermittent as discussed in §206.7; the services must meet the definition of home health aide services of this section; and the services must be reasonable and necessary to the treatment of the beneficiary's illness or injury.

The reason for the visits by the home health aide must be to provide hands-on personal care of the beneficiary or services which are needed to maintain the beneficiary's health or to facilitate treatment of the beneficiary's illness or injury.

1. Must meet qualifying criteria:

° homebound;

° under a physician's plan of care; and

° needs skilled nursing care on an intermittent basis, or PT, ST, or continued need for OT.

2. Home health aide services provided must be part-time or intermittent. When skilled nursing services are provided, both the home health aide and skilled nursing visits/hours are combined to determine part-time or intermittent.

Home health aide visits may be to furnish personal care, OR to maintain a beneficiary's health, OR to facilitate treatments.

The physician's order should indicate the frequency of the home health aide services required by the beneficiary. These services may include but are not limited to:

Physician orders for aide services must specify the type of service furnished, i.e., "HHA for personal care," "HHA to assist with maintenance exercise program."

A. Personal Care.—Personal care means:

° Bathing, dressing, grooming, caring for hair, nail and oral hygiene which are needed to facilitate treatment or to prevent deterioration of the beneficiary's health, changing the bed linens of an incontinent beneficiary, shaving, deodorant application, skin care with lotions and/or powder, foot care, and ear care.

A home health aide may furnish a single service (e.g., assist with ADLs) or several services on a visit.

° Feeding, assistance with elimination (including enemas unless the skills of a licensed nurse are required due to the patient's condition, routine catheter care, and routine colostomy care), assistance with ambulation, changing position in bed, assistance with transfers.

EXAMPLE 1: A physician has ordered home health aide visits to assist the beneficiary in personal care because the beneficiary is recovering from a stroke and continues to have significant right side weakness which causes him to be unable to bathe, dress, or perform hair and oral care. The plan of care established by the home health agency nurse sets forth the specific tasks with which the beneficiary needs assistance. Home health aide visits at an appropriate frequency would be reasonable and necessary to assist in these tasks.

EXAMPLE 2: A physician ordered four home health aide visits per week for personal care for a multiple sclerosis patient who is unable to perform these functions because of increasing debilitation. The home health aide gave the beneficiary a bath twice per week and washed hair on the other two visits each week. Only two visits are reasonable and necessary since the services could have been provided in the course of two visits.

EXAMPLE 3: A physician ordered seven home health aide visits per week for personal care for a bed-bound, incontinent patient. All visits are reasonable and necessary because the patient has extensive personal care needs.

EXAMPLE 4: A beneficiary with a well-established colostomy forgets to change the bag regularly and has difficulty changing it. Home health aide services at an appropriate frequency to change the bag would be considered reasonable and necessary to the treatment of the illness or injury.

Other services which may be covered when provided by home health aides include, but are not limited to:

B. Simple dressing changes which do not require the skills of a licensed nurse.

EXAMPLE: A beneficiary who is confined to the bed has developed a small reddened area on the buttocks. The physician has ordered home health aide visits for more frequent repositioning, bathing, and the application of a topical ointment and a gauze 4×4. Home health aide visits at an appropriate frequency would be reasonable and necessary.

C. Assistance with medications which are ordinarily self-administered and which do not require the skills of a licensed nurse to be provided safely and effectively.

NOTE: Prefilling of insulin syringes is ordinarily performed by the diabetic as part of the self-administration of the insulin and, unlike the injection of the insulin, does not require the skill of a licensed nurse to be performed properly. Therefore, if the prefilling of insulin syringes is performed by home health agency staff, it is considered to be a home health aide service. However, where State law precludes the provision of this service by other than a licensed nurse or physician, Medicare will make payment for this service, when covered, as though it were a skilled nursing service. Where the beneficiary needs only prefilling of insulin syringes and does not need skilled nursing care on an intermittent basis, or physical therapy or speech therapy or have a continuing need for occupational therapy, then Medicare cannot cover any home health services to the beneficiary (even if State law requires that the insulin syringes be filled by a licensed nurse).

D. Assistance with activities which are directly supportive of skilled therapy services but do not require the skills of a therapist to be safely and effectively performed such as routine maintenance exercises, and repetitive speech routines to support speech therapy.

E. Routine care of prosthetic and orthotic devices.

When a home health aide visits a patient to provide a health-related service as discussed above, the home health aide may also perform some incidental services which do not meet the definition of a home health aide service (e.g., light cleaning, preparation of a meal, taking out the trash, shopping). However, the purpose of a home health aide visit may not be to provide these incidental services since they are not health-related services, but rather are necessary household tasks that must be performed by anyone to maintain a home.

EXAMPLE 1: A home health aide visits a recovering stroke patient whose right side weakness and poor endurance cause her to be able to leave the bed and chair only with extreme difficulty. The physician has ordered physical therapy and speech therapy for the beneficiary and has ordered home health aide services three or four times per week for personal care, assistance with ambulation as mobility increases, and assistance with repetitive speech exercises as her impaired speech improves. The home health aide also provides incidental household services such as preparation of meals, light cleaning, and taking out the trash. The beneficiary lives with an elderly frail sister who is disabled and who cannot perform either the personal care or the incidental tasks. The home health aide visits at a frequency appropriate to the performance of the health-related services would be covered, notwithstanding the incidental provision of noncovered services (i.e., the household services) in the course of the visits.

EXAMPLE 2: A physician orders home health aide visits 3 times per week. The only services provided are light housekeeping, meal preparation, and trash removal. The home health aide visits cannot be covered, notwithstanding their importance to the beneficiary, because the services provided do not meet Medicare's definition of "home health aide services."

> The purpose of a home health aide visit must be to perform a health-related service even though some incidental services may be performed during the visit.

206.3 <u>Medical Social Services</u>.—Medical social services which are provided by a qualified medical social worker or a social work assistant under the supervision of a qualified medical social worker may be covered as home health services where the beneficiary meets the qualifying criteria specified in §204, and:

° The services of these professionals are necessary to resolve social or emotional problems which are or are expected to be an impediment to the effective treatment of the beneficiary's medical condition or his or her rate of recovery, and

° The plan of care indicates how the services which are required necessitate the skills of a qualified social worker or a social work assistant under the supervision of a qualified medical social worker to be performed safely and effectively.

Documentation must indicate:

° A clear and specific link between the social and emotional needs of the beneficiary and the beneficiary's medical condition and/or rate of recovery.

° The services furnished require the skills of a qualified social worker.

Where both of these requirements for coverage are met, services of these professionals which may be covered include, but are not limited to:

° Assessment of the social and emotional factors related to the beneficiary's illness, need for care, response to treatment, and adjustment to care,

° Assessment of the relationship of the beneficiary's medical and nursing requirements to the individual's home situation, financial resources, and availability of community resources,

° Appropriate action to obtain available community resources to assist in resolving the beneficiary's problem. (Note: Medicare does not cover the services of a medical social worker to complete or assist in the completion of an application for Medicaid because Federal regulations require the State to provide assistance in completing the application to anyone who chooses to apply for Medicaid), and

This is a clarification of existing coverage policy.

° Counseling services which are required by the beneficiary. Counseling of beneficiaries' families is covered only when such services are incidental to other covered medical social services being provided to the beneficiary, and when they are reasonable and necessary to treat the beneficiary's illness or injury. Visits by a medical social worker are not covered when the only reason for the visit is to counsel the beneficiary's family.

If the only reason to visit is to counsel the beneficiary's family, this visit is not covered.

NOTE: Participating in the development of the plan of treatment, preparing clinical and progress notes, participating in discharge planning and inservice programs, and acting as a consultant to other agency personnel are appropriate administrative costs to the home health agency.

EXAMPLE 1: The physician has ordered a medical social worker assessment of a diabetic beneficiary who has recently become insulin dependent and is not yet stabilized. The skilled nurse, who is providing skilled observation and evaluation to try to restabilize the beneficiary notices during her visits that the supplies left in the home for the beneficiary's use appear to be frequently missing, and that the beneficiary is not compliant with the regimen although she refuses to discuss the matter. The assessment by a medical social worker would be reasonable and necessary to determine if there are underlying social or emotional problems which are impeding the beneficiary's treatment.

EXAMPLE 2: A physician ordered an assessment by a medical social worker for a multiple sclerosis patient who was unable to move anything but her head and who had an indwelling catheter. The beneficiary had experienced recurring urinary tract infections and multiple infected ulcers. The physician ordered medical social services after the home health agency indicated to him that the home was not well cared for, and that the beneficiary appeared to be neglected much of the time and that the relationship between the beneficiary and family was very poor. The physician and home health agency were concerned that social problems created by family caregivers were impeding the treatment of the recurring infections and ulcers. The assessment and follow-up for counseling both the beneficiary and the family by a medical social worker were reasonable and necessary.

EXAMPLE 3: A physician is aware that a beneficiary with arteriosclerosis and hypertension is not taking medications as ordered and is not adhering to dietary restrictions because he is unable to afford the medication and is unable to cook. The physician orders several visits by a medical social worker to assist in resolving these problems. The visits by the medical social worker to review the beneficiary's financial status, to discuss options, and to make appropriate contacts with social services agencies or other community resources to arrange for medications and meals would be a reasonable and necessary medical social service.

EXAMPLE 4: A physician has ordered counseling by a medical social worker for a beneficiary with cirrhosis of the liver who has recently been discharged from a 28-day inpatient alcohol treatment program to her home which she shares with an alcoholic and neglectful adult child. The physician has ordered counseling several times per week to assist the beneficiary in remaining free of alcohol and in dealing with the adult child. The services of the medical social worker would be covered until the beneficiary's social situation ceased to impact on her recovery and/or treatment.

EXAMPLE 5: A physician has ordered medical social services for a beneficiary who is worried about her financial arrangements and payment for medical care. The services ordered are to arrange Medicaid if possible and resolve unpaid medical bills. There is no evidence that the beneficiary's concerns are adversely impacting recovery or treatment of her illness or injury. Medical social services cannot be covered.

EXAMPLE 6: A physician has ordered medical social services for a beneficiary of extremely limited income who has incurred large unpaid hospital and other medical bills following a significant illness. The beneficiary's recovery is adversely affected because the beneficiary is not maintaining a proper therapeutic diet, and cannot leave the home to acquire the medication necessary to treat his illness. The medical social worker reviews the beneficiary's financial status, arranges meal service to resolve the dietary problem, arranges for home-delivered medications, gathers the information necessary for application to Medicaid to acquire coverage for the medications the beneficiary needs, files the application on behalf of the beneficiary, and follows up repeatedly with the Medicaid State agency.

The medical social services which are necessary to review the financial status of the beneficiary, to arrange for meal service, to arrange for the medications to be delivered to the home, and to arrange for the Medicaid State agency to assist the beneficiary with the application for Medicaid would be covered. The services related to the assistance in filing the application for Medicaid, and the follow-up on the application are not covered since they must be provided by the State agency free of charge, and hence the beneficiary has no obligation to pay for such assistance.

> If the only documented service provided is calling "Meals on Wheels," this would not be a covered MSS visit (absent any other service requiring the skills of a MSW), since this call could be placed by any individual.

206.4 Medical Supplies (Except for Drugs and Biologicals) and the Use of Durable Medical Equipment

> The manual provisions are unchanged in this section. Note that for a medical supply to be covered the following criteria must be met:
>
> ° There must be a therapeutic or diagnostic use for the supply;
> ° The supply must be ordered by a physician as part of a prescribed treatment;
> ° It must be essential for agency personnel carrying out the plan of care; and
> ° Ordered supplies should be identified in locator 14 of the HCFA-485 or locator 16 of the HCFA-486.
>
> Some routine supplies might also meet this criteria but would not be separately billable, e.g., thermometer.

A. Medical Supplies.—Medical supplies are items which, due to their therapeutic or diagnostic characteristics, are essential in enabling home health agency personnel to carry out effectively the care which the physician has ordered for the treatment or diagnosis of the patient's illness or injury. Certain items which, by their very nature, are designed only to serve a medical purpose are obviously considered to be medical supplies; e.g., catheters, needles, syringes, surgical dressings and materials used for dressings such as cotton gauze and adhesive bandages, and materials used for aseptic techniques. Other medical supplies include, but are not limited to, irrigating solutions and intravenous fluids.

Other items which are often used by persons who are not ill or injured may be considered medical supplies but only where (1) the item is recognized as having the capacity to serve a therapeutic or diagnostic purpose in a specific situation, and (2) the item is required as a part of the actual physician-prescribed treatment of a patient's existing illness or injury. For example, items which generally serve a routine hygienic purpose, such as soaps and shampoos, and items which generally serve as skin conditioners, such as baby lotion, baby oil, skin softeners, powders, lotions, etc., would not be considered medical supplies unless the particular item is recognized as serving a specific therapeutic purpose in the physician's prescribed treatment of the patient's existing skin (scalp) disease or injury.

Limited amounts of medical supplies may be left in the home between visits where repeated applications are required and will be rendered by the patient or by family members. Such supplies as needles, syringes, and catheters which require administration by a nurse should not be left in the home between visits.

B. Drugs and Biologicals.—Drugs and biologicals are excluded from coverage as items or services administered by home health agencies, under both hospital insurance and medical insurance. They may, in certain cases, be covered under medical insurance, when administered by a physician as a part of his professional service, and are not capable of being self-administered.

C. Durable Medical Equipment.—Durable medical equipment which meets the requirements of §220ff may be covered under the home health benefit, with the beneficiary responsible for payment of a 20 percent coinsurance.

206.5 Services of Interns and Residents.—Home health services include the medical services of interns and residents-in-training under an approved hospital teaching program (if the agency has an affiliation with or is under common control of a hospital providing such medical services). "Approved" means approved by the Council on Medical Education of the American Medical Association, or in the case of an osteopathic hospital, the Committee on Hospitals of the Bureau of Professional Education of the American Osteopathic Association and, in the case of an intern or resident-in-training in the field of dentistry, approved by the Council on Dental Education of the American Dental Association. Reimbursement is provided under Part B for other services hospital interns and residents furnish to beneficiaries receiving home health services.

The services of interns and residents-in-training in the field of podiatry under a teaching program approved by the Council on Podiatry Education of the American Podiatry Association are covered under Part A on the same basis as the services of other interns and residents-in-training in approved teaching programs.

206.6 Outpatient Services.—Outpatient services include any of the items or services described above which are provided under arrangements on an outpatient basis at a hospital, skilled nursing facility, rehabilitation center, or outpatient department affiliated with a medical school, and (1) which require equipment which cannot readily be made available at the patient's place of residence, or (2) which are furnished while he is at the facility to receive the services described in (1). The hospital, skilled nursing facility, or outpatient department affiliated with a medical school must all be qualified providers of services. However, there are special provisions for the use of the facilities of rehabilitation centers (see §200.3). The cost of transporting an individual to a facility cannot be reimbursed as home health services.

> This section is unchanged from the previous manual guidelines.

206.7 Part-time or Intermittent Home Health Aide and Skilled Nursing Services.—Where a beneficiary qualifies for coverage of home health services, Medicare covers either part-time or intermittent home health aide services and skilled nursing services.

> This section applies to SN when the beneficiary qualifies for home health benefits on the basis of a need for PT, ST, or a continuing need for OT. It always applies to aide services.
>
> Where the average number of SN and aide visits per day are 2 or greater, hours will be reviewed. In other cases review of hours will be performed on postpayment review.

A. Definition of "Part-time."—"Part-time" means any number of days per week:

° Up to and including 28 hours per week of skilled nursing and home health aide services combined for less than 8 hours per day; or

° Up to 35 hours per week of skilled nursing and home health aide services combined for less than 8 hours per day subject to review by fiscal intermediaries on a case by case basis, based upon documentation justifying the need for and reasonableness of such additional care.

B. Definition of "Intermittent."—"Intermittent" means:

° Up to and including 28 hours per week of skilled nursing and home health aide services combined provided on a less than daily basis;

° Up to 35 hours per week of skilled nursing and home health aide services combined which are provided on a less than daily basis, subject to review by fiscal intermediaries on a case by case basis, based upon documentation justifying the need for and reasonableness of such additional care; or

° Up to and including full-time (i.e., 8 hours per day) skilled nursing and home health aide services combined which are provided and needed 7 days per week for temporary, but not indefinite, periods of time of up to 21 days with allowances for extensions in exceptional circumstances where the need for care in excess of 21 days is finite and predictable.

C. Impact on Care Provided in Excess of "Intermittent" or "Part-time" Care.—Home health aide and/or skilled nursing care in excess of the amounts of care which meet these definitions of part time or intermittent may be provided to a home care beneficiary or purchased by other payers without bearing on whether the home health aide and skilled nursing care meets the Medicare definitions of part time or intermittent.

EXAMPLE: A beneficiary needs skilled nursing care monthly for a catheter change and the home health agency also renders needed daily home health aide services 24 hours per day which will be needed for a long and indefinite period of time. The HHA bills Medicare for the skilled nursing and home health aide services which were provided before the 35th hour of service each week and bills the beneficiary (or another payer) for the remainder of the care. If the intermediary determines that the 35 hours of care are reasonable and necessary, Medicare would therefore cover the 35 hours of skilled nursing and home health aide visits.

D. Application of This Policy Revision.—A beneficiary must meet the long-standing and unchanged qualifying criteria for Medicare coverage of home health services, before this policy revision becomes applicable to skilled nursing services and/or home health aide services. The definition of "intermittent" with respect to the need for skilled nursing care where the beneficiary qualifies for coverage based on the need for "skilled nursing care on an intermittent basis" remains unchanged. Specifically:

° This policy revision always applies to home health aide services when the beneficiary qualifies for coverage;

° This policy revision applies to skilled nursing care only when the beneficiary needs physical therapy or speech therapy or continued occupational therapy, and also needs skilled nursing care; and

° If the beneficiary needs skilled nursing care but does not need physical therapy or speech therapy or occupational therapy, the beneficiary must still meet the long-standing and unchanged definition of "intermittent" skilled nursing care in order to qualify for coverage of any home health services.

Additional Resources

American Public Health Association. (1991). *Healthy communities 2000: Model standards* (3rd ed.). Washington, DC: Author.

Barr, P. (Ed.). (1991). *Diabetes educational resources for minority and low literacy populations.* Southfield, MI: Coalition for Diabetes Education and Minority Health.

Bedrosian, C.A. (1989). *Home health nursing: Nursing diagnoses and care plans.* E. Norwalk, CT: Appleton & Lange.

Berwick, D.M., Godfrey, A., & Roessner, J. (1990). *Curing health care,* San Francisco: Jossey-Bass.

Bohnet, N., Ilcyn, J., Milanovich, P.S., Ream, M.A., & Wright, K. (1993). Continuous quality improvement: Improving quality in your home care organization, *Journal of Nursing Administration, 23*(2), 42–48.

Buhler-Wilkerson, K. (1985). Public health nursing: In sickness or in health? *American Journal of Public Health, 75*(10), 1155–1161.

Buhler-Wilkerson, K. (1987). Left carrying the bag: Experiments in visiting nursing, 1877–1909. *Nursing Research, 36*(1), 42–47.

Coleman, J., & Haga, E. (1991, October). Collaborative practice: Case managers and home care nurses. *The Case Manager,* 64–72.

Crosby, P.B. (1984). *Quality without tears: The art of hassle-free management.* New York: New American Library.

Crosby, P.B. (1989). *Let's talk quality: 96 questions you always wanted to ask Philip Crosby.* New York: McGraw-Hill.

Davis, J.H., Berry, R.K., Lettow, J., & Foltin, J.J. (1993). An innovative preceptor program for intravenous home care nursing. *Journal of Intravenous Nursing, 16*(5), 287–292.

Dellasega, C. (1991). Caregiving stress among community caregivers for the elderly: Does institutionalization make a difference? *Journal of Community Health Nursing, 8*(4), 197–205.

Deming, W.E. (1986). *Out of the crisis.* Cambridge, MA: Massachusetts Institute of Technology, Center for Advanced Engineering Study.

Edwardson, S.R., & Nardone, P. (1991). Resource use in home care agencies. *Applied Nursing Research, 4*(1), 25–30.

Ethridge, D. (1989). Professional nursing case management improves quality, access and costs. *Nursing Management, 20,* 30–35.

Feinburg, E. (1985). Family stress in pediatric home care. *Caring, 5,* 38–41.

Friedman, J. (1986). *Home healthcare: A complete guide for patients and their families.* New York: Norton.

Friedman, M. (1993). Sample quality plan. *Quality improvement in home care* (pp. 195–210). Oakbrook Terrace, IL: Joint Commission on Accreditation of Healthcare Organizations.

Friedman, M. (1995). *Performance improvement systems.* Marietta, GA: Home Health Systems.

Frisch, N. (1993). Home care nursing and psychosocial-emotional needs. How nursing diagnosis helps to direct and inform practice. *Home Healthcare Nurse, 11*(2), 64–65, 70.

Gingerich, B.S., & Ondeck, D.A. (1994). Clinical pathway for the muldisciplinary home care team. Gaithersburg, MD: Aspen Publishers.

Giuliano, K., & Poirier, C. (1991). Nursing case management: Critical pathways to desirable outcomes. *Nursing Management, 22*(3), 52–55.

Goodwin, D. (1992). Critical pathways in home healthcare. *Journal of Nursing Administration, 22*(2), 35–40.

Harris, M. (1994). *Handbook of home healthcare administration.* Gaithersburg, MD: Aspen Publishers.

Hass-Beckert, B., & Heyman, M. (1993). Comparison of two skin-level gastrostomy feeding tubes for infants and children. *Pediatric Nursing, 19*(4), 351–354.

Heinrich, J. (1983). Historical perspectives on public health nursing. *Nursing Outlook, 31*(6), 317–320.

Heiser, C. (1987). Home phototherapy. *Pediatric Nursing, 13,* 425–427.

Hekelman, F. P., Stricklin, M.L., Brown, K., & Alemagno, S. (1992). Clinical research in home care. *Journal of Nursing Administration, 22*(1), 29–32.

Helberg, J.L. (1993). Factors influencing home care nursing problems and nursing care. *Research in Nursing & Health, 16*(5), 363–370.

Helberg, J.L. (1993). Patients' status at home care discharge. *Journal of Nursing Scholarship.* 25(2), 93–99.

Hellwig, K. (1993). Psychiatric home care nursing: Managing patients in the community setting. *Journal of Psychosocial Nursing & Mental Health Services, 31*(12), 21–24.

Hughes, K.K., & Marcantonio, R.J. (1992). Practice patterns among home health, public health, and hospital nurses. *Nursing & Health Care, 13*(10), 532–536.

Humphrey, C.J., & Milone-Nuzzo, P. (1992). Home care nursing orientation model. Justification and structure. *Home Healthcare Nurse, 10*(3), 18–25.

Joint Commission on Accreditation of Healthcare Organizations. (1991). *An introduction to quality improvement in health care.* Oakbrook Terrace, IL: Author.

Joint Commission on Accreditation of Healthcare Organizations. (1992). *Striving toward improvement: Six hospitals in search of quality.* Oakbrook Terrace, IL: Author.

Joint Commission on Accreditation of Healthcare Organizations. (1992). *Using quality improvement tools in a health care setting.* Oakbrook Terrace, IL: Author.

Joint Commission on Accreditation of Healthcare Organizations. (1993). *The management mandate: On the road to performance in health care.* Oakbrook Terrace, IL: Author.

Joint Commission on Accreditation of Healthcare Organizations. (1993). *Process improvement models: Case studies in health care.* Oakbrook Terrace, IL: Author.

Joint Commission on Accreditation of Healthcare Organizations. (1993). *Quality improvement in home care.* Oakbrook Terrace, IL: Author.

Joint Commission on Accreditation of Healthcare Organizations. (1994). *Framework for improving performance: From principles to practice.* Oakbrook Terrace, IL: Author.

Joint Commission on Accreditation of Healthcare Organizations. (1994). *Primer on indicator development and application: Measuring quality in health care.* Oakbrook Terrace, IL: Author.

Joint Commission on Accreditation of Healthcare Organizations. (1995). Improving organizational performance. In *Accreditation manual for home care: Volume II. Scoring guidelines.* Oakbrook Terrace, IL: Author.

Juran Institute. (1992). *Quality improvement tools: Desk guide.* Washington, DC: Department of Treasury, Internal Revenue Service.

Juran, J.M. (1988). *Juran on planning for quality.* New York: Free Press.

Juran, J.M. (1989). *Juran on leadership for quality: An executive handbook.* New York: Free Press.

Juran, J.M. (1991). *Juran's new quality road map: Planning, setting and researching quality goals.* New York: Free Press.

Kennedy, A.H., Johnson, W., & Sturdevant, E. (1982). An educational program for families of children with tracheostomies. *The American Journal of Maternal-Child Nursing, 7,* 42–49.

Kilajonowicz, A. (1985). Home apnea monitoring. *NAACOG Update Series, 3* (Lesson 15), 2–7.

Knollmueller, R. (1993). The role of prevention in home healthcare nursing practice. *Home Healthcare Nurse, 11*(1), 21–23.

Kouzes, J.M. (1987). *The leadership challenge: How to get extraordinary things done in organizations.* San Francisco: Jossey-Bass.

Kun, S., & Brennan, K. (1985). Pediatric discharge planning: Challenges and rewards. *Caring, 4,* 37.

Leonard, B.J., Brust, J.D., & Sielaff, B.H. (1991). Determinants of home care nursing hours for technology-assisted children. *Public Health Nursing, 8*(4), 239–244.

Lynch, S.A. (1994). Job satisfaction of home health nurses. *Home Healthcare Nurse, 12*(5), 21–28.

Malloy, C., & Hartshorn, J. (1989). *Acute care nursing in the home: A holistic approach.* Philadelphia: J.B. Lippincott.

Marquis, B., & Huston, C. (1987). *Management decision making for nurses.* Philadelphia: J.B. Lippincott.

Marszalek-Gaucher, E., & Coffey, R. (1990). *Transforming health care organizations: How to achieve and sustain organizational excellence.* San Francisco: Jossey-Bass.

Martin, K., & Scheet, N. (1992). *The Omaha system.* Philadelphia: Saunders.

Melum, M.M., & Sinioris, M.K. (1992). *Total quality management: The health care pioneers,* Chicago: American Hospital Publishing.

Milone-Nuzzo, P., & Humphrey, C.J. (1992). Home care nursing orientation model: Content and strategies. *Home Healthcare Nurse, 10*(6), 24–30.

Mitchell, M.K. (1992). Nursing's legacy of leadership. *Nursing and Health Care, 13*(6), 295–297.

Morgan, K.J. (1991). National certification for home care RNs. *Nursing Management, 22*(9), 63–64.

Nadler, G. (1990). *Breakthrough thinking: Why we must change the way we solve problems, and the seven principles to achieve this.* Rocklin, CA: Prima Publishers.

Nadwairski, J.A. (1992). Inner-city safety for home care providers. *Journal of Nursing Administration, 22*(9), 42–47.

Peters, D. (1992). Consumer-oriented quality assurance in home care. *Pride Institute Journal of Long Term Home Care, 10*(2), 8–13.

Phaneuf, M. (1976). Documentation of the side effects of medication. *Home Health Care Nurse, 5,* 36–38.

Ralph, I. (1993). Infectious medical waste management: A home care responsibility. *Home Healthcare Nurse, 11*(3), 25–33.

Rohrer, K.S., Poppe, M., & Noel, L. (1993). Staff preparation for managed care. *Nursing Administration Quarterly, 17*(3), 74–78.

Rooney, A.L., & Biere, D.M. (1992). Demonstrating excellence in home care through Joint Commission accreditation. *Journal of Nursing Administration, 22*(9), 31–36.

Scholtes, P. (1991). *The team handbook: How to use teams to improve quality.* Madison, WI: Joiner Associates.

Senge, P. (1990). *The fifth discipline: The art and practice of the learning organization.* New York: Doubleday.

Sherman, C.V. (1991). Total management, not total quality management. *Journal of Quality Assurance, 27*(1), 26–31.

Stulginsky, M. (1993). Nurses' home health experience: Part I. The practice setting. *Nursing and Health Care, 14*(8), 402–407.

Stulginsky, M. (1993). Nurses' home health experience: Part II. The unique demands of home visits. *Nursing and Health Care, 14*(9), 476–485.

U.S. Department of Health and Human Services. (1990). *Healthy people 2000: National health promotion and disease prevention objectives.* Washington, DC: U.S. Government Printing Office.

Walton, M. (1988). *The Deming management method.* New York: Putnam.

Walton, M. (1990). *Deming management at work.* New York: Putnam.

Watterworth, B., & Podrasky, D. (1989). Meeting the learning needs of the person discharged home with an open wound. *Journal of Enterostomal Therapy, 16,* 12–15.

Index